Back and Neck Disorders
SOURCEBOOK
THIRD EDITION

Health Reference Series

Back and Neck Disorders SOURCEBOOK

THIRD EDITION

Basic Consumer Health Information about Spinal Pain, Spinal Cord Injuries, and Related Disorders, Such as Fractures, Osteoarthritis, Scoliosis, Spina Bifida, Spinal Stenosis, Ankylosing Spondylitis, and Cancers, and Featuring Facts about Maintaining Spinal Health, Self-Care, Pain Management, Rehabilitative Care, Chiropractic Care, Spinal Surgeries, and Clinical Trials

Along with Suggestions for Preventing Back and Neck Pain, a Glossary of Related Terms, and a Directory of Resources

OMNIGRAPHICS
615 Griswold, Ste. 520, Detroit, MI 48226

Bibliographic Note

Because this page cannot legibly accommodate all the copyright notices, the Bibliographic Note portion of the Preface constitutes an extension of the copyright notice.

* * *

OMNIGRAPHICS
Angela L. Williams, *Managing Editor*

* * *

ISBN 978-0-7808-1705-0
E-ISBN 978-0-7808-1706-7

Library of Congress Cataloging-in-Publication Data

Names: Omnigraphics, Inc., issuing body.

Title: Back and neck disorders sourcebook: basic consumer health information about spinal pain, spinal cord injuries, and related disorders, such as degenerative disc disease, osteoarthritis, scoliosis, sciatica, spina bifida, and spinal stenosis, and featuring facts about maintaining spinal health, self-care, pain management, rehabilitative care, chiropractic care, and spinal surgeries, along with suggestions for preventing back and neck pain, a glossary of related terms, and a directory of resources.

Description: Third edition. | Detroit, MI: Omnigraphics, Inc., [2019] | Series: Health reference series | Includes bibliographical references and index.

Identifiers: LCCN 2019013653 (print) | LCCN 2019018896 (ebook) | ISBN 9780780817067 (ebook) | ISBN 9780780817050 (hard cover: alk. paper)

Subjects: LCSH: Spine--Diseases--Popular works. | Spinal cord--Wounds and injuries--Popular works. | Spine--Abnormalities--Popular works. | Neck--Diseases--Popular works.

Classification: LCC RD768 (ebook) | LCC RD768.B28 2019 (print) | DDC 617.4/71044--dc23

LC record available at https://lccn.loc.gov/2019013653

This book is printed on acid-free paper meeting the ANSI Z39.48 Standard. The infinity symbol that appears above indicates that the paper in this book meets that standard.

Printed in the United States

Table of Contents

Preface xi

Part I: Understanding Back and Neck Problems

Chapter 1 — Anatomy and Functions of the Spine 3

Chapter 2 — Understanding Pain 11

Chapter 3 — Overview of the Causes and Risk Factors for Back Pain 21

Chapter 4 — How Aging Affects the Spine 29

Chapter 5 — Facts about Low Back Pain 33

Chapter 6 — Neck Pain 41

Chapter 7 — Diagnosis and Treatment for Back Pain 47

Part II: Maintaining Spinal Health

Chapter 8 — Understanding Neutral Spine Posture 57

Section 8.1 — Getting It Straight: Looking after Your Back 58

Section 8.2 — Guide to Good Posture 61

Chapter 9 — The Importance of Proper Body Mechanics 67

Chapter 10 — Ergonomics for a Healthy Spine 71

Chapter 11—Work-Related Musculoskeletal Disorders of Spine 77
Section 11.1—Spinal Pain at Work 78
Section 11.2—Risk Factors for Occupational Musculoskeletal Disorders 84

Chapter 12—Back Pain Prevention at Work 87
Section 12.1—Safe Lifting Techniques 88
Section 12.2—Ergonomics for Computer Workstations 92

Chapter 13—Preventing Back Injury among Caregivers 101

Chapter 14—Compensatory Workplace Exercises for a Healthy Back 105

Chapter 15—Ergonomic Tips for Driving 111

Chapter 16—Do Back Belts Really Work? 115

Chapter 17—When Wearing Backpacks, Are Kids Ergonomically Safe? 121

Chapter 18—Back Pain during Pregnancy 125

Chapter 19—Exercises for Low Back Pain 129

Chapter 20—Pilates Promotes Back Health 133

Part III: Acute Injuries to the Back and Neck

Chapter 21—Neck Injuries 139
Section 21.1—Whiplash 140
Section 21.2—Cervical Fracture 141

Chapter 22—Fractures of the Thoracic and Lumbar Spine 145

Chapter 23—Osteoporosis and Fractures 151

Chapter 24—Understanding Spinal Cord Injury 173

Part IV: Chronic Disorders Associated with Back and Neck Pain

Chapter 25—Skeletal Deformities of Spine 187

Section 25.1—Kyphosis 188

Section 25.2—Lordosis 192

Section 25.3—Scoliosis 196

Chapter 26—Inflammatory Joint Disease of the Spine 199

Section 26.1—Arthritis 200

Section 26.2—Ankylosing Spondylitis 203

Chapter 27—Osteoarthritis: Degenerative Spinal Joint Disease 211

Chapter 28—Intervertebral Disc Disease 219

Chapter 29—Slipped (Herniated) Disc 223

Chapter 30—Spinal Stenosis 229

Chapter 31—Radiculopathy 243

Section 31.1—Pinched Nerve (Compressed Nerve) 244

Section 31.2—Cauda Equina Syndrome 245

Chapter 32—Spina Bifida and Tethered Spinal Cord Syndrome 247

Section 32.1—Spina Bifida 248

Section 32.2—Living with Spina Bifida at Different Ages 254

Section 32.3—Tethered Spinal Cord Syndrome 271

Chapter 33—Spinal Tumors and Cysts 273

Section 33.1—Facts about Spinal Tumors 274

Section 33.2—Syringomyelia 288

Section 33.3—Tarlov Cysts 293

Chapter 34—Cervical Disc Disease 297

Chapter 35—Other Musculoskeletal Conditions of Back and Neck 301

Section 35.1—Sacroiliac Joint Syndrome........ 302

Section 35.2—Spondylolisthesis 305

Section 35.3—Torticollis 309

Section 35.4—Chronic Myofascial Pain........ 312

Section 35.5—Klippel-Feil Syndrome........ 315

Part V: Medications and Rehabilitative Therapies for Spinal Problems

Chapter 36—Managing Chronic Pain........ 323

Chapter 37—All about Medications for Spinal Pain........ 327

Chapter 38—What You Need to Know about Nonsteroidal Anti-Inflammatory Medications........ 333

Chapter 39—Spinal Injections 337

Chapter 40—Physical Therapy for Back and Neck Disorders 341

Chapter 41—Back and Neck Braces 345

Chapter 42—Spinal Manipulation for Low Back Pain........ 349

Chapter 43—Spinal Manipulation or Home Exercise Is More Effective than Medication for Acute Neck Pain 353

Chapter 44—Chiropractic Care for Back Pain........ 355

Section 44.1—Overview of Chiropractic Care 356

Section 44.2—What to Expect at Your First Chiropractic Visit 360

Chapter 45—Meditation and Cognitive-Behavioral Therapy to Ease Low Back Pain 365

Chapter 46—Yoga May Help Treat Back Pain 367

Chapter 47—Acupuncture for Back Pain 369

Section 47.1—The Use of Acupuncture to Treat Pain 370

Section 47.2—Acupuncture and Low Back Pain 373

Chapter 48—M6-C™ Artificial Cervical Disc 375

Part VI: Information about Spinal Surgeries

Chapter 49—What You Should Know before Your Surgery 379

Chapter 50—Questions to Ask Your Doctor before You Have Surgery 383

Chapter 51—Minimally Invasive Spinal Surgery 387

Chapter 52—Neck Surgery 391

Chapter 53—Low Back Surgery 395

Section 53.1—What Is Lumbar Spinal Surgery? 396

Section 53.2—Surgical versus Nonsurgical Therapy for Chronic Low Back Pain 399

Chapter 54—Spinal Fusion Surgery 403

Chapter 55—Bone Graft and Bone Allografts 407

Part VII: Cancers of the Back and Neck

Chapter 56—Childhood Brain and Spinal Cord Tumors 413

Chapter 57—Metastatic Squamous Neck Cancer 423

Chapter 58—Nasopharyngeal Cancer 431

Chapter 59—Hypopharyngeal Cancer 439

Chapter 60—Oropharyngeal Cancer 447

Part VIII: Clinical Trials and Research Studies

Chapter 61—Understanding Clinical Trials and Observational Studies 461

Chapter 62—Ongoing Clinical Trials for Back and Neck Related Problems 465

Section 62.1—Change of Lumbar Symptom after Surgical Treatment for Patients with Cervical Stenosis (LBP).......................... 466

Section 62.2—Behavior of the Upper Cervical Spine in Rugby Players (Cervistab) 467

Section 62.3—Dosing of Methadone for Spine Surgery 468

Section 62.4—Postoperative Pain Management Following Spine Surgery (EXPAREL) 469

Section 62.5—Outcome Analysis for Minimally Invasive Spine Surgery.................................... 471

Section 62.6—The Effects of Thoracic Spine Mobilizations in Individuals with Neck Pain...... 473

Chapter 63—Research Studies on Spinal Cord Injuries 475

Part IX: Additional Help and Information

Chapter 64—Glossary of Terms Related to Back and Neck Care.. 487

Chapter 65—Directory of Back and Neck Organizations and Resources.............................. 497

Index 509

Preface

About This Book

Back and neck pains may range from mild discomfort to severe disabling health conditions. Such pains can adversely affect the mobility and daily activities. According to the National Institute of Neurological Disorders and Stroke (NINDS), about 80 percent of adults experience low back pain at some point in their lifetimes. All told, low back pain is the second most common neurological ailment in the United States after headache. Although back and neck disorders are responsible for significant suffering, new treatments, medications, exercise programs, and surgical advances are bringing hope to many patients with spinal concerns.

Back and Neck Disorders Sourcebook, Third Edition provides information about diseases, disorders, and injuries that affect the spinal column, including fractures, osteoarthritis, scoliosis, spina bifida, spinal stenosis, ankylosing spondylitis, and cancers that occur in the back and neck regions. It also describes proper spine function and includes suggestions for maintaining spinal health. For patients with back and neck problems, it offers helpful information about medications and rehabilitative therapies, along with facts about surgical techniques, and presents facts about clinical trials. A glossary, directory of resources for further help and information, and suggestions for additional reading are also provided.

How to Use This Book

This book is divided into parts and chapters. Parts focus on broad areas of interest. Chapters are devoted to single topics within a part.

Part I: Understanding Back and Neck Problems presents information about the anatomy and function of the spine and explains how aging affects the spine. It talks about causes and risk factors of various spinal disorders. It also provides an overview of different diagnostic techniques and treatments available for back and neck pain.

Part II: Maintaining Spinal Health focuses on methods of pain and disability prevention with the use of good body mechanics and proper posture. It gives an insight into the incidence and prevention of spinal pain at home and work and also offers tips for easing spinal pain during pregnancy. Information about exercises, including yoga and Pilates, for preventing back and neck pain are also provided.

Part III: Acute Injuries to the Back and Neck identifies acutely painful back and neck injuries, including whiplash; osteoporosis; and cervical, thoracic, and lumbar spinal fractures. In addition, it offers guidance on understanding and adapting to spinal cord injuries that cause permanent disability.

Part IV: Chronic Disorders Associated with Back and Neck Pain includes chapters on spinal conditions, such as ankylosing spondylitis, cauda equina syndrome, scoliosis, osteoarthritis, sacroiliac joint syndrome, spina bifida, spinal stenosis, and spinal tumors and cysts.

Part V: Medications and Rehabilitative Therapies for Spinal Problems identifies common medications used to reduce the pain associated with spinal disorders, such as nonsteroidal anti-inflammatory medications and spinal injections. It also deals with other nonsurgical pain relief treatments, including physical therapy, back and neck braces, chiropractic care, yoga, and acupuncture.

Part VI: Information about Spinal Surgeries details traditional surgical treatments for spinal disorders, including spinal fusion surgery, bone grafts, and minimally invasive spinal surgery. It also deals with the recovery and complications associated with the spinal surgeries.

Part VII: Cancers of the Back and Neck explains in detail about the causes, symptoms, diagnosis, and treatment for the cancers that affect the spine, such as brain and spinal cord tumors, metastatic squamous neck cancer, nasopharyngeal cancer, hypopharyngeal cancer, and oropharyngeal cancer.

Part VIII: Clinical Trials and Research Studies deals with the ongoing clinical trials and research studies involving back and neck problems.

Part IX: Additional Help and Information offers a glossary of important terms and directory of government agencies and private organizations that provide help and information to patients with spinal disorders.

Bibliographic Note

This volume contains documents and excerpts from publications issued by the following U.S. government agencies: Agency for Healthcare Research and Quality (AHRQ); Centers for Disease Control and Prevention (CDC); Division of Occupational Health and Safety (DOHS); *Eunice Kennedy Shriver* National Institute of Child Health and Human Development (NICHD); Genetic and Rare Diseases Information Center (GARD); Genetics Home Reference (GHR); *Go4Life*; National Cancer Institute (NCI); National Center for Complementary and Integrative Health (NCCIH); National Institute of Arthritis and Musculoskeletal and Skin Diseases (NIAMS); National Institute of Neurological Disorders and Stroke (NINDS); National Institute on Aging (NIA); National Institutes of Health (NIH); *NIH News in Health*; Occupational Safety and Health Administration (OSHA); Office of the Assistant Secretary for Planning and Evaluation (ASPE); Office on Women's Health (OWH); U.S. Department of Agriculture (USDA); U.S. Department of Veterans Affairs (VA); and U.S. Food and Drug Administration (FDA).

It may also contain original material produced by Omnigraphics and reviewed by medical consultants.

About the Health Reference Series

The *Health Reference Series* is designed to provide basic medical information for patients, families, caregivers, and the general public. Each volume takes a particular topic and provides comprehensive coverage. This is especially important for people who may be dealing with a newly diagnosed disease or a chronic disorder in themselves or in a family member. People looking for preventive guidance, information about disease warning signs, medical statistics, and risk factors for health problems will also find answers to their questions in the *Health Reference Series*. The *Series*, however, is not intended to serve as a tool for diagnosing illness, in prescribing treatments, or as a substitute for the physician/patient relationship. All people concerned about medical symptoms or the possibility of disease are encouraged to seek professional care from an appropriate healthcare provider.

A Note about Spelling and Style

Health Reference Series editors use *Stedman's Medical Dictionary* as an authority for questions related to the spelling of medical terms and the *Chicago Manual of Style* for questions related to grammatical structures, punctuation, and other editorial concerns. Consistent adherence is not always possible, however, because the individual volumes within the *Series* include many documents from a wide variety of different producers, and the editor's primary goal is to present material from each source as accurately as is possible. This sometimes means that information in different chapters or sections may follow other guidelines and alternate spelling authorities. For example, occasionally a copyright holder may require that eponymous terms be shown in possessive forms (Crohn's disease vs. Crohn disease) or that British spelling norms be retained (leukaemia vs. leukemia).

Medical Review

Omnigraphics contracts with a team of qualified, senior medical professionals who serve as medical consultants for the *Health Reference Series*. As necessary, medical consultants review reprinted and originally written material for currency and accuracy. Citations including the phrase "Reviewed (month, year)" indicate material reviewed by this team. Medical consultation services are provided to the *Health Reference Series* editors by:

Dr. Vijayalakshmi, MBBS, DGO, MD
Dr. Senthil Selvan, MBBS, DCH, MD
Dr. K. Sivanandham, MBBS, DCH, MS (Research), PhD

Our Advisory Board

We would like to thank the following board members for providing initial guidance on the development of this series:

- Dr. Lynda Baker, Associate Professor of Library and Information Science, Wayne State University, Detroit, MI
- Nancy Bulgarelli, William Beaumont Hospital Library, Royal Oak, MI

- Karen Imarisio, Bloomfield Township Public Library, Bloomfield Township, MI
- Karen Morgan, Mardigian Library, University of Michigan-Dearborn, Dearborn, MI
- Rosemary Orlando, St. Clair Shores Public Library, St. Clair Shores, MI

Health Reference Series *Update Policy*

The inaugural book in the *Health Reference Series* was the first edition of *Cancer Sourcebook* published in 1989. Since then, the *Series* has been enthusiastically received by librarians and in the medical community. In order to maintain the standard of providing high-quality health information for the layperson the editorial staff at Omnigraphics felt it was necessary to implement a policy of updating volumes when warranted.

Medical researchers have been making tremendous strides, and it is the purpose of the *Health Reference Series* to stay current with the most recent advances. Each decision to update a volume is made on an individual basis. Some of the considerations include how much new information is available and the feedback we receive from people who use the books. If there is a topic you would like to see added to the update list, or an area of medical concern you feel has not been adequately addressed, please write to:

Managing Editor
Health Reference Series
Omnigraphics
615 Griswold, Ste. 520
Detroit, MI 48226

Part One

Understanding Back and Neck Problems

Chapter 1

Anatomy and Functions of the Spine

The spine, or the backbone, is a characteristic feature of vertebrates and forms the central support structure for the body. Also known as the "vertebral column," the spine in human beings is a complex construct of 33 interlocking bones called the "vertebrae," which extend from the base of the skull to the coccyx, or the tailbone (representative of the vestigial tail).

The spine is a flexible structure that forms the longitudinal axis of the human skeleton, and it encloses and protects the spinal cord. The spine also helps carry the weight of the head, arms, and torso; maintains posture; provides an attachment site for ribs; and assists in movement and locomotion.

The bones of the vertebrae are stacked on top of each other, and adjacent vertebrae are separated by cushioning material called the "intervertebral discs." These fibrocartilaginous discs permit limited movement of the spine and also serve as shock absorbers for the spine. The vertebrae are associated with muscles, joints, tendons, ligaments, and nerves woven together to form a remarkable and complex system of structural and functional importance.

Anatomy of the Spine

The lateral view of a normal spine shows an almost S-shaped curvature formed by 4 distinct areas of the vertebral column. These curves are extremely important in terms of load-bearing capacity and strength of the vertebral column. The uppermost region of the spine, which makes up the neck, is composed of 7 bones and constitutes the cervical region. The cervical vertebrae are numbered C1 to C7, from top to bottom. The next set of 12 vertebrae (numbered T1 to T12) constitutes the thoracic curve.

The lumbar curve, formed by a set of 5 vertebrae, constitutes the lower back and is followed by the sacral curve, which is also made up of 5 vertebrae. The vertebrae of the lumbar region are numbered from L1 to L5, and those of the sacral region are numbered S1 to S5. The coccyx forms the final segment of the vertebral column and is composed of 3 to 5 smaller vertebrae, which fuse together to form a single bone. The cervical and lumbar regions of the spine curve inward, which is termed the "lordotic curve," while the thoracic and sacral spine curve outward, which is termed the "kyphotic curve."

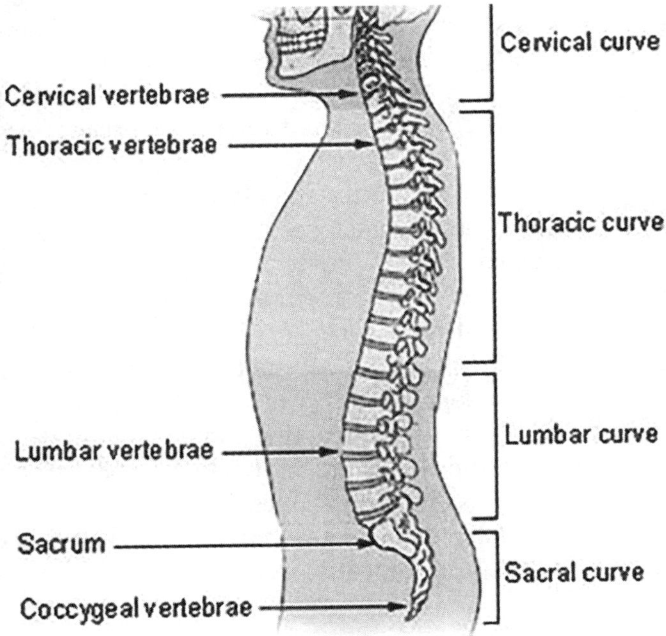

Figure 1.1. *Anatomy of the Spine* (Source: National Institute of Arthritis and Musculoskeletal and Skin Diseases (NIAMS).)

Structure of a Typical Vertebra

Anatomically, the vertebrae show considerable variation in shapes and sizes in different regions of the spine, but they also share certain common structural features. A typical vertebra has a vertebral body, which forms its anterior part, and a bony projection called the "vertebral arch" on the lateral and posterior sides. The body is the main load-bearing part of the spine and progressively increases in size and thickness as it goes down the spine. Intervertebral discs separate the bodies of adjacent vertebra. Each vertebral arch is associated with three types of bony processes, which serve as attachment sites for muscles and soft tissues and assist in articulation. The processes are classified as spinous, transverse, and articular processes. The vertebral body and arch form a central canal called the "vertebral foramen," through which the spinal cord passes.

The posterior part of each vertebra is made up of a single spinous process, which is the bony ridge you can feel when you run your hand over your spine. This serves as a lever to effect movement of the vertebrae. Laterally, there is a pair of bony elements called the "pedicles." Posteriorly, a pair of broad bony plates flares out from the pedicles of the vertebral arches and is called the "laminae." The laminae fuse together to form the flattened, posterior portion of the vertebral arch and the dorsal wall of the vertebral foramen.

A pair of small bony processes, called the "transverse processes," arises laterally from the vertebral arch at the junction of the pedicle and lamina. These serve as an attachment site for muscles and ligaments.

The articular processes form a point of contact between adjacent vertebrae and are located in the intersection of the pedicles and laminae. There are two pairs of articular processes: a pair of superior processes (which project upward from a lower vertebra) and a pair of inferior processes (which project downward from a vertebra above). The actual point of contact is termed the "articular facet." The articular processes provide limited movement and vary in orientation and shape depending on the type and range of motion of the particular spinal region in which they are present.

Facet Joints

The facet joint, also referred to as the "zygapophyseal joint," plays an important role in spinal movement and spinal stability. It is highly susceptible to degenerative changes and is one of the leading causes of pain and disability in the neck, lower back, and mid-back. It comprises a cartilage-covered surface enclosed in a tough connective tissue called the "synovial capsule." The inner surface of the capsule is lined by a thin synovial membrane, which secretes a fluid called the "synovium." The synovial fluid reduces friction between the articulating surfaces of the bones and nourishes the avascular (lacking blood supply) cartilage. The facet joints have different orientations, depending on the area, and allow a range of movements, including flexion (forward bending, backward bending) and rotation. They can also restrict excessive movement of the spine (hyperflexion and hyperextension), as in the case of whiplash injuries.

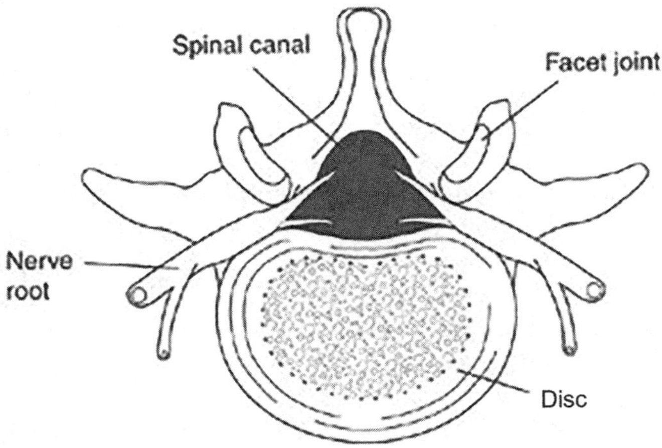

Figure 1.2. *Facet Joints* (Source: National Institute of Arthritis and Musculoskeletal and Skin Diseases (NIAMS).)

Intervertebral Discs

Adjacent vertebral bodies are cushioned by intervertebral discs that are made of a multi-layer cartilage. A tough ring of ligament fibers, called the "annulus fibrosus," surrounds the soft inner core of the disc called the "nucleus pulposus." The nucleus pulposus is a gelatinous material that is composed of water and loose collagen fibers. The pulposus behaves like a pressurized fluid and helps the disc to withstand compression and torsion forces.

The annulus seals this pressurized fluid and helps to evenly distribute forces or pressure across the intervertebral disc. Aging reduces the water content of the pulposus, causing the discs to become thinner.

This impacts one's range of motion and the flexibility of their joints, and it also explains the slight decline of body height as we age. If the annulus fibrosus is weakened by trauma or age, the pulposus can prolapse through a tear in the annulus fibrosus and lead to a ruptured or herniated disc, a common degenerative condition of the spine.

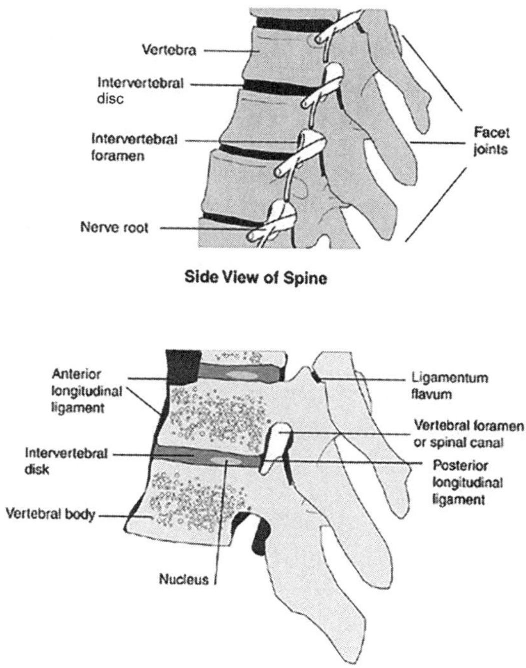

Figure 1.3. *Intervertebral Discs* (Source: National Institute of Arthritis and Musculoskeletal and Skin Diseases (NIAMS).)

Spinal Cord and Nerves

The spinal cord is the tight bundle of nerve cells and nerve pathways that extends from the brainstem to the lumbar region. It is an important part of the central nervous system (CNS), which controls and coordinates most of the body functions and serves as an information highway for transmitting sensory information from the sense organs, internal organs, and muscles to the brain. It also has a descending tract, which transmits impulses in the reverse direction—from the brain to the body systems. The spinal cord is protected by the bony elements of the vertebral column and comprises 31 pairs of spinal nerves, which arise from both sides of the spinal cord.

Also called the "peripheral nerves," the spinal nerves are in pairs, and each nerve branches off into two roots—the dorsal and ventral. The spinal nerves are mixed nerves, as they are composed of both afferent (sensory) and efferent (motor) components. The dorsal root is the afferent component and includes sensory nerves that carry impulses from sense organs to the spinal cord, while the ventral root is the efferent component and comprises motor nerves whose function is to transmit impulses from the spinal cord to the muscles.

The spinal nerves are classified depending on the corresponding regions of the vertebral column they arise from.

Cervical nerves: 8 pairs of cervical nerves transmit impulses to the head, neck, diaphragm, and arms.

Thoracic nerves: 12 pairs of thoracic nerves control motor and sensory signals for the upper back, chest, abdomen, and other internal organs.

Lumbar nerves: 5 pairs of lumbar nerves control signals to the lower abdomen, lower back, legs, and certain parts of the legs and external genitalia.

Sacral nerves: 5 pairs of sacral nerves control signals to the feet, lower parts of the leg, the thighs, and a major part of the external genital organs.

Coccygeal nerve: A single pair that forms the final nerve of the spinal cord and is composed of axons from the last sacral nerve (S4-S5), innervating the muscles supporting the pelvic organs.

Additional Structures Associated with the Spine

Muscles, Tendons, and Ligaments

A system of soft tissues, such as muscles, ligaments, and tendons, provides structural stability to the spine and assists with movement. It also protects the spine from injury. Muscle groups associated with the vertebral column occur in pairs, and they play a pivotal role in maintaining posture by supporting it upright against gravity. Spinal muscles are both extrinsic (superficial) and intrinsic (deep-seated). They connect the trunk to the limbs, and they control movement of the limbs and the vertebral column. Some of the muscles also control respiratory movements. A group of muscles, called the "erector spinae," helps to extend the spine and maintain posture.

Ligaments are tough bands of connective tissue, which link two or more bones or cartilages together. The main ligaments are anterior longitudinal ligament and posterior longitudinal ligament. They provide stability to a joint during rest and prevent movement in certain directions. They also prevent excessive movements, such as hyperextension or hyperflexion. The ligaments stabilize the spine and protect the discs.

Tendons, as with ligaments, are tough bands of fibrous connective tissue composed of collagen protein. They fasten muscles to the bones of the vertebral column and possess high tensile strength that is capable of withstanding mechanical stresses generated by muscle contraction.

References

1. "Anatomy and Physiology—The Vertebral Column," Rice University, n.d.
2. "Axial Skeleton (80 bones)," Surveillance, Epidemiology, and End Results Program (SEER), National Cancer Institute (NCI), n.d.
3. "Spinal Stenosis," National Institute of Arthritis and Musculoskeletal and Skin Diseases (NIAMS), n.d.

Chapter 2

Understanding Pain

Pain, in its most benign form, warns us that something is not quite right, that we should take medicine, or see a doctor. At its worst, however, pain robs us of our productivity, our well-being, and, for many of us suffering from extended illness, our lives. Pain is a complex perception that differs enormously among individual patients, even those who appear to have identical injuries or illnesses.

The burden of pain in the United States is astounding. More than 100 million Americans have pain that persists for weeks to years. The financial toll of this epidemic costs $560 billion to $635 billion per year according to "Relieving Pain in America: A Blueprint for Transforming Prevention, Care, Education, and Research," a report from the Institute of Medicine (IOM). Pain is ultimately a challenge for family, friends, and healthcare providers who must give support to the individual suffering from the physical, and emotional, consequences of pain.

A Pain Primer: What Is Known about Pain?

What is pain? The International Association for the Study of Pain (IASP) defines "pain" as: "an unpleasant sensory and emotional experience associated with actual or potential tissue damage or described in terms of such damage." The IASP definition means that pain is a subjective experience—one that cannot be objectively measured and depends on the person's self-report. As will be discussed later, there

---

This chapter includes text excerpted from "Pain: Hope through Research," National Institute of Neurological Disorders and Stroke (NINDS), August 8, 2018.

can be a wide variability in how a person experiences pain to a given stimulus or injury.

Pain can be classified as acute or chronic, and the two kinds differ greatly.

Acute pain, for the most part, results from disease, inflammation, or injury to tissues. This type of pain generally comes on suddenly, such as after trauma or surgery, and may be accompanied by anxiety or emotional distress. The cause of acute pain can usually be diagnosed and treated. The pain is self-limiting, which means it is confined to a given period of time and severity. It can become chronic.

Chronic pain is now believed to be a chronic disease condition in the same manner as diabetes and asthma. Chronic pain can be made worse by environmental and psychological factors. By its nature, chronic pain persists over a long period of time and is resistant to many medical treatments. It can—and often does—cause severe problems. People with chronic pain often suffer from more than one painful condition. It is thought that there are common mechanisms that put some people at higher risk of developing multiple pain disorders. It is not known whether these disorders share a common cause.

We may experience pain as a prick, tingle, sting, burn, or ache. Normally, acute pain is a protective response to tissue damage resulting from injury, disease, overuse, or environmental stressors. To sense pain, specialized receptors (called "nociceptors"), which are found throughout the body, trigger a series of events in response to a noxious (painful) stimulus. The events begin with conversion of the stimulus to an electrical impulse, which then travels through nerves from the site of injury or disease and to the spinal cord. These signals are transmitted to a specialized part of the spinal cord called the "dorsal horn," where they can be dampened or amplified before being relayed to the brain.

Anatomy of Pain

Pain signals from the head and face directly enter the brain stem, which is where they join the pain pathways that travel from the spinal cord to the brain. One central place these signals travel to is the thalamus. The thalamus is a relay station that distributes sensory signals to many other brain regions, including the anterior cingulate cortex, somatosensory cortex, insular cortex, and prefrontal cortex. These cortical brain regions process the nociceptive (pain causing or reacting to pain) information from the body and generate the complex experience of pain. This pain experience has multiple components that include the:

- **Sensory-discriminative aspect**, which helps us localize where on our body the injury occurs
- **Affective-motivational aspect**, which conveys just how unpleasant the experience is
- **Cognitive-evaluative aspect**, which involves thoughtful planning on what to do to get away from the pain

Many of these characteristics of pain have been associated with specific brain systems; although, much remains to be learned. Additionally, researchers have found that many of the brain systems involved with the experience of pain overlap with the experience of basic emotions. Consequently, when people experience negative emotions (e.g., fear, anxiety, anger), the same brain systems responsible for these emotions also amplify the experience of pain.

Fortunately, there are systems in the brain that help to dampen or decrease pain. Descending signals from the brain are sent back to the spinal cord and can inhibit the intensity of incoming nociceptive signals, thereby reducing the pain experience.

Neurochemistry of Pain

This complicated process by which we perceive pain involves intricate connections among multifaceted brain regions. The nervous system uses a set of chemicals, called "neurotransmitters," to communicate between neurons within and across these stations in the pain pathway. These chemicals are released by neurons in tiny packets (vesicles) into the space between two cells. When they reach their target cell, they bind to special proteins on the surface of the cells called "receptors." The transmitter then activates the receptor, which functions much like a gate. The gate will either close to block (inhibitory receptor) the signal or open to send (excitatory receptor) the signal along to the next station.

There are many different neurotransmitters in the human body, and they play a role in normal function, as well as in disease. In the case of nociception and pain, they act in various combinations at all levels of the nervous system to transmit and modify signals generated by noxious stimuli.

One excitatory neurotransmitter of special interest to pain researchers is glutamate, which plays a major role in nervous system function and in pain pathophysiology. The modulation of glutamate neurotransmission is complex, but it plays a key role in heightening the sensitivity to pain through increased responsiveness of excitatory receptors in the spinal cord dorsal horn and in the brain. This is part of a process called "central sensitization" and contributes to making pain persist. A great deal of attention has been given to developing molecules/drugs that block certain receptors for glutamate for their potential in reducing pain.

Unlike glutamate, gamma-aminobutyric acid (GABA) is predominantly an inhibitory neurotransmitter, as it generally decreases or blocks the activity of neurons. Most of what we know of its role in pain is related to its function in inhibiting spinal cord neurons from transmitting pain signals and, therefore, dampening pain. Chemicals that are similar to GABA have been explored as possible analgesics, but because GABA is so widespread in the nervous system, it is difficult to make a GABA-like drug without affecting other nervous system functions. As we learn more about the specific roles of GABA receptors, drug development may be accelerated.

Norepinephrine and serotonin are neurotransmitters used by the descending pain pathways from the brain stem to dampen the incoming signals from painful stimuli from the site of the injury or inflammation. Drugs that modulate the activity of these transmitters, such as some antidepressants, are effective in treating some chronic pain conditions, likely by enhancing the availability of the transmitters through a recycling and reuse process. Serotonin receptors also are present on the nerves that supply the surface of the brain involved in migraines, and their modulation by a class of drugs called "triptans" is effective in acutely treating migraine.

The opioids are another important class of neurotransmitters that are involved in pain control, as well as pleasure and addiction. Their receptors are found throughout the body and can be activated by endogenous (produced by our bodies) opioid peptides that are released by neurons in the brain. The enkephalins, dynorphins, and endorphins are some of the body's own natural pain killers. They may be more familiar for the role of endorphins in the feeling of well-being during exercise—the runner's high. Opioid receptors also can be activated by morphine, which mimics the effect of our endogenous opioids. Morphine is a natural product and is a very potent, but potentially addictive, painkiller that is used broadly for severe acute and chronic pain management. Together, the opioids provide effective pain relief for many people with pain. Other peptides also transmit neuronal signals and play a role in pain responses. Scientists have shown that mice bred experimentally to lack a gene for two peptides, called "tachykinins-neurokinin A" and "substance P," have a reduced response to severe pain.

When exposed to mild pain, these mice react in the same way as mice that carry the missing gene. But when exposed to more severe pain, the mice exhibit a reduced pain response. This suggests that the two peptides are involved in the perception of pain sensations, especially moderate-to-severe pain.

Genetics of Pain

Differences in our genes highlight how different we are in respect to pain. Scientists believe that genetic variations can determine our risk for developing chronic pain, how sensitive we are to painful stimuli, whether or not certain therapies will ease our pain, and how we respond to acute or chronic pain. Many genes contribute to pain perception, and mutations in one or more pain-related genes account for some of the variability of each individual's pain experiences. Some people born genetically insensate to pain—meaning they cannot feel pain—have a mutation in part of a gene that plays a role in electrical activity of nerve cells. A different mutation in that same gene can cause a severe and disabling pain condition. Scientists have identified many genes involved in pain by screening large numbers of people with pain conditions for shared gene mutations. While genes play a role in determining our sensitivity to pain, they only account for a portion of this variability. Ultimately, our individual sensitivity to pain is governed by a complex interaction of genes, cognitions, mood, our environment, and early life experiences.

Inflammation and Pain

The link between the nervous and immune systems also is important. Cytokines, a group of proteins found in the nervous system, are also part of the immune system—the body's shield for fighting off disease and responding to tissue injury. Cytokines can trigger pain by promoting inflammation, even in the absence of injury or damage. After trauma, cytokine levels rise in the brain and spinal cord and at the site where the injury occurred. Improvements in our understanding of the precise role of cytokines in producing pain may lead to new classes of drugs that can block the action of these substances to produce analgesia.

Neural Circuits and Chronic Pain

The pain that we perceive when we have an injury or infection alerts us to the potential for tissue damage. Sometimes, this protective pain persists after the healing occurs or may even appear when there was no apparent cause. This persistent pain is linked to changes in our nervous system, which responds to internal and external change by reorganizing and adapting throughout life. This phenomenon is known as "neuronal plasticity," a process that allows us to learn, remember, and recover from brain injury. Following an injury or disease process, the nervous system sometimes undergoes a structural and functional reorganization that is not a healthy form of plasticity. Long-term, maladaptive changes in both the peripheral and central nervous system can make us hypersensitive to pain and can make pain persist after injuries have healed. For example, sensory neurons in the peripheral nervous system, which normally detect noxious/painful stimuli, may alter the electrical or molecular signals that they send to the spinal cord. This in turn triggers genes to alter production of receptors and chemical transmitters in spinal cord neurons, setting up a chronic pain state. Scientists have methods to identify which genes' activities change with injury and chronic pain. Knowledge of the proteins that ultimately are synthesized by these genes are providing new targets for therapy development. Increased physiological excitation of neurons in the spinal cord enhance pain signaling pathways to the brain stem and in the brain. This hypersensitivity of the central nervous system is called "central sensitization." It is difficult to reverse and makes pain persist beyond its protective role.

Gender and Pain

It is widely believed that pain affects men and women differently. In fact, according to the Institute of Medicine's 2011 report "Relieving Pain in America," women often report a higher prevalence of chronic pain than men and are at a greater risk for many pain conditions. Women are likely to have more pain from certain diseases, such as cancer. Also, a number of chronic pain disorders occur only in women and others occur predominantly in women. These include chronic fatigue syndrome (CFS), endometriosis, fibromyalgia, interstitial cystitis, vulvodynia, and temporomandibular disorders.

The Institute of Medicine (IOM) report mentions at least three theories that may explain the differences in pain experience by gender:

- A gender-role theory that assumes it is more socially acceptable for women to report pain
- An exposure theory that suggests women are exposed to more pain risk factors

- A vulnerability theory that proposes that women are more vulnerable to developing certain types of pain, such as musculoskeletal pain

Of these, the vulnerability theory is best supported by scientific evidence.

A greater understanding of gender differences in pain may lead to better avenues of pain management.

How Is Pain Treated?

The goal of pain management is to improve function, enabling individuals to work, attend school, and participate in day-to-day activities. People with pain and their physicians have a number of options for treatment; some are more effective than others. Sometimes, relaxation and the use of imagery as a distraction provide relief. These methods may be powerful and effective, according to those who advocate their use. Whatever the treatment regime, it is important to remember that, while not all pain is curable, all pain is treatable. The following treatments are among the most common.

Treatment varies depending on the duration and type of pain. For the most part, the medications listed below have been shown in clinical trials to relieve or prevent pain associated with a specific condition(s), but none have been proven fully effective in relieving all types of pain. A healthcare professional should be consulted to determine which medication is effective for a given pain condition and what to expect for pain relief and side effects. Evidence for the procedures listed below is variable in its quality. In some cases, evidence suggesting that some treatments are effective is anecdotal—or based on personal experience—and in other cases it is collected from well-designed clinical trials.

Acetaminophen is the basic ingredient found in Tylenol® and its many generic equivalents. It is sold over the counter, in a prescription-strength preparation, and in combination with codeine (also by prescription).

Acupuncture involves the application of needles to precise points on the body. It is part of a general category of healing called "traditional Chinese medicine." The mechanism by which acupuncture provides pain relief remains controversial but is quite popular and may one day prove to be useful for a variety of conditions as it continues to be explored. Evidence of the effectiveness of acupuncture for pain relief is conflicting and clinical studies to investigate its benefits are ongoing.

Analgesic refers to the classes of drugs that includes most painkillers. This includes classes of nonsteroidal anti-inflammatory agents such as aspirin, ibuprofen, and naproxen, as well as acetaminophen and opioids. The word "analgesic" is derived from ancient Greek and means to reduce or stop pain. Nonprescription or over-the-counter (OTC) pain relievers (e.g., aspirin, ibuprofen, acetaminophen) are generally used for mild to moderate pain. Prescription opioid pain relievers, sold through a pharmacy under the direction of a physician, are used for moderate to severe pain.

Biofeedback is used to treat many common pain problems, most notably headache and back pain. Using a special electronic machine, individuals are trained to become aware of, follow, and gain control over certain bodily functions, including muscle tension, heart rate, and skin temperature. The individual can then learn to change his or her responses to pain, for example, by using relaxation techniques. Eventually, these changes can be maintained without using the machine. Biofeedback is often used in combination with other treatment methods, generally without side effects. Similarly, the use of relaxation techniques to treat pain can increase a person's feeling of well-being.

Chiropractic care may ease back pain, neck pain, headaches, and musculoskeletal conditions. It involves "hands-on" therapy that is designed to adjust the relationship between the body's structure (mainly the spine) and its functioning. Chiropractic spinal manipulation includes the adjustment and manipulation of the joints and adjacent tissues. Such care may also involve therapeutic and rehabilitative exercises. Numerous clinical trials have been done to assess the effectiveness of spinal manipulations. A review of these trials concludes that evidence of their benefit for acute and subacute low back pain is of low quality. For chronic back pain, however, there is evidence for small to moderate treatment relief.

Cognitive-behavioral therapy is a well-established treatment for pain that involves helping the person improve coping skills, address negative thoughts and emotions that can amplify pain, and learn relaxation methods to help prepare for and cope with pain. It is used for chronic pain, postoperative pain, cancer pain, and the pain of childbirth. Many clinical studies provide evidence for the effectiveness of this form of treatment in pain management.

Counseling can give an individual suffering from pain much-needed support, whether it comes from family, group, or individual counseling. Support groups can provide an important supplement to drug or surgical treatment. Psychological treatment can also help people learn about the physiological changes produced by pain.

Electrical stimulation, including transcutaneous electrical stimulation (TENS), implanted electrical nerve stimulation, and deep brain or spinal cord stimulation, is the modern-day extension of age-old practices in which the nerves or muscles are subjected to a variety of stimuli, including heat or massage. The following techniques each require specialized equipment and personnel trained in the specific procedure being used:

- **TENS** uses tiny electrical pulses, delivered through the skin to nerve fibers, to cause changes in muscles, such as numbness or contractions. This produces temporary pain relief. There is also evidence that TENS can activate subsets of peripheral nerve fibers that can block pain transmission at the spinal cord level, in the same way that shaking your hand can reduce pain.
- **Peripheral nerve stimulation** uses electrodes placed surgically or percutaneously (through the skin using a needle) on a peripheral nerve. The individual is then able to deliver an electrical current as needed to the affected nerve, using a controllable electrical generator.
- **Spinal cord stimulation** uses electrodes surgically or percutaneously inserted within the epidural space of the spinal cord. The individual is able to deliver a pulse of electricity to the spinal cord, using an implanted electrical pulse generator that resembles a cardiac pacemaker.
- **Deep brain stimulation** is considered a more extreme treatment and involves surgical stimulation of the brain, usually the thalamus or motor cortex. It is used to treat chronic pain in cases that do not respond to less invasive or conservative treatments.

Exercise also may be part of the pain treatment regime for some people with pain. Because there is a known link between many types of chronic pain and tense, weak muscles, exercise—even light to moderate exercise such as walking or swimming—can contribute to an overall sense of well-being by improving blood and oxygen flow to muscles.

Just as we know that stress contributes to pain, we also know that exercise, sleep, and relaxation can all help reduce stress, thereby helping to alleviate pain. Exercise has been proven to help many people with low back pain. It is important, however, to work with a physician or physical therapist to create an appropriate routine.

Ibuprofen is a member of the aspirin family of analgesics, the so-called "nonsteroidal anti-inflammatory drugs." It is sold over the counter and also comes in prescription-strength preparations.

Physical therapy and rehabilitation date back to the ancient practice of using physical techniques and methods, such as heat, cold, exercise, massage, and manipulation, in the treatment of certain conditions. These may be applied to increase function, control pain, and gain full recovery.

Placebo is not a treatment for pain but is an effect generally used in clinical studies as a control factor to help determine the effectiveness of an active treatment. Placebos are inactive substances, such as sugar pills, or harmless procedures, such as saline injections or sham surgeries. Placebos offer some individuals pain relief although how they have an effect is mysterious and somewhat controversial. Although placebos have no direct effect on the underlying causes of pain, evidence from clinical studies suggests that many pain conditions, such as migraine headache, back pain, postsurgical pain, rheumatoid arthritis, angina, and depression, sometimes respond well to them. This positive response is known as the "placebo response," which is defined as the observable or measurable change that can occur in people after administration of a placebo. One large component responsible for the effect of placebo is the degree to which people expect the treatment to work. Placebos work, in part, by stimulating the brain's own analgesics.

RICE—Rest, Ice, Compression, and Elevation (RICE)—are four components prescribed by many orthopedists, coaches, trainers, nurses, and other professionals for temporary muscle or joint injuries, such as sprains or strains. Ice is used to reduce the inflammation associated with painful and acute injuries. Ice or heat may be recommended to relieve subacute and chronic pain, allowing for reduced inflammation and increased mobility. While many common orthopedic problems can be controlled with these four simple steps, especially when combined with OTC pain relievers, more serious conditions may require surgery or physical therapy, including exercise, joint movement or manipulation, and stimulation of muscles.

Chapter 3

Overview of the Causes and Risk Factors for Back Pain

Back pain is one of the most common medical problems in the United States. It can range from a dull, constant ache to a sudden, sharp pain that puts you out of action. Sometimes, it can come on suddenly—from an accident, a fall, or lifting something heavy. In other cases, it can develop slowly due to age-related changes to the spine.

Who Gets Back Pain

Although anyone can have back pain, a number of factors increase your risk. They include:

- **Age**. Back pain becomes more common with age, with the first attack typically between the ages of 30 and 40.
- **Fitness level**. Back pain is more common among people who are not physically fit. For example, weak back and stomach muscles may not properly support the spine. Back pain is also more likely if you exercise a lot after being inactive for a while.
- **Diet**. A diet high in calories and fat, combined with an inactive lifestyle, can lead to obesity. This can put stress on the back.

This chapter includes text excerpted from "Back Pain," National Institute of Arthritis and Musculoskeletal and Skin Diseases (NIAMS), August 30, 2016.

- **Heredity**. Genetics play a role in some disorders that cause back pain.
- **Race**. African American women are more likely to develop spondylolisthesis, a condition in which bones in the lower spine slip out of place, than White women.
- **Other diseases**. Back pain may be caused or worsened by some diseases, such as certain types of arthritis and cancers that spread to the spine.
- **Job-related risk factors**. Jobs that require heavy lifting, pushing, pulling, or twisting can injure the back. A desk job may also play a role, especially if you have poor posture or sit all day in an uncomfortable chair.
- **Cigarette smoking**. Although smoking may not directly cause back pain, it increases your risk of developing low back pain and sciatica, which is back pain that travels to the hip and/or leg. Smoking can also slow healing from back injuries or surgeries.

Types of Back Pain

There are two types of back pain: acute and chronic pain.

- **Acute pain** is pain that hits you suddenly after an accident, a fall, or lifting something heavy. Acute pain is the most common type of back pain and lasts no longer than six weeks.
- **Chronic pain** may come on either quickly or slowly and lasts a long time, generally longer than three months. This type of back pain is much less common.

Causes of Back Pain

Back pain can be caused by many different things, including:

- **Mechanical problems** in the way your spine moves or the way you feel when you move your spine in certain ways. Mechanical causes of back pain include the breakdown of the discs between the bones of the spine, ruptured discs, spasms, and muscle tension.
- **Injuries**, such as sprains and fractures, can cause either short-lived or chronic pain. Sprains are tears in the ligaments that support the spine, and they can occur from twisting or

lifting improperly. Fractured vertebrae are often the result of osteoporosis. Less commonly, back pain may be caused by more severe injuries that result from accidents or falls.

- **Medical conditions** can cause or contribute to back pain. They include:
  - Scoliosis, curving of the spine that does not usually cause pain until middle age
  - Spondylolisthesis, where a bone in the spine slips out of place
  - Various forms of arthritis
  - Spinal stenosis, a narrowing of the spinal column that puts pressure on the spinal cord and nerves
  - Osteoporosis, which can lead to painful fractures of the vertebrae
  - Pregnancy
  - Kidney stones or infections
  - Endometriosis, which is the buildup of uterine tissue in places outside the uterus
  - Fibromyalgia, a condition of widespread muscle pain and fatigue
  - Infections can cause pain when they involve the bones of the spine or the discs between these bones.
  - Tumors can cause back pain in rare cases. Tumors may appear in the back or be the result of cancer that has spread from other parts of the body.
- **Stress** can worsen pain by causing back muscles to become tense and painful.

Treatment of Back Pain

Treatment for back pain generally depends on how long your pain lasts.

Acute (short-term) back pain usually gets better on its own. Exercises or surgery are usually not recommended for acute back pain. There are some things you may try while you wait for your pain to get better.

- Acetaminophen, aspirin, or ibuprofen will help ease the pain.
- Get up and move around to ease stiffness and relieve pain in order to return to your regular activities sooner.

Chronic (long-term) back pain is typically treated with nonsurgical options before surgery is recommended.

Nonsurgical treatments include:

- **Hot or cold packs** can be soothing to constantly sore, stiff backs.
- **Exercise** can help ease chronic pain and may reduce the risk of it returning. Check with your doctor before starting a new exercise routine.
- **Medications** to treat chronic back pain are available over-the-counter (OTC) or by prescription.
    - **Pain relievers** that are taken by mouth or applied to the skin. Examples include acetaminophen and aspirin.
    - **Nonsteroidal anti-inflammatory drugs (NSAIDs)** relieve pain and inflammation. Examples include ibuprofen, ketoprofen, and naproxen sodium.
    - **Muscle** relaxants and some antidepressants may be prescribed for some types of chronic back pain.
    - Your doctor may suggest **steroid** or numbing shots to lessen your pain.
- **Traction** involves using pulleys and weights to stretch the back, which may allow a bulging disc to slip back into place. Your pain may be relieved while in traction, but pain returns once you are not in traction.
- **Behavioral modification** teaches you to:
    - Move your body properly while you do daily activities, especially those involving heavy lifting, pushing, or pulling.
    - Practice healthy habits, such as exercise, relaxation, regular sleep, proper diet, and quitting smoking.
- **Complementary and alternative treatments** are an option when medications and other therapies do not relieve pain. Examples include:

- **Manipulation**. Professionals use their hands to adjust or massage the spine or nearby tissues.
- **Transcutaneous electrical nerve stimulation (TENS)**. A small box over the painful area sends mild electrical pulses to nerves. TENS treatments are not always effective for reducing pain.
- **Acupuncture**. This Chinese practice uses thin needles to relieve pain and restore health. Acupuncture may be effective when used as a part of a comprehensive treatment plan for low back pain.
- **Acupressure**. A therapist applies pressure to certain places in the body to relieve pain. Acupressure has not been well studied for back pain.

Surgical treatments may be necessary in some cases, including:

- **Herniated (ruptured) discs** are when one or more of the discs that cushion the bones of the spine are damaged. The jelly-like center of the disc leaks, causing pain. Common surgeries include:
  - **Laminectomy/discectomy**, which removes a portion of spinal bone as well as the damaged disc
  - **Microdiscectomy,** which removes a damaged disc but through a smaller incision when compared to laminectomy/discectomy
  - **Laser surgery** uses a needle that produces bursts of laser energy to reduce the size of the damaged disc. This relieves pressure on the nerves. The usefulness of this procedure is still being debated.
- **Spinal stenosis**, a narrowing of the spinal column that puts pressure on the spinal cord and nerves, is treated by laminectomy. This is a major surgery that opens up the spinal column. A short hospital stay and physical therapy will be required after the surgery.
- **Spondylolisthesis**, where one or more bones in the spine slip out of place. This is treated by laminectomy and spinal fusion, which joins two of the spinal bones together so that they do not move.
- **Vertebral fractures** caused by injury to the bones in the spine or by osteoporosis. This is treated by:

    - **Vertebroplasty** involves injecting a cement-like mixture into the fractured bone to relieve pain and stabilize the spine.
    - **Kyphoplasty** relieves pain and stabilizes the spine following fractures caused by osteoporosis. Doctors insert a balloon-device to help restore the height and shape of the spine and then inject a cement-like mixture to repair the fractured bone.
- **Degenerative disc disease** or damage to the spine's discs as a person gets older. This can be treated by:
    - **Intradiscal electrothermal therapy (IDET)** is one of the least invasive therapies for low back pain. Doctors insert a heating wire into the damaged disc and pass an electrical current through the wire to strengthen the fibers that hold the disc together. The effectiveness of IDET is not clear.
    - **Spinal fusion**, which involves removing and fusing the damaged disc to help with the pain
    - **Disc replacement** replaces the damaged disc with a synthetic one.

Back pain is a symptom of a medical condition, not a diagnosis itself. In rare cases, back pain is caused by a tumor, an infection, or a nerve-root problem called "cauda equina syndrome." In these cases, surgery is needed right away to ease the pain and prevent more problems.

You probably do not need to see your doctor for back pain, unless you have:

- Numbness and tingling
- Severe back pain that does not improve with medication
- Back pain after a fall or injury
- Back pain along with:
    - Trouble urinating
    - Weakness, pain, or numbness in your legs
    - Fever
    - Unintended weight loss

Who Treats Back Pain

Many different types of doctors treat back pain:

- Family or primary care doctors (usually seen first)
- Doctors who specialize in disorders of the nerves, muscles, or skeleton

Living with Back Pain

There are a few things you can do to help you live with back pain:

- **Hot or cold** packs can be soothing to constantly sore, stiff backs. Heat dilates the blood vessels to increase blood supply to the back and reduce muscle spasms. Cold may reduce inflammation and numb deep pain.
- **Exercise** can help ease chronic pain and may reduce the risk of it returning. Check with your doctor before starting a new exercise routine, which may include the following:
    - Flexion exercises have you bending forward to reduce pressure on the nerves, stretch the back and hip muscles, and strengthen the stomach and buttock muscles.
    - The extension involves bending backward, such as lying on your stomach while you lift your leg or raise your trunk. These exercises may help reduce spreading pain and develop muscles that support the spine.
    - Stretching improves the extension of muscles and other soft tissues of the back. These exercises can reduce back stiffness and improve range of motion.
    - Aerobic exercise gets your heart pumping faster and includes brisk walking, jogging, and swimming. Avoid exercise that requires twisting and bending forward quickly, such as aerobic dancing and rowing. Avoid high-impact activities if you have a disc disease.

Prevention of Back Pain

Work with your doctor to develop a plan to help prevent many types of back pain. The plan should include:

- **Regular exercise** that keeps your back muscles strong. Exercises that increase balance and strength can decrease your risk of falling and injuring your back or breaking bones. Exercises such as tai chi and yoga—or any weight-bearing exercise that challenges your balance—are good ones to try.

- **Eating a healthy diet** that includes enough calcium and vitamin D, nutrients that keep your spine strong. A healthy diet also helps in controlling weight to avoid putting unnecessary and injury-causing stress and strain on your back.
- **Practicing good posture**, supporting your back properly, and avoiding heavy lifting when possible.

Chapter 4

How Aging Affects the Spine

Is your back hurting? You are in good company. In any three-month period, about one in four adults in the United States has at least one day of back pain, a majority of these cases occurring in the lower back.

The back is a complicated structure. Its center is the spine, which is made up of 33 bones, called "vertebrae," stacked in a column. The nerves of the spinal cord run in a tunnel through the middle of those bones. Spongy discs between the vertebrae act as cushions. Ligaments and tendons hold everything together.

A lot of things can go wrong with your back. A strained muscle or a problem with a disc or a bone can cause pain. Back pain might also arise from a fracture or tumor. Most of the time, though, it is impossible to tell what is making your back hurt.

"We rarely find out exactly what it is," says Dr. Gunnar Andersson, an orthopedic surgeon at Rush University Medical Center in Chicago. "As long as it stays as back pain, we are typically not that concerned."

Your back naturally changes as you get older. Discs degenerate, and arthritis may develop in the small joints of the back. Those changes may show up on a magnetic resonance imaging (MRI) scan or other types of imaging scans. But such changes to the back are also seen in

---

This chapter contains text excerpted from the following sources: Text in this chapter begins with excerpts from "When Your Back Hurts, Don't Let Back Pain Knock You Flat," National Institute of Arthritis and Musculoskeletal and Skin Diseases (NIAMS), December 4, 2014. Reviewed April 2019; Text under the heading "Spinal Stenosis" is excerpted from "Spinal Stenosis," MedlinePlus, National Institutes of Health (NIH), January 3, 2017.

a lot of people who do not have back pain. Therefore, it is hard to know if the changes are actually what is causing the pain.

People that are obese are more likely to have low back pain, as are people who smoke. Back pain is also more common in people who do not exercise often, or in people who are mostly inactive but have occasional bursts of exercise.

The good news is that most back pain goes away by itself. For a new pain in the back, Andersson says he usually advises taking over-the-counter (OTC) medications for the pain and staying away from activity that is hard on the back, such as lifting, carrying, bending, and twisting. "Then, wait for the problem to disappear, which it will in the great majority of people over a few weeks," he says.

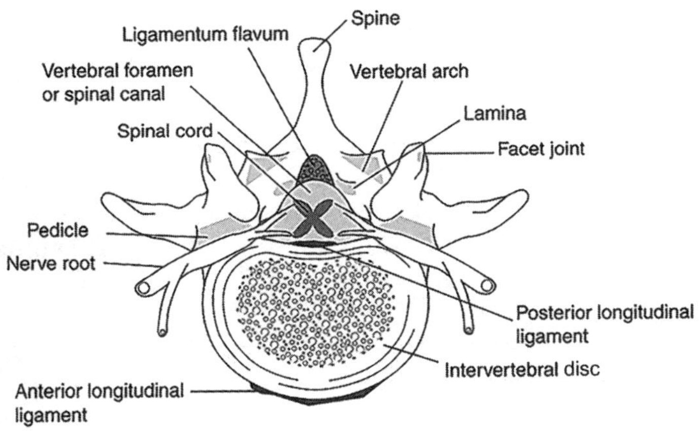

Figure 4.1. *Structures of Spine* (Source: "Structures of Spine," National Institute of Arthritis and Musculoskeletal and Skin Diseases (NIAMS).)

But for some people, the pain continues. If your back hurts most of the time for more than three months, you have chronic back pain.

What doctors do about chronic pain depends on the source of the pain. Some chronic back pain requires prolonged medical attention. If the pain comes from a fracture or tumor, those problems can be treated. Surgery can help if the pain is caused by a ruptured (herniated) disc or certain other conditions, such as spinal stenosis (narrowing of the spinal column, which can put pressure on the nerves) or degenerative spondylolisthesis (when one vertebra slips over another). But, surgery is not the right choice for everyone.

There are many treatment options for back pain, so be sure to talk to your healthcare provider about which approach is right for you. For most people, even chronic pain eventually clears up without surgery. The most important thing, Andersson says, is not to let the pain take over. Research has shown that patients who stay active are better off. Just be sure to avoid activities that might strain the back. "It is important not to succumb to the pain and become afraid of moving," Andersson says. "It does not seem to make much difference what you do, as long as you stay active."

Spinal Stenosis

Your spine, or backbone, protects your spinal cord and allows you to stand and bend. Spinal stenosis causes narrowing in your spine. The narrowing puts pressure on your nerves and spinal cord and can cause pain.

Spinal stenosis occurs mostly in people older than 50 years of age. Younger people with a spine injury or a narrow spinal canal are also at risk. Diseases such as arthritis and scoliosis can cause spinal stenosis too. Symptoms might appear gradually or not at all. They include:

- Pain in your neck or back
- Numbness, weakness, cramping, or pain in your arms or legs
- Pain going down the leg
- Foot problems

Doctors diagnose spinal stenosis with a physical exam and imaging tests. Treatments include medications, physical therapy (PT), braces, and surgery.

Chapter 5

Facts about Low Back Pain

If you have lower back pain, you are not alone. About 80 percent of adults experience low back pain at some point in their lifetimes. It is the most common cause of job-related disability and a leading contributor to missed work days. In a large survey, more than a quarter of adults reported experiencing low back pain during the past 3 months.

Men and women are equally affected by low back pain, which can range in intensity from a dull, constant ache to a sudden, sharp sensation that leaves the person incapacitated. Pain can begin abruptly as a result of an accident or by lifting something heavy, or it can develop over time due to age-related changes of the spine. Sedentary lifestyles also can set the stage for low back pain, especially when a weekday routine of getting too little exercise is punctuated by strenuous weekend workout.

Most low back pain is acute, or short term, and lasts a few days to a few weeks. It tends to resolve on its own with self-care, and there is no residual loss of function. The majority of acute low back pain is mechanical in nature, meaning that there is a disruption in the way the components of the back (the spine, muscle, intervertebral discs, and nerves) fit together and move.

Subacute low back pain is defined as pain that lasts between 4 and 12 weeks.

This chapter includes text excerpted from "Low Back Pain Fact Sheet," National Institute of Neurological Disorders and Stroke (NINDS), December 19, 2014. Reviewed April 2019.

Chronic back pain is defined as pain that persists for 12 weeks or longer, even after an initial injury or underlying cause of acute low back pain has been treated. About 20 percent of people affected by acute low back pain develop chronic low back pain with persistent symptoms within 1 year. In some cases, treatment successfully relieves chronic low back pain, but in other cases, pain persists despite medical and surgical treatment.

In 1990, a study ranking the most burdensome conditions in the United States in terms of mortality or poor health as a result of disease put low back pain in sixth place; in 2010, low back pain jumped to third place, with only ischemic heart disease and chronic obstructive pulmonary disease (COPD) ranking higher.

What Causes Lower Back Pain

The vast majority of low back pain is mechanical in nature. In many cases, low back pain is associated with spondylosis, a term that refers to the general degeneration of the spine associated with normal wear and tear that occurs in the joints, discs, and bones of the spine as people get older. Some examples of mechanical causes of low back pain include:

- **Sprains and strains** account for most acute back pain. Sprains are caused by overstretching or tearing ligaments, and strains are tears in tendon or muscle. Both can occur from twisting or lifting something improperly, lifting something too heavy, or overstretching. Such movements may also trigger spasms in back muscles, which can also be painful.
- **Intervertebral disc degeneration** is one of the most common mechanical causes of low back pain, and it occurs when the usually rubbery discs lose integrity as a normal process of aging. In a healthy back, intervertebral discs provide height and allow bending, flexion, and torsion of the lower back. As the discs deteriorate, they lose their cushioning ability.
- **Herniated or ruptured discs** can occur when the intervertebral discs become compressed and bulge outward (herniation) or rupture, causing low back pain.
- **Radiculopathy** is a condition caused by compression, inflammation, and/or injury to a spinal nerve root. Pressure on the nerve root results in pain, numbness, or a tingling sensation that travels or radiates to other areas of the body that are served

by that nerve. Radiculopathy may occur when spinal stenosis or a herniated or ruptured disc compresses the nerve root.

- **Sciatica** is a form of radiculopathy caused by compression of the sciatic nerve, the large nerve that travels through the buttocks and extends down the back of the leg. This compression causes shock-like or burning low back pain, combined with pain through the buttocks and down one leg, occasionally reaching the foot. In the most extreme cases, when the nerve is pinched between the disc and the adjacent bone, the symptoms may involve not only pain, but numbness and muscle weakness in the leg because of interrupted nerve signaling. The condition may also be caused by a tumor or cyst that presses on the sciatic nerve or its roots.
- **Spondylolisthesis** is a condition in which a vertebra of the lower spine slips out of place, pinching the nerves exiting the spinal column.
- **A traumatic injury**—such as from playing sports, car accidents, or a fall—can injure tendons, ligaments, or muscle and result in low back pain. Traumatic injury may also cause the spine to become overly compressed, which in turn can cause an intervertebral disc to rupture or herniate, exerting pressure on any of the nerves rooted to the spinal cord. When spinal nerves become compressed and irritated, back pain and sciatica may result.
- **Spinal stenosis** is a narrowing of the spinal column that puts pressure on the spinal cord and nerves that can cause pain or numbness with walking and over time leads to leg weakness and sensory loss.
- **Skeletal irregularities** include scoliosis, a curvature of the spine that does not usually cause pain until middle age; lordosis, an abnormally accentuated arch in the lower back; and other congenital anomalies of the spine.

Low back pain is rarely related to serious underlying conditions, but when these conditions do occur, they require immediate medical attention. Serious underlying conditions include:

- **Infections** are not a common cause of back pain. However, infections can cause pain when they involve the vertebrae, a condition called "osteomyelitis;" the intervertebral discs, called "discitis;" or the sacroiliac joints connecting the lower spine to the pelvis, called "sacroiliitis."

- **Tumors** are a relatively rare cause of back pain. Occasionally, tumors begin in the back, but more often they appear in the back as a result of cancer that has spread from elsewhere in the body.
- **Cauda equina syndrome (CES)** is a serious but rare complication of a ruptured disc. It occurs when disc material is pushed into the spinal canal and compresses the bundle of lumbar and sacral nerve roots, causing loss of bladder and bowel control. Permanent neurological damage may result if this syndrome is left untreated.
- **Abdominal aortic aneurysms (AAAs)** occur when the large blood vessel that supplies blood to the abdomen, pelvis, and legs becomes abnormally enlarged. Back pain can be a sign that the aneurysm is becoming larger and that the risk of rupture should be assessed.
- **Kidney stones** can cause sharp pain in the lower back, usually on one side.

Other underlying conditions that predispose people to low back pain include:

- **Inflammatory diseases** of the joints—such as arthritis, including osteoarthritis and rheumatoid arthritis, as well as spondylitis, an inflammation of the vertebrae—can also cause low back pain. Spondylitis is also called "spondyloarthritis" or "spondyloarthropathy."
- **Osteoporosis** is a metabolic bone disease marked by a progressive decrease in bone density and strength, which can lead to painful fractures of the vertebrae.
- **Endometriosis** is the buildup of uterine tissue in places outside the uterus.
- **Fibromyalgia**, a chronic pain syndrome involving widespread muscle pain and fatigue

What Are the Risk Factors for Developing Low Back Pain?

Beyond underlying diseases, certain other risk factors may elevate one's risk for low back pain, including:

- **Age.** The first attack of low back pain typically occurs between the ages of 30 and 50, and back pain becomes more common with advancing age. As people grow older, loss of bone strength from osteoporosis can lead to fractures, and at the same time, muscle elasticity and tone decrease. The intervertebral discs begin to lose fluid and flexibility with age, which decreases their ability to cushion the vertebrae. The risk of spinal stenosis also increases with age.

- **Fitness level.** Back pain is more common among people who are not physically fit. Weak back and abdominal muscles may not properly support the spine. "Weekend warriors"—people who go out and exercise a lot after being inactive all week—are more likely to suffer painful back injuries than people who make moderate physical activity a daily habit. Studies show that low-impact aerobic exercise is beneficial for maintaining the integrity of intervertebral discs.
- **Pregnancy** is commonly accompanied by low back pain, which results from pelvic changes and alterations in weight loading. Back symptoms almost always resolve postpartum.
- **Weight gain.** Being overweight, obese, or quickly gaining significant amounts of weight can put stress on the back and lead to low back pain.
- **Genetics.** Some causes of back pain, such as ankylosing spondylitis, a form of arthritis that involves fusion of the spinal joints and leads to some immobility of the spine, have a genetic component.
- **Occupational risk factors.** Having a job that requires heavy lifting, pushing, or pulling, particularly when it involves twisting or vibrating the spine, can lead to injury and back pain. An inactive job or a desk job may also lead to or contribute to pain, especially if you have poor posture or sit all day in a chair with inadequate back support.
- **Mental-health factors:** Preexisting mental-health issues, such as anxiety and depression, can influence how closely one focuses on their pain, as well as their perception of its severity. Pain that becomes chronic also can contribute to the development of such psychological factors. Stress can affect the body in numerous ways, including causing muscle tension.
- **Backpack overload in children.** Low back pain unrelated to injury or another known cause is unusual in preteen children. However, a backpack overloaded with school books and supplies

can strain the back and cause muscle fatigue. The American Academy of Orthopaedic Surgeons (AAOS) recommends that a child's backpack should weigh no more than 15 to 20 percent of the child's body weight.

Can Back Pain Be Prevented?

Recurring back pain resulting from improper body mechanics is often preventable by avoiding movements that jolt or strain the back, maintaining correct posture, and lifting objects properly. Many work-related injuries are caused or aggravated by stressors, such as heavy lifting, contact stress (repeated or constant contact between soft body tissue and a hard or sharp object), vibration, repetitive motion, and awkward posture. Using ergonomically designed furniture and equipment to protect the body from injury at home and in the workplace may reduce the risk of back injury.

The use of lumbar supports in the form of wide elastic bands that can be tightened to provide support to the lower back and abdominal muscles to prevent low back pain remains controversial. Such supports are widely used despite a lack of evidence showing that they actually prevent pain. Multiple studies have determined that the use of lumbar supports provides no benefit in terms of the prevention and treatment of back pain. Although, there have been anecdotal case reports of injury reduction among workers using lumbar support belts, many companies that have back belt programs also have training and ergonomic awareness programs. The reported injury reduction may be related to a combination of these or other factors. Furthermore, some caution is advised given that wearing supportive belts may actually lead to or aggravate back pain by causing back muscles to weaken from lack of use.

Recommendations for Keeping One's Back Healthy

Following any period of prolonged inactivity, a regimen of low-impact exercises is advised. Speed walking, swimming, or stationary bike riding for 30 minutes each day can increase muscle strength and flexibility. Yoga also can help stretch and strengthen muscles and improve posture. Consult a physician for a list of low-impact, age-appropriate exercises that are specifically targeted to strengthening lower back and abdominal muscles.

- Always stretch before exercise or other strenuous physical activity.

- Do not slouch when standing or sitting. The lower back can support a person's weight most easily when the curvature is reduced. When standing, keep your weight balanced on your feet.
- At home or work, make sure work surfaces are at a comfortable height.
- Sit in a chair with good lumbar support and proper position and height for the task. Keep shoulders back. Switch sitting positions often and periodically walk around the office or gently stretch muscles to relieve tension. A pillow or rolled-up towel placed behind the small of the back can provide some lumbar support. During prolonged periods of sitting, elevate feet on a low stool or a stack of books.
- Wear comfortable, low-heeled shoes.
- Sleeping on one's side with the knees drawn up in a fetal position can help open up the joints in the spine and relieve pressure by reducing the curvature of the spine. Always sleep on a firm surface.
- Do not try to lift objects that are too heavy. Lift from the knees, pull the stomach muscles in, and keep the head down and in line with a straight back. When lifting, keep objects close to the body. Do not twist when lifting.
- Maintain proper nutrition and diet to reduce and prevent excessive weight gain, especially weight around the waistline that taxes lower back muscles. A diet with sufficient daily intake of calcium, phosphorus, and vitamin D helps to promote new bone growth.
- Quit smoking. Smoking reduces blood flow to the lower spine, which can contribute to spinal disc degeneration. Smoking also increases the risk of osteoporosis and impedes healing. Coughing due to heavy smoking also may cause back pain.

Chapter 6

Neck Pain

The neck (cervical spine) consists of seven vertebrae that starts from the base of the skull and extends to the upper torso. The cervical spine is one of the most flexible regions of the spine. It allows motion and supports the weight of your head. The cervical spine consists of bones that are linked together by small facet joints. There are cervical discs located in between the vertebrae, and these discs act as a shock absorber and protect bone from wearing away.

People sometimes experience pain and stiffness around the neck, which usually happens due to poor posture and stressing the neck.

Types

The neck pain is categorized into three types, and they are as follows:

- **Acute pain:** Acute pain lasts for four weeks or less. There is no specific cause, but it can be due to one's posture, sleeping position, stress level, etc.
- **Subacute pain:** Subacute pain lasts anywhere from 4 to 12 weeks and requires medical attention to alleviate the neck pain.
- **Chronic pain:** Chronic pain lasts for three months or longer, and it may cause other problems if left untreated for a long time.

Causes

Since the cervical spine is less protected than the rest of the spine, it is more vulnerable to disorders and injuries that can cause pain and restrain motion. The most common causes of neck pain are:

- Sleeping in a bad position
- Involvement in high-intensity sports
- Working at a desk for a long time
- Lifting heavy weights
- Wearing heavy necklaces

Severe injury or the presence of any disease—such as cervical disc degeneration, which causes worn joints—can lead to neck pain.

Symptoms

The symptoms of neck pain are as follows:

- A stiff neck
- Sharp pain in one area or spot in the neck
- Soreness or tenderness
- Pain around the arms, shoulders, and hands
- Headache

The other symptoms associated with neck pain are:

- Difficulty with gripping or holding objects
- Problems with walking
- Loss of bladder control

Neck pain is not a serious condition, and it can be relieved with medication within a few days. But in some cases, neck pain might be an indication of a serious problem and requires immediate medical attention.

When to See Your Doctor

If you have continuous and severe neck pain for a long time, visit your doctor to discuss your symptoms. In case of a sudden neck injury, such as a car accident (whiplash injury) or a fall from a great height, call 911 immediately. Trained professionals will temporarily immobilize the person who is injured to avoid further injury or casualties.

Diagnosis

The diagnosis of neck pain starts with identifying the location, duration, and severity of pain in the neck. The doctor also reviews your medical history in order to find previous neck injuries and surgeries, if any. Questions about the workplace, lifestyle, and sleeping habits are also asked by your doctor.

After the physical examination, the doctor orders for imaging tests, such as X-rays, magnetic resonance imaging (MRI), computerized tomography (CT) scan, myelogram, electromyograph (EMG), and nerve conduction velocity (NCV) test.

Based on the results, the doctor will decide on the best treatment for your condition.

Treatment

Nonsurgical Treatment

Treatment for neck pain normally begins with nonsurgical treatment and does not move to surgical treatment until the nonsurgical treatment is proven ineffective.

Nonsurgical treatment includes the following:

- **Physical exercises** are recommended by the doctor. These exercises consist of specific movements for the neck and other parts of the body.
- **Massaging** of the neck muscles with heat and cold applications can alleviate the pain for a short period of time.
- **Better posture** while standing, sitting, and sleeping are suggested by the physiotherapist in order to avoid a worsening of the condition.
- **Over-the-counter (OTC) medications** are prescribed by the doctor to relieve excess pain and to prevent that pain from spreading around the arms, hands, and fingers.
- **Cervical braces** are worn in order to decrease pain and to restore motion of the neck muscles.
- **Chiropractic adjustments** are done on the spine, which involves controlled and abrupt force to a joint. This can give a short-term pain relief.
- **Alternative treatments,** including acupuncture, are useful for managing neck pain.

Surgical Treatment

The surgical treatment is done for three reasons, and they are as follows:

- To relieve pain around your neck
- To remove and replace the damaged disc/structure
- To decompress the spinal cord compression

Some of the surgeries that are used to treat neck pain are:

- **Anterior cervical discectomy and fusion (ACDF)** is the surgery used to remove the damaged discs from the cervical spine. This is done in the front part of the neck in conjunction with spinal fusion.
- **Posterior cervical fusion (PCF)** is performed to relieve pain and to release the compression in nerve roots or spinal cord. It involves fusing the damaged vertebrae with the adjacent one from a posterior (back) incision.
- **Artificial cervical disc replacement (ACDR)** is done as an alternative to ACDF. This procedure includes replacing the problematic disc with an artificial disc. The purpose of this surgical procedure is to restore the neck's flexibility.

Prognosis

Neck pain can be a result of poor posture and the regular wear and tear of the vertebrae associated with aging. Precautions that may prevent neck pain from occurring are:

- Maintaining good posture
- Taking breaks during a long journey
- Avoiding lifting heavy objects
- Quitting smoking
- Sleeping in a good position

References

1. "Neck pain," Mayo Clinic, December 19, 2018.
2. Shim, John H. "Chronic Neck Pain: What Condition Is Causing My Neck Pain?" SPINE-health, June 22, 2016.

3. "Neck Pain," OrthoInfo, February 1, 2001.
4. Pietrangelo, Ann. "Neck Pain: Possible Causes and How to Treat It," Healthline, July 31, 2017.
5. "Neck Pain," Versus Arthritis, September 19, 2018.

Chapter 7

Diagnosis and Treatment for Back Pain

How Is Low Back Pain Diagnosed?

A complete medical history and physical exam can usually identify any serious conditions that may be causing the pain. During the exam, a healthcare provider will ask about the onset, site, and severity of the pain; duration of symptoms and any limitations in movement; and history of previous episodes or any health conditions that might be related to the pain. Along with a thorough back examination, neurologic tests are conducted to determine the cause of pain and appropriate treatment. The cause of chronic lower back pain is often difficult to determine even after a thorough examination.

Imaging tests are not warranted in most cases. Under certain circumstances, however, imaging may be ordered to rule out specific causes of pain, including tumors and spinal stenosis. Imaging and other types of tests include:

- **X-ray** is often the first imaging technique used to look for broken bones or an injured vertebra. X-rays show the bony structures and any vertebral misalignment or fractures. Soft tissues,

---

This chapter includes text excerpted from "Low Back Pain Fact Sheet," National Institute of Neurological Disorders and Stroke (NINDS), August 7, 2018.

such as muscles, ligaments, or bulging discs, are not visible on conventional X-rays.

- **Computed tomography (CT) scan** is used to see spinal structures that cannot be seen on conventional X-rays, such as disc rupture, spinal stenosis, or tumors. Using a computer, the CT scan creates a three-dimensional image from a series of two-dimensional pictures.
- **Myelograms** enhance the diagnostic imaging of X-rays and CT scans. In this procedure, a contrast dye is injected into the spinal canal, allowing spinal cord and nerve compression caused by herniated discs or fractures to be seen on an X-ray or CT scans.
- **Discography** may be used when other diagnostic procedures fail to identify the cause of pain. This procedure involves the injection of a contrast dye into a spinal disc thought to be causing low back pain. The fluid's pressure in the disc will reproduce the person's symptoms if the disc is the cause. The dye helps to show the damaged areas on CT scans taken following the injection. Discography may provide useful information in cases where people are considering lumbar surgery or when their pain has not responded to conventional treatments.
- **Magnetic resonance imaging (MRI)** uses a magnetic force instead of radiation to create a computer-generated image. Unlike X-rays, which show only bony structures, MRI scans also produce images of soft tissues, such as muscles, ligaments, tendons, and blood vessels. An MRI may be ordered if a problem such as infection, tumor, inflammation, disc herniation or rupture, or pressure on a nerve is suspected. MRI is a noninvasive way to identify a condition requiring prompt surgical treatment. However, in most instances, unless there are "red flags" in the history or physical exam, an MRI scan is not necessary during the early phases of low back pain.
- **Electrodiagnostics** are procedures that, in the setting of low back pain, are primarily used to confirm whether a person has lumbar radiculopathy. The procedures include electromyography (EMG), nerve conduction studies (NCS), and evoked potential (EP) studies. EMG assesses the electrical activity in a muscle and can detect if muscle weakness results from a problem with the nerves that control the muscles. Very fine needles are inserted in muscles to measure electrical activity transmitted

from the brain or spinal cord to a particular area of the body. NCSs are often performed along with EMG to exclude conditions that can mimic radiculopathy. In NCSs, two sets of electrodes are placed on the skin over the muscles. The first set provides a mild shock to stimulate the nerve that runs to a particular muscle. The second set records the nerve's electrical signals, and from this information, nerve damage that slows conduction of the nerve signal can be detected. EP tests also involve two sets of electrodes—one set to stimulate a sensory nerve and the other placed on the scalp to record the speed of nerve signal transmissions to the brain.

- **Bone scans** are used to detect and monitor infection, fracture, or disorders in the bone. A small amount of radioactive material is injected into the bloodstream and will collect in the bones, particularly in areas with some abnormality. Scanner-generated images can be used to identify specific areas of irregular bone metabolism or abnormal blood flow, as well as to measure levels of joint disease.
- **Ultrasound imaging,** also called "ultrasound scanning" or "sonography," uses high-frequency sound waves to obtain images inside the body. The sound wave echoes are recorded and displayed as a real-time visual image. Ultrasound imaging can show tears in ligaments, muscles, tendons, and other soft tissue masses in the back.
- **Blood tests** are not routinely used to diagnose the cause of back pain; however, in some cases, they may be ordered to look for indications of inflammation, infection, and/or the presence of arthritis. Potential tests include complete blood count, erythrocyte sedimentation rate, and C-reactive protein. Blood tests may also detect HLA-B27, a genetic marker in the blood that is more common in people with ankylosing spondylitis or reactive arthritis (a form of arthritis that occurs following infection in another part of the body, usually in the genitourinary tract).

How Is Back Pain Treated?

Treatment for low back pain generally depends on whether the pain is acute or chronic. In general, surgery is recommended only if there is evidence of worsening nerve damage and when diagnostic tests indicate structural changes for which corrective surgical procedures have been developed.

Conventionally used treatments and their level of supportive evidence include:

Hot or cold packs have never been proven to quickly resolve low back injury; however, they may help ease pain and reduce inflammation for people with acute, subacute, or chronic pain, allowing for greater mobility among some individuals.

Activity. Bed rest should be limited. Individuals should begin stretching exercises and resume normal daily activities as soon as possible, while avoiding movements that aggravate pain. Strong evidence shows that persons who continue their activities without bed rest following onset of low back pain appeared to have better back flexibility than those who rested in bed for a week. Other studies suggest that bed rest alone may make back pain worse and can lead to secondary complications, such as depression, decreased muscle tone, and blood clots in the legs.

Strengthening exercises, beyond general daily activities, are not advised for acute low back pain, but may be an effective way to speed recovery from chronic or subacute low back pain. Maintaining and building muscle strength is particularly important for persons with skeletal irregularities. Healthcare providers can provide a list of beneficial exercises that will help improve coordination and develop proper posture and muscle balance. Evidence supports short- and long-term benefits of yoga to ease chronic low back pain.

Physical therapy programs to strengthen core muscle groups that support the low back, improve mobility and flexibility, and promote proper positioning and posture are often used in combinations with other interventions.

Medications. A wide range of medications are used to treat acute and chronic low back pain. Some are available over-the-counter (OTC); others require a physician's prescription. Certain drugs, even those available OTC, may be unsafe during pregnancy; may interact with other medications; cause side effects; or lead to serious adverse effects, such as liver damage or gastrointestinal ulcers and bleeding. Consultation with a healthcare provider is advised before use. The following are the main types of medications used for low back pain.

- **Analgesic medications** are those specifically designed to relieve pain. They include OTC acetaminophen and aspirin, as well as prescription opioids, such as codeine, oxycodone, hydrocodone, and morphine. Opioids should be used only for a short period of time and under a physician's supervision. People can develop a tolerance to opioids and require increasingly higher dosages to achieve the same effect. Opioids can also be addictive. Their side effects can include drowsiness, constipation, decreased reaction time, and impaired judgment. Some specialists are concerned that chronic use of opioids is detrimental to people with back pain because they can aggravate depression, leading to a worsening of the pain.
- **Nonsteroidal anti-inflammatory drugs (NSAIDs)** relieve pain and inflammation and include OTC formulations (ibuprofen, ketoprofen, and naproxen sodium). Several others, including a type of NSAID called "COX-2 inhibitors," are available only by prescription. Long-term use of NSAIDs has been associated with stomach irritation, ulcers, heartburn, diarrhea, fluid retention, and in rare cases, kidney dysfunction and cardiovascular disease. The longer a person uses NSAIDs, the more likely they are to develop side effects. Many other drugs cannot be taken at the same time a person is treated with NSAIDs because they alter the way the body processes or eliminates other medications.
- **Anticonvulsants**—drugs primarily used to treat seizures—may be useful in treating people with radiculopathy and radicular pain.
- **Antidepressants,** such as tricyclics and serotonin and norepinephrine reuptake inhibitors, have been commonly prescribed for chronic low back pain, but their benefit for nonspecific low back pain is unproven, according to a review of studies assessing their benefit.
- **Counter-irritants,** such as creams or sprays applied topically, stimulate the nerves in the skin to provide feelings of warmth or cold in order to dull the sensation of pain. Topical analgesics reduce inflammation and stimulate blood flow.

Spinal manipulation and spinal mobilization are approaches in which professionally licensed specialists (doctors of chiropractic care) use their hands to mobilize, adjust, massage, or stimulate the spine and the surrounding tissues. Manipulation involves a rapid movement over which the individual has no control; mobilization involves slower adjustment movements. The techniques have been shown to provide small to moderate short-term benefits in people with chronic low back pain. Evidence supporting their use for acute or subacute low back pain is generally of low quality. Neither technique is appropriate when a person has an underlying medical cause for the back pain, such as osteoporosis, spinal cord compression, or arthritis.

Traction involves the use of weights and pulleys to apply constant or intermittent force to gradually "pull" the skeletal structure into better alignment. Some people experience pain relief while in traction, but that relief is usually temporary. Once traction is released, the back pain tends to return. There is no evidence that traction provides any long-term benefits for people with low back pain.

Acupuncture is moderately effective for chronic low back pain. It involves the insertion of thin needles into precise points throughout the body. Some practitioners believe this process helps clear away blockages in the body's life force known as "Qi." Others who may not believe in the concept of Qi theorize that when the needles are inserted and then stimulated (by twisting or passing a low-voltage electrical current through them), naturally occurring painkilling chemicals, such as endorphins, serotonin, and acetylcholine, are released. Evidence of acupuncture's benefit for acute low back pain is conflicting, and clinical studies continue to investigate its benefits.

Biofeedback is used to treat many acute pain problems, most notably back pain and headache. The therapy involves the attachment of electrodes to the skin and the use of an electromyography machine that allows people to become aware of and self-regulate their breathing, muscle tension, heart rate, and skin temperature. People regulate their response to pain by using relaxation techniques. Biofeedback is often used in combination with other treatment methods, generally without side effects. Evidence is lacking that biofeedback provides a clear benefit for low back pain.

Nerve block therapies aim to relieve chronic pain by blocking nerve conduction from specific areas of the body. Nerve block approaches range from injections of local anesthetics, botulinum toxin, or steroids into affected soft tissues or joints to more complex nerve-root blocks and spinal cord stimulation. When extreme pain is involved, low doses of drugs may be administered by catheter directly into the spinal cord. The success of a nerve block approach depends on the ability of a practitioner to locate and inject precisely the correct nerve. Chronic use of steroid injections may lead to increased functional impairment.

Epidural steroid injections are a commonly used short-term option for treating low back pain and sciatica associated with inflammation. Pain relief associated with the injections, however, tends to be temporary, and the injections are not advised for long-term use. A National Institutes of Health (NIH)-funded randomized controlled trial assessing the benefit of epidural steroid injections for the treatment of chronic low back pain associated with spinal stenosis showed that long-term outcomes were worse among those people who received the injections compared with those who did not.

Transcutaneous electrical nerve stimulation (TENS) involves wearing a battery-powered device, consisting of electrodes, on the skin and over the painful area; the device generates electrical impulses that are designed to block incoming pain signals from the peripheral nerves. The theory is that stimulating the nervous system can modify the perception of pain. Early studies of TENS suggested that it elevated levels of endorphins, the body's natural pain-numbing chemicals. More recent studies, however, have produced mixed results on its effectiveness for providing relief from low back pain.

Surgery

When other therapies fail, surgery may be considered an option to relieve pain caused by serious musculoskeletal injuries or nerve compression. It may be months following surgery before the patient is fully healed, and he or she may suffer permanent loss of flexibility.

Surgical procedures are not always successful, and there is little evidence to show which procedures work best for their particular indications. Patients considering surgical approaches should be fully informed of all related risks. Surgical options include:

- Vertebroplasty and kyphoplasty
- Spinal laminectomy (also known as "spinal decompression")
- Discectomy or microdiscectomy
- Foraminotomy
- Intradiscal electrothermal therapy (IDET)

- Nucleoplasty
- Radiofrequency denervation
- Spinal fusion
- Artificial disc replacement

Part Two

Maintaining Spinal Health

Chapter 8

Understanding Neutral Spine Posture

Chapter Contents

Section 8.1—Getting It Straight: Looking after Your Back 58
Section 8.2—Guide to Good Posture 61

Section 8.1

Getting It Straight: Looking after Your Back

This section includes text excerpted from "Getting It Straight: Improve Your Posture for Better Health," *NIH News in Health*, National Institutes of Health (NIH), August 2017.

Sit up straight! This common request may have been how you first heard about posture, the way you hold your body. Posture is not just about how you look. How you position yourself can help or hurt your health over your lifetime.

"Posture is not only about how well you sit, but how well you move and go about your daily life," says Dr. George Salem, a National Institutes of Health (NIH)-funded researcher at the University of Southern California (USC) who studies how movement affects health and quality of life (QOL).

How you hold yourself when you are not moving—such as when you are sitting, standing, or sleeping—is called "static posture." Dynamic posture is how you position your body while you are moving, such as walking or bending over to pick something up. "It's important to consider both static and dynamic components of posture," Salem says.

Posture can be affected by many things: your age, the situations you find yourself in, and your daily choices. For instance, children may have to adjust to carry heavy backpacks to school. Pregnant women move differently to accommodate the change in their center of gravity.

Your posture involves your musculoskeletal system. This includes your bones, muscles, joints, and other tissues that connect the parts of your body together. It is what provides form, support, stability, and movement to your body.

How you hold yourself can either align or misalign your musculoskeletal system. Throughout life, this system must adapt to the type of work you do, the hobbies you enjoy, how you use electronic devices, injuries, and even the kind of shoes you wear.

You may think that sitting with slumped shoulders or bending at your back instead of your knees sometimes will not hurt you. But, small changes in how you hold yourself and move can add up over a lifetime.

Years of slouching wears away at your spine to make it more fragile and prone to injury. Holding your body and moving in unhealthy ways often leads to neck, shoulder, and back pain. In any three-month period, about one in four adults in the United States has at least one day of back pain.

Poor posture can also decrease your flexibility, how well your joints move, and your balance. It can impact your ability to do things for yourself and increase your risk for falls. Slumped posture can even make it more difficult to digest the food you eat and breathe comfortably.

Some research suggests a link between posture and mental health as well. "Someone with depression may appear more closed in, curved, and tend to look down," says National Institutes of Health (NIH) physical therapist Dr. Cris Zampieri. "When people feel anxious, they may raise their shoulders." Scientists are now exploring the connections between posture and how we think and process information in the brain.

Our bodies change as we age. These natural changes make it especially important for older adults to maintain good posture, strength, flexibility, and balance. "Older adults tend to adopt a progressively hunched posture," says Salem. "When shoulders continue to round forward over time, it creates excessive loading on the shoulder joint. This can create injury and limit the independence of older adults."

An extremely hunched posture, or hyperkyphosis, affects up to two-thirds of senior women and half of senior men. This posture has been associated with back pain, weakness, and trouble breathing. It can also limit everyday activities, such as brushing your hair and dressing yourself.

Salem and other researchers have been studying the possible health benefits of yoga, particularly for older adults. Yoga is a mind and body practice that typically combines physical postures, breathing exercises, and meditation or relaxation. In one study, older adults with hyperkyphosis showed significant improvement and less rounded shoulders after a six-month yoga program.

"More people are participating in yoga," Salem says. "We're using innovative tools—like motion analysis with high-speed cameras and platforms that measure force—to understand what yoga is actually doing and how it is targeting the biological processes of our body." Ultimately, Salem says these findings will help therapists and yoga instructors design programs that are safe and effective for older adults. The team also plans to study other age groups and people with disabilities.

It is never too early or late in life to work on improving your posture and how you move.

"One way to improve your posture is to be aware of it in the first place," Zampieri says. "It's important to take a look at your posture before it becomes a problem. Yoga, tai chi, and other types of classes that focus on body awareness and mindfulness can help you learn to feel what's wrong in your own posture. They also help you connect your physical posture with your emotional state, offering benefits in both areas."

Classes are not the only way to improve your posture. "Be mindful of your posture and how you're moving," Salem says. "Think about lifting your head, pulling your shoulders back, and tightening your abdominal muscles in everyday situations." Be aware of repetitive postures, such as regularly lifting heavy objects, and holding positions for a long time, such as sitting at a computer all day at work.

"If you spend a lot of time in front of a computer, make sure you have a good setup," says NIH physical therapist Dr. Jesse Matsubara. "It's important that your workstation fits you the best it can. You should also switch sitting positions often, take brief walks around the office, and gently stretch your muscles every so often to help relieve muscle tension."

The foundation of good posture is having a body that can support it. This means having strong abdominal and back muscles, flexibility, and a balanced body over your life. Another way to improve posture is to lose weight, especially around your gut. More than two out of three Americans are either overweight or obese. Extra weight weakens your abdominal muscles, causes problems for your pelvis and spine, and contributes to low back pain.

"It's easy to develop suboptimal movement patterns after an injury or from years of pain," Salem explains, "but people can learn to distribute their weight evenly and balance their bodies again."

It is important to work with a doctor to find the types of physical activity that can help you maintain your health and mobility. Talk to your healthcare providers if you feel pain, have an injury, or have had surgery. They can give you feedback on how you are moving, help you avoid unhealthy movement patterns, and work with you to create a plan that is best for you.

Improve Your Posture

- Be mindful of your posture during everyday activities, such as watching television, washing dishes, or walking.
- Take frequent breaks for stretching and moving your body in different ways.
- Stay active.

- Maintain a healthy weight.
- Make sure work surfaces are at a comfortable height for you, whether you are working in an office, doing a hobby, preparing dinner, or eating a meal.
- Wear comfortable, low-heeled shoes.

Section 8.2

Guide to Good Posture

This section includes text excerpted from "Guide to Good Posture," MedlinePlus, National Institutes of Health (NIH), October 25, 2017.

Good posture is about more than standing up straight so you can look your best. It is an important part of your long-term health. Making sure that you hold your body the right way, whether you are moving or still, can prevent pain, injuries, and other health problems.

What Is Posture?

Posture is how you hold your body. There are two types:

- **Dynamic posture** is how you hold yourself when you are moving, such as when you are walking, running, or bending over to pick up something.
- **Static posture** is how you hold yourself when you are not moving, such as when you are sitting, standing, or sleeping.

It is important to make sure that you have good dynamic and static posture.

The key to good posture is the position of your spine. Your spine has three natural curves—at your neck, mid-back, and low back. Correct posture should maintain these curves but not increase them. Your head should be above your shoulders, and the top of your shoulder should be over the hips.

How Can Posture Affect Your Health?

Poor posture can be bad for your health. Slouching or slumping over can:

- Misalign your musculoskeletal system
- Wear away at your spine, making it more fragile and prone to injury
- Cause neck, shoulder, and back pain
- Decrease your flexibility
- Affect how well your joints move
- Affect your balance and increase your risk of falling
- Make it harder to digest your food
- Make it harder to breathe

How Can You Improve Your Posture in General?

To improve your posture in general, you can:

- **Be mindful** of your posture during everyday activities, such as watching television, washing dishes, or walking.
- **Stay active**. Any kind of exercise may help improve your posture, but certain types of exercises can be especially helpful. They include yoga, tai chi, and other classes that focus on body awareness. It is also a good idea to do exercises that strengthen your core (muscles around your back, abdomen, and pelvis).
- **Maintain a healthy weight**. Extra weight can weaken your abdominal muscles, cause problems for your pelvis and spine, and contribute to low back pain. All of these can hurt your posture.
- **Wear comfortable, low-heeled shoes**. High heels, for example, can throw off your balance and force you to walk differently. This puts more stress on your muscles and harms your posture.
- **Make sure work surfaces are at a comfortable height for you**, whether you are sitting in front of a computer, making dinner, or eating a meal.

How Can You Improve Your Posture When Sitting?

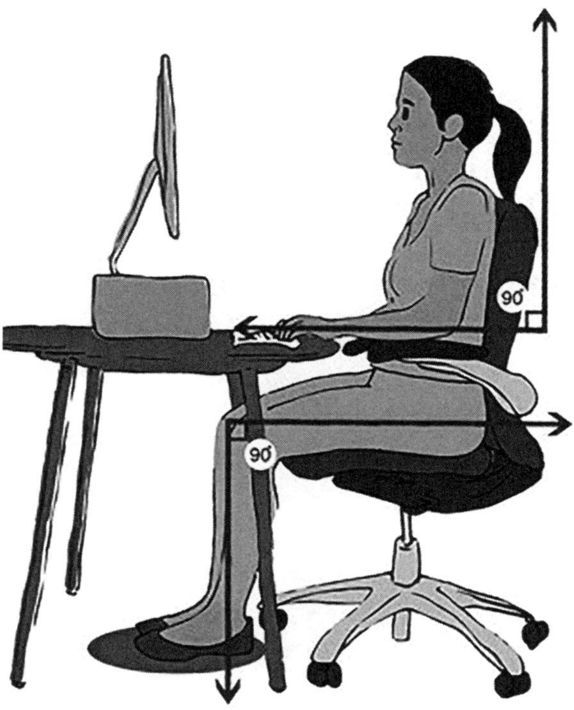

Figure 8.1. *The Ideal Sitting Posture*

Many Americans spend a lot of their time sitting—either at work, at school, or at home. It is important to sit properly, and to take frequent breaks:

- Switch sitting positions often.
- Take brief walks around your office or home.
- Gently stretch your muscles every so often to help relieve muscle tension.
- Do not cross your legs; keep your feet on the floor, with your ankles in front of your knees.
- Make sure that your feet touch the floor or, if that is not possible, use a footrest.
- Relax your shoulders; they should not be rounded or pulled backward.

- Keep your elbows in close to your body. They should be bent between 90 and 120 degrees.
- Make sure that your back is fully supported. Use a back pillow or other back support if your chair does not have a backrest that can support your lower back's curve.
- Make sure that your thighs and hips are supported. You should have a well-padded seat, and your thighs and hips should be parallel to the floor.

How Can You Improve Your Posture When Standing?

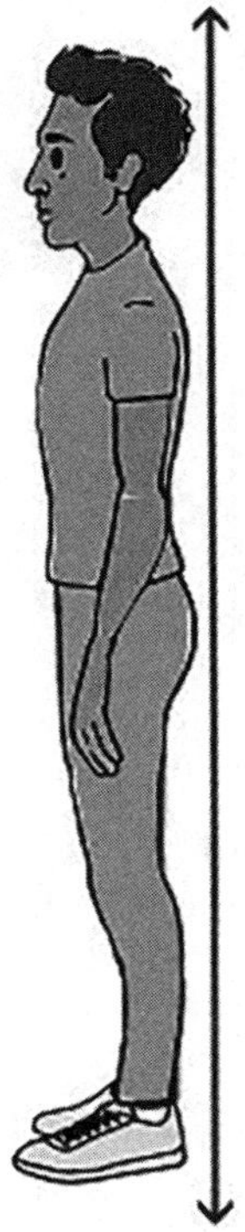

Figure 8.2. *The Ideal Standing Posture*

While standing you should:

- Stand up straight and tall.
- Keep your shoulders back.
- Pull your stomach in.

- Put your weight mostly on the balls of your feet.
- Keep your head level.
- Let your arms hang down naturally at your sides.
- Keep your feet about shoulder-width apart.

With practice, you can improve your posture; you will look and feel better.

Chapter 9

The Importance of Proper Body Mechanics

Think about all the movements you do every day: walking, climbing stairs, typing, turning doorknobs, and lifting. Your bones, muscles, and joints all work together to make your body an amazingly movable machine. As with any machine, your body can suffer some wear and tear. It needs regular care and maintenance to keep moving with ease.

Scientists are studying the mechanical movements of our bodies to help us be as strong, flexible, and mobile as possible throughout our lives. This type of research is called "biomechanics." These studies are finding that the way you move—including walking, standing, and bending—can affect your future mobility and overall health.

"All systems, whether in traditional mechanics or in the human body, are governed by the same basic physical laws," says Dr. Jeffrey Weiss, a biomechanics expert at the University of Utah. Body movements involve force, balance, gravity, and motion. "Biomechanics is effectively applying the physics of mechanics to problems in biology and medicine," Weiss says.

The main moving parts of your body include the solid bones, the joint tissues that link bones together, and the muscles that attach to your bones. Your body has about 200 bones and more than 600 muscles. These parts all work together to help you move throughout the day.

This chapter includes text excerpted from "Healthy Movements," *NIH News in Health*, National Institutes of Health (NIH), July 2013. Reviewed April 2019.

National Institutes of Health (NIH)-funded studies of biomechanics have already led to better ways to prevent muscle and joint injuries in kids during sports and play and to help older people stay more mobile and independent. Some researchers are working to develop better artificial joints. Others have devised improved treatments for movement disorders, such as cerebral palsy (CP) and Parkinson disease (PD).

Joints are a common source of problems and pain. Some joints, such as your shoulder joint, can move in many directions. But others, such as your knee joint, can only bend one way. Any movements outside a joint's natural range might cause injury.

Dr. Timothy Hewett, head of sports medicine research at Ohio State University, has long studied a part of the knee joint known as the "anterior cruciate ligament" (ACL). The ACL connects the thigh bone to the shin bone. When it stretches or tears, some people hear or feel a "pop." Athletes who need to make sudden stops or quickly change direction—as in basketball, tennis, and soccer—are at risk for damaging the ACL.

Hewett and other biomechanics researchers use motion capture tools to study how people move. Reflective markers—about the size of coins—are attached to the skin or clothing over people's joints and muscles to make it easy to visualize their movements on a computer screen. A series of cameras around the lab can then track how people run, jump, walk, and twist. Feeding these data into computers allows scientists to create three dimensional (3-D) animations of full-body motions. It is the same type of technology used to make animated characters in Hollywood movies, such as *Shrek* or *Avatar*.

"Using the tools of biomechanics, we can tell what is normal and what is abnormal in movement, and we can measure the forces on the body," Hewett says. "We use biomechanics as a screening tool to figure out which athletes are at greater risk for injury and why."

Hewett and his colleagues have identified certain movements that make some people more likely to get ACL injuries. For instance, athletes who allow their knees to collapse inward when landing from a jump are at risk for ACL tears. Once at-risk people are identified, coaches and physical therapists can develop exercises to help them strengthen certain muscles and learn to land and pivot in healthier, safer ways. "We've shown that we can use this information to reduce the relative risk of an ACL injury by 60 to 65 percent," says Hewett.

Motion-tracking tools are also being used to learn how older people might avoid injury from falls. Dr. Clive Pai, a physical therapist and researcher at the University of Illinois at Chicago, explains, "We are studying how older adults can learn to modify their movements to adapt to an unexpected environment, such as a slippery floor."

Falls are serious at any age, but especially for older adults, who are more likely to break a bone. Each year, more than 1.6 million older Americans go to emergency rooms for fall-related injuries. "Falling causes a lot of suffering and is a huge problem for society," says Pai.

Exercises that improve your balance and strengthen your muscles can help to prevent falls. Pai and his colleagues have also found that people can be trained to avoid falls if they practice walking over unstable, but safe, surfaces in the laboratory. "People age 65 and older can adapt and remember remarkably well how to keep their body posture upright when disturbances occur in the environment if they have encountered similar situations 2 or 3 times before," Pai says.

Biomechanics can also be used to guide treatments for movement problems. Weiss used computer models to look at how hip joints are stressed when someone walks or travels up and down stairs. He analyzed both normal hips and those with a condition called "hip dysplasia." "Hip dysplasia produces an instability that can lead to early onset of arthritis over time," Weiss says. Eventually, these computer models might help doctors choose appropriate treatments and figure out which patients would benefit from surgery.

People with cerebral palsy, Parkinson disease, and multiple sclerosis (MS) could also benefit from biomechanical analysis. "We use motion tracking to look at how well these patients are walking and what might be wrong, so we can try to do something about it," says Dr. Diane Damiano, a physical therapist who heads biomechanics research at the NIH Clinical Center in Bethesda, Maryland. "We focus on helping patients to strengthen their muscles and work to improve their balance and coordination. We are also looking at brain activation while they are moving. That can give us clues to how these movements are controlled by the brain."

Muscle strengthening and proper joint alignment are important for just about anyone who wants to stay flexible and mobile. "The bottom line is that everybody needs to be active," Damiano says. "We want to make it so that all people can move better, regardless of their age or health condition."

Body Maintenance

- Maintain a healthy weight. Too much weight can make your knees and hips ache.

- Engage in muscle-strengthening (resistance) activities that involve all your major muscle groups two or more times a week.
- Stay active all week long. Aim for 150 minutes of moderate intensity activity a week, such as brisk walking.
- Wear comfortable, properly fitting shoes.
- Eat a well-balanced diet. Get enough calcium and vitamin D daily to protect your bones.
- Try to avoid lifting heavy objects. If you need to lift something heavy, bend your knees and keep your back straight.

Chapter 10

Ergonomics for a Healthy Spine

Whole health is an approach to healthcare that empowers and enables you to take charge of your health and well-being and live your life to the fullest. Whole health starts with you. It is fueled by the power of knowing yourself and what will really work for you in your life. Only you have these insights, this knowledge.

What Is Ergonomics and How Does It Affect Me?

Ergonomics is the way you position your body. This includes whether you are sitting at a desk, in front of a computer, walking, driving, or standing. Often, people develop new aches and pains seemingly for no reason. In reality, they may have been carrying their bodies in less than ideal ways every day of their lives. Your body is very adaptable. It creates a balance even if your body is not positioned well. And your body tries to compensate by tightening muscles or using muscles differently to keep you moving. Yet when these actions continue to happen, it throws your balance off. You may then develop a new ache or pain.

This chapter includes text excerpted from "Ergonomics—Positioning Your Body for Whole Health," U.S. Department of Veterans Affairs (VA), April 30, 2018.

What Should My Body Be Like?

This question becomes very difficult because it is unique to each person's body. Your body has adjusted to fit your life, so what works for your neighbor might worsen or cause pain for you. To start with, your spine has some natural curves. This causes your center of gravity (where you focus your weight) to be in the middle of your body. Your body will make adjustments so your center of gravity does not change too much.

People who do bodywork (such as osteopathic doctors, chiropractors, physical therapists, and massage therapists) may talk about ears, shoulders, hips, and ankle alignment. If your body has not made changes to make up for an imbalance, then when you stand straight you should be able to draw a straight line from your ears to your shoulders to your hips to your ankles and the ground. If you are not in this alignment, your body has likely made an adjustment to fix an imbalance.

What Gets Me Out of Alignment?

To name a few causes of imbalance, you might have weak or tight muscles, have been in an accident, or not have ideal daily habits. Often, it is due to bad posture and habits. For example, at work or home your computer might not be positioned well. As a result, your neck sticks forward to see the screen better. To adjust, your body tips the pelvis and/or moves the lumbar spine (the lower part). The next thing you know, you have low back or neck pain.

In real life, pain does not develop fast. Your body was made to tilt and adjust. When you do this every day for six to eight hours, your muscles change, your bones move, and more. Then, one day you step off the curb funny or lift a box badly, and you think that is caused your back pain. Really, the back pain has been in the works every day you spend at work.

If you are on your feet all day, your posture also changes. This is similar to people who sit at a desk all day. Even constantly looking at your iPad or phone changes your posture. That is because your head is always looking down. Many people feel that tension on the neck muscles and low back.

So What Can I Do Then?

The first step is mindful awareness. Just pay attention to your posture and habits. Identify situations when your body goes out of alignment. Often, you can correct minor habits yourself by just being aware that you are doing them.

This can be difficult though, especially if you have developed these habits for a decade or more. Because some of your muscles are weak, or others are tense, it may be quite overwhelming to start. Ask for help! Physical therapists are fantastic at noting muscle imbalances and working with you to improve this. If you are not moving the best nor have the greatest posture, then you might choose an occupational therapist. These therapists focus on day-to-day movements that you might do at home or at your job.

Another group who can help are bodyworkers. They can help to physically put the body back in alignment. Just remember the imbalance in your body likely happened over years of poor habits, so you will need to stretch and tone the weak muscles in your body. Or else your body will return to the imbalance. This process takes time, so be patient with your body and your healthcare team.

You might consider yoga or Pilates (or many other types of movement therapies) to strengthen the muscles of your core and pelvic floor. (Your core muscles are those in the trunk of your body including your belly and chest. Your pelvic floor muscles are those in your lower belly.) These are usually underworked and weak in the average person. The added bonus of working the core muscles is that you might trim your waistline. Also, strong pelvic floor muscles can improve sexual health and function.

I Sit at a Desk All Day, and I Cannot Quit My Job. What Do I Do?

Let Us Start with Things That You Might Do to Help Yourself at Your Computer

- As mentioned above, make sure you are not leaning forward with your head to see the computer monitor. Aim for the top of the monitor to be just below eye level. Also, have your monitor less than arm's length away.
- Keep the computer screen glare low. Consider a glare guard. Also, do not forget to wipe the screen clean.
- If you wear glasses, you may need to change pairs depending on if you are near-sighted, far-sighted, or wearing bifocals.
- Your keyboard should be placed at a level where your elbows are bent about 90 degrees and close to the body.

- Your wrist should be in a neutral position when using a mouse or keyboard. This often means that your wrists and hands are in line with your forearms.

Let Us Talk about How You Are Seated in Your Chair

- As discussed above, aim for your head to be over your shoulders, which should be over your hips when seated. Your knees should be over your ankles, and your feet flat on the floor.
- Try to find a chair that supports the natural curve of your spine.
- Armrests should allow your shoulders to be relaxed while keeping the elbows close to the body and supported.
- Adjustable chairs make all the above easier to achieve.

I Have a Standing Desk at Work, So I Am Fine—Right?

Standing desks help people not to remain in the same position all day and to get more activity in the day. But, unless you adjust your workstation to be more ergonomic, it might hurt your posture. Remember, when you stand in front of your computer, you still want to try to have your ears, shoulders, hips, and ankles in alignment. Often "soft knees" or knees slightly bent and not locked helps your back.

Another thing to consider is how you stand, both at work and while waiting in line at the grocery store. Think about where the pressure is on each foot. Are you more often on the balls of your feet (leaning forward), on your heels, or is the pressure mainly on one foot? Keeping both feet on the ground helps to spread out your center of gravity. Having the pressure on both heels and balls help too.

I Have Started Stretching and Correcting My Posture, and My Pain Is Worse. What Is Going On?

To start, it is a good idea to check with your healthcare team to make sure nothing more serious is happening. If you have the pain to begin with, as mentioned earlier, your body has probably made a lot of changes to compensate over the years. This is why mindful awareness is the first step to correct things.

Things must be done slowly. When most of us think of fixing our posture, we force ourselves into positions that our bodies are not used to. In the long term, these new positions may be ideal. But this forces us to use muscles that are not ready yet to do the job that they are needed for. This will often cause pain flares. This is also why some people have pain flares after physical therapy or massage therapy session. It is because an imbalance has been found, and your body is not used to that imbalance being brought to light. It is important to find the balance, to strengthen and stretch muscles, and to allow yourself time to do so.

Ergonomics is something that you can work on both if you have already developed chronic pain and if you want to take preventative measures. If you think that you would like to know more, then do not be afraid to ask your healthcare team, because there are many people trained to help you. Consider making an appointment with any of the following clinicians: osteopathic doctors, chiropractors, physical therapists, occupational therapists, and massage therapists.

Chapter 11

Work-Related Musculoskeletal Disorders of Spine

Chapter Contents

Section 11.1—Spinal Pain at Work 78

Section 11.2—Risk Factors for Occupational Musculoskeletal Disorders 84

Section 11.1

Spinal Pain at Work

This section includes text excerpted from "Work-Related Musculoskeletal Disorders and Ergonomics," Centers for Disease Control and Prevention (CDC), February 1, 2018.

Work-Related Musculoskeletal Disorders

Musculoskeletal disorders (MSDs) are injuries or disorders of the muscles, nerves, tendons, joints, cartilage, and spinal discs. Work-related musculoskeletal disorders (WMSDs) are conditions in which:

1. The work environment and performance of work contribute significantly to the condition.
2. The condition is made worse or persists longer due to work conditions.

In 1997, the Centers for Disease Control and Prevention's (CDC) National Institute for Occupational Safety and Health (NIOSH) released a review of evidence for work-related MSDs. Examples of work conditions that may lead to a WMSD include routine lifting of heavy objects, daily exposure to whole-body vibration, routine overhead work, work with the neck in chronic flexion position, or performing repetitive forceful tasks. This report identified positive evidence for relationships between work conditions and MSDs of the neck, shoulder, elbow, hand, wrist, and back.

The U.S. Bureau of Labor Statistics (BLS) of the U.S. Department of Labor (DOL) defines "MSDs" as "musculoskeletal system and connective tissue diseases and disorders when the event or exposure leading to the case is bodily reaction (e.g., bending, climbing, crawling, reaching, and twisting), overexertion, or repetitive motion." MSDs do not include disorders caused by slips, trips, falls, or similar incidents. Examples of MSDs include:

- Sprains, strains, and tears
- Back pain
- Carpal tunnel syndrome (CTS)
- Hernia

Musculoskeletal disorders are associated with high costs to employers, such as absenteeism; lost productivity; and increased healthcare, disability, and worker's compensation costs. MSD cases are more severe than the average nonfatal injury or illness.

- In 2001, MSDs involved a median of 8 days away from work compared with 6 days for all nonfatal injury and illness cases (e.g., hearing loss, occupational skin diseases, such as dermatitis, eczema, or rash).
    - 3 age groups (25 to 34 year olds, 35 to 44 year olds, and 45 to 54 year olds) accounted for 79 percent of cases,
    - More male than female workers were affected, as were more White, non-Hispanic workers.
    - Operators; fabricators; laborers; and persons in technical, sales, and administrative support occupations accounted for 58 percent of the MSD cases.
    - The manufacturing and services industry sectors together accounted for about half of all MSD cases.
- Musculoskeletal disorders account for nearly 70 million physician office visits in the United States annually, and an estimated 130 million total healthcare encounters including outpatient, hospital, and emergency room visits.
- In 1999, nearly 1 million people took time away from work to treat and recover from work-related musculoskeletal pain or impairment of function in the low back or upper extremities.
- The Institute of Medicine (IOM) estimates the economic burden of WMSDs as measured by compensation costs, lost wages, and lost productivity, are between $45 and $54 billion annually.
- According to Liberty Mutual, the largest workers' compensation insurance provider in the United States, overexertion injuries—lifting, pushing, pulling, holding, carrying or throwing an object—cost employers $13.4 billion every year.

Common Work-Related Musculoskeletal Disorders

Carpal Tunnel Syndrome

The U.S. Department of Labor defines "CTS" as "a disorder associated with the peripheral nervous system (PNS), which includes nerves and ganglia located outside the spinal cord and brain." Carpal tunnel syndrome is the compression of the median nerve at the wrist, which may result in numbness, tingling, weakness, or muscle atrophy in the hand and fingers.

- Carpal tunnel syndrome may affect as many as 1.9 million people, and 300,000 to 500,000 surgeries are performed each year to correct this condition.
- The U.S. Bureau of Labor Statistics reported 26,794 CTS cases involving days away from work in 2001, representing a median of 25 days away from work compared with 6 days for all nonfatal injury and illness cases. Most cases involved workers who were between the ages of 25 and 54 (84%), female, and White, non-Hispanic (75%)
- Two occupational groups accounted for more than 70 percent of all CTS cases in 2001: operators, fabricators, and laborers; and technical, sales, and administrative support.

Back Injury and Back Pain

Back symptoms are among the top 10 reasons for medical visits. For 5 to 10 percent of patients, the back pain becomes chronic.

- In 2001, the BLS reported 372,683 back injury cases involving days away from work. Most cases involved workers who were between the ages of 25 and 54 (79%); male (64%); and White, non-Hispanic (70%).
- Two occupational groups accounted for more than 54 percent of back injury cases: operators, fabricators, and laborers (38%); and precision production, craft, and repair (17%).

Data from scientific studies of primary and secondary interventions indicate that low back pain can be reduced by:

- Engineering controls (e.g., ergonomic workplace redesign)
- Administrative controls (specifically, adjusting work schedules and workloads)
- Programs designed to modify individual factors, such as employee exercise
- Combinations of these approaches

Arthritis

The term "arthritis" is used to describe more than 100 rheumatic diseases and conditions that affect joints, the tissues which surround the joint and other connective tissue. The pattern, severity, and location of symptoms can vary depending on the specific form of the disease. 46 million Americans report that a doctor told them they have arthritis or other rheumatic conditions. Arthritis is the most common cause of disability in the United States. Arthritis limits the activities of nearly 19 million adults. Two-thirds of individuals with arthritis are under the age of 65.

The National Arthritis Data Working Group (NADW) estimates that 27 million adults have osteoarthritis. 9 million adults report symptomatic knee osteoarthritis, and 13 million reports symptomatic hand osteoarthritis. Persons are considered to have symptomatic osteoarthritis if they have frequent pain in a joint (e.g., pain in a joint on most days of a recent month) and radiographic (e.g., X-ray) evidence of osteoarthritis in that joint; although, sometimes this pain may not actually emanate from arthritis seen on the radiograph. Other forms of arthritis include rheumatoid arthritis (RA) and gout. Arthritis is a concern in the workplace both because it may develop from work-related conditions and because it may require worksite adaptations for employees with limitations or disabilities.

Certain occupations are associated with increased prevalence of arthritis, specifically osteoarthritis, most often of the knee and/or hip. These occupations include mining, construction, agriculture, and sectors of the service industry. Common features of these occupations are physically demanding/heavy labor tasks; lifting or carrying heavy loads; exposure to vibration; high risk of joint or tissue injury; and prolonged periods of working in awkward or unnatural postures, such as kneeling and crawling.

- In 2003, the total cost for arthritis conditions was $128 billion—$81 billion in direct costs and $47 billion in indirect costs.
- Persons who are limited in their work by arthritis are said to have arthritis-attributable work limitations (AAWL). AAWL affects 1 in 20 working-age adults (between the ages of 18 and 64) in the United States and 1 in 3 working-age adults with self-reported, doctor-diagnosed arthritis.
- The National Business Group on Health (NBGH) recommends that employers address arthritis by encouraging workers

to avoid obesity and providing ergonomically appropriate workplace design.

Early diagnosis and appropriate management of arthritis can help people with arthritis decrease pain, improve function, stay productive, and lower healthcare costs. Appropriate management includes consulting with a doctor and self-management education programs to help teach people with arthritis techniques to manage arthritis on a day-to-day basis. Physical activity and weight management programs are also important self-management activities for persons with arthritis.

Developing and Implementing Workplace Controls

A three-tier hierarchy of controls is widely accepted as an intervention strategy for reducing, eliminating, or controlling workplace hazards, including ergonomic hazards. The three tiers are:

Use of Engineering Controls

- The preferred approach to prevent and control WMSDs is to design the job to take account of the capabilities and limitations of the workforce using engineering controls. Some examples include:
  - Changing the way materials, parts, and products can be transported. For example, using mechanical assist devices to relieve heavy load lifting and carrying tasks or using handles or slotted hand holes in packages requiring manual handling.
  - Changing the workstation layout, which might include using height-adjustable workbenches or locating tools and materials within short reaching distances.

Use of Administrative Controls (Changes in Work Practices and Management Policies)

- Administrative control strategies are policies and practices that reduce WMSD risk, but they do not eliminate workplace hazards. Although engineering controls are preferred, administrative controls can be helpful as temporary measures until engineering controls can be implemented or when engineering controls are not technically feasible. Some examples include:

- Reducing shift length or limiting the amount of overtime
- Changes in job rules and procedures, such as scheduling more breaks to allow for rest and recovery
- Rotating workers through jobs that are physically tiring
- Training in the recognition of risk factors for WMSDs and instructions in work practices and techniques that can ease the task demands or burden (e.g., stress and strain)

Use of Personal Protective Equipment

- Personal protective equipment (PPE) generally provides a barrier between the worker and the hazard source. Respirators, ear plugs, safety goggles, chemical aprons, safety shoes, and hard hats are all examples of PPE.
- Whether braces, wrist splints, back belts, and similar devices can be regarded as offering personal protection against ergonomic hazards remains an open question. Although these devices may, in some situations, reduce the duration, frequency, or intensity of exposure, evidence of their effectiveness in injury reduction is inconclusive. In some instances, these devices may decrease one exposure but increase another because the worker has to "fight" the device to perform the work. An example is the use of wrist splints while engaging in work that requires wrist bending.

Ergonomics

Ergonomics is the science of fitting workplace conditions and job demands to the capability of the working population. The goal of ergonomics is to reduce stress and eliminate injuries and disorders associated with the overuse of muscles, bad posture, and repeated tasks. A workplace ergonomics program can aim to prevent or control injuries and illnesses by eliminating or reducing worker exposure to WMSD risk factors using engineering and administrative controls. PPE is also used in some instances but it is the least effective workplace control to address ergonomic hazards. Risk factors include awkward postures, repetition, material handling, force, mechanical compression, vibration, temperature extremes, glare, inadequate lighting, and duration of exposure. For example, employees who spend many hours at a workstation may develop ergonomic-related problems resulting in MSDs.

Section 11.2

Risk Factors for Occupational Musculoskeletal Disorders

This section includes text excerpted from "Back Disorders and Injuries," Occupational Safety and Health Administration (OSHA), February 1, 2001. Reviewed April 2019.

Back disorders can develop gradually as a result of microtrauma brought about by repetitive activity over time or can be the product of a single traumatic event. Because of the slow and progressive onset of this internal injury, the condition is often ignored until the symptoms become acute, often resulting in disabling injury. Acute back injuries can be the immediate result of improper lifting techniques and/or lifting loads that are too heavy for the back to support. While the acute injury may seem to be caused by a single well-defined incident, the real cause is often a combined interaction of the observed stressor coupled with years of weakening of the musculoskeletal support mechanism by repetitive microtrauma. Injuries can arise in muscle, ligament, vertebrae, and discs, either singly or in combination.

Incidence

Although back injuries account for no work-related deaths, they do account for a significant amount of human suffering, loss of productivity, and economic burden on compensation systems. Back disorders are one of the leading causes of disability for people in their working years. The frequency and economic impact of back injuries and disorders on the workforce are expected to increase over the next several decades as the average age of the workforce increases and medical costs go up.

Contributing Factors

These factors usually account for very few work-related back injuries.

- Congenital defects of the spine
- Increase in static standing or sitting tasks
- An aging workforce

- Decreases in physical conditioning and exercise
- Increased awareness of workplace hazards
- Job dissatisfaction

Manual Materials Handling

Manual materials handling is the principal source of compensable injuries in the American workforce, and four out of five of these injuries will affect the lower back.

Factors Associated with Back Disorders

Back disorders result from exceeding the capability of the muscles, tendons, discs, or the cumulative effect of several contributors:

- Reaching while lifting
- Poor posture—how one sits or stands
- Stressful living and working activities—staying in one position for too long
- Bad body mechanics—how one lifts, pushes, pulls, or carries objects
- Poor physical condition—losing the strength and endurance to perform physical tasks without strain
- Poor design of job or work station
- Repetitive lifting of awkward items, equipment, or (in healthcare facilities) patients
- Twisting while lifting
- Bending while lifting
- Maintaining bent postures
- Heavy lifting
- Fatigue
- Poor footings, such as slippery floors, or constrained posture
- Lifting with forceful movement
- Vibration, such as with lift truck drivers, delivery drivers, etc.

Signs and Symptoms of Work-Related Back Injury

Signs and symptoms include pain when attempting to assume normal posture, decreased mobility, and pain when standing or rising from a seated position.

Chapter 12

Back Pain Prevention at Work

Chapter Contents

Section 12.1—Safe Lifting Techniques 88
Section 12.2—Ergonomics for Computer Workstations 92

Section 12.1

Safe Lifting Techniques

This section contains text excerpted from the following sources: Text in this section begins with excerpts from "Safe Lifting Techniques," U.S. Department of Agriculture (USDA), August 3, 2003. Reviewed April 2019; Text under the heading "Good Posture" is excerpted from "Back Health," Division of Occupational Health and Safety (DOHS), National Institutes of Health (NIH), February 1, 2001. Reviewed April 2019.

Experts do not often agree as to what constitutes a truly safe lifting method, and in reality, there is no single correct way to lift. The method espoused for the past several decades (bend the knees and not the back) has not been particularly effective in reducing the incidence or severity of low back injury by itself. Lifting, in practice, is highly dependent on the particulars of the task at hand.

Expert opinions differ as to which lifting methodology poses the least physical threat to the handler. The biomechanical approach indicates that a squat lift (knees and hips bent with the back more or less straight) places the least stress on the back. Proponents of the physiological approach to lifting argue that the stoop lift (legs straight with the back bent) is less physiologically stressful than the squat lift. And the psychophysical approach to lifting indicates that a freestyle lift is least taxing. A freestyle lift is described as a semi-squat posture, which allows the handler to rest the load on the thigh(s) during the lift.

However, there is general agreement on some fundamental principles that should help protect materials handlers when lifting under most circumstances.

Typically, when lifting the handler should:

1. Test the weight of the load, its weight distribution, and stability within the container. This minimizes the chance of being surprised by an unexpectedly heavy weight or having to contend with a shifting load.
2. Get help from someone or use a mechanical assist device whenever very heavy or awkward loads must be handled. When lifting with a partner, the team should communicate and coordinate the task (when lifting, moving, and lowering the object).

3. Know where the load is going. Make sure the path is free from obstructions or hazards, and ensure that space is available at the destination to set the object down.
4. Be positioned close to the load, with the feet flat and stable. Keep the load as close to the body as possible so that the center of gravity is as close to the spine as possible. Moving the load away from the torso (horizontally and/or vertically) greatly increases the load to the back, shoulders, and arms, and, therefore, increases the risk of injury.
5. Grasp the object with the whole hand, using a power grip whenever possible. Avoid pinching with the fingertips to hold an object. Ideally, the handler should be able to use both hands on handles or handholds to pick up the load.
6. Move with natural, smooth, continuous, and balanced motions while avoiding rapid, jerky, or unbalanced lifts. Move the feet to avoid twisting the torso and to maintain balance and stability during the lift, if necessary.
7. Minimize twisting, bending, stretching, and reaching with the trunk during the lift. These movements greatly increase the risk of developing low back pain (LBP).

These principles should make it clear that we need to lift with our head before we lift with our back. Taking a couple of seconds to help ensure our safety and health is time well spent.

Body Mechanics

All of the problems in the last exercise had something to do with body mechanics. Lifting, carrying, and reaching—remember it is not how much you lift or carry as much as it is how you do it. Once you have factored in the upper body weight due to posture or position of the object to be lifted or carried, you can consider the following examples of how you can overcome the lifting hazard by using proper body mechanics.

Remember the five general lifting rules:

1. Plan the lift.
2. Both squat and stoop lifting is now considered acceptable for jobs requiring repetitive lifting. The term used to describe this is "free-form lifting." No matter what type of lift is used, it is

never permissible to exceed the maximum acceptable load of the worker.

3. Keep the load as close to the body as possible.
4. Lift the load with a smooth body motion (avoid jerking).
5. When turning, do not twist. Turn with the feet rather than twisting of the trunk.

Pushing, Pulling, Carrying, and Transporting Loads

Generally speaking, lowering is preferable to lifting, and pushing is preferable to pulling; however, all these activities have the potential to be stressful to the arms, shoulders, back, and legs.

Factors that influence the ease or difficulty of pushing and pulling are the initial (or breaking) and sustaining forces necessary to move the device, steering, and controlling the unit while in motion, the frequency with which the push/pull task is performed, and the terrain and distance over which the task takes place.

In pushing and pulling tasks, it is harder to start a body moving (the initial forces) than it is to keep the body in motion (the sustaining forces). When pushing or pulling, the handler should use her or his own weight to advantage. When pushing, the person should lean into the push, and when pulling, the person should lean in the direction of travel.

All push/pull tasks require adequate friction between the floor and the operator's shoes to provide adequate traction and avoid slipping.

When pushing, arms should be flexed at the elbow, extended to about half their length, thereby allowing the operator to regulate effort as necessary by flexing and extending the arms. When pulling, arms should be extended, then effort to move the load is transferred to the lower extremities.

Carrying tasks have the potential to stress the arms, shoulders, and back in particular. To help minimize these stressors, keep the weight of the load acceptable, keep the load as close to the body as possible, and use both hands in a power grip (rather than a pinch grip) to hold the load.

Other factors that influence the ease of a carrying task are the width (side-to-side) and height of the load, the frequency with which the task takes place, and the distance over which the load is carried.

Ideally, the width of the load should be about as wide as the person's torso. The height of the load should allow the handler a clear view of the travel path. Carrying distances should be minimized.

"The easiest way of carrying a load like a crate or a box is holding it by the front corners, with the arms straight, at hip height, so that it does not interfere with the movements of the lower limbs."

Loads to be carried to the side of the body (suitcases, grocery bags, briefcases, etc.) should be equipped with suitable top mounted handles, "should be as slim as possible," and "should clear the ground when the carriers' arm hangs by their side."

Good Posture

"Neutral spine" is a term used when your back and, therefore, your spinal column, is in its natural, neutral posture. First, what is good posture?

Three Natural Curves

In order to assure the spine is working efficiently, we must keep the bones in the best alignment. Otherwise, the stress and forces are magnified. Ligaments will be overstretched and muscles fatigued, causing pain and possible injury. In any activity, these three curves should be maintained but not increased. The head should be above the shoulders so that the ear is inline with the top of the shoulder. The top of the shoulder should be over the hips.

Section 12.2

Ergonomics for Computer Workstations

This section contains text excerpted from the following sources: Text in this section begins with excerpts from "Office Technology and Musculoskeletal Disorders: Building an Ecological Model," Centers for Disease Control and Prevention (CDC), April 12, 2019; Text under the heading "Good Working Positions" is excerpted from "Computer Workstations eTool," Occupational Safety and Health Administration (OSHA), August 29, 2003. Reviewed April 2019.

There are no accurate statistics on the number of workers in the United States who routinely use computers in their jobs. Estimates of the number of people engaged in computer-mediated work also are difficult to determine. However, based on the number of workers in occupations known to use computers to some degree, a conservative estimate is that about half of the 120 million workers in the United States are now spending some time during the workday at a computer keyboard.

With the continued rapid expansion of computer technology to all sectors of the economy, the numbers will only increase. The effects of the physical aspects of the computer work environment on worker health have long been a concern; Studies since the 1970s have indicated a link between ergonomic aspects of the work environment and musculoskeletal and other problems. Although this research has prompted significant improvements in the design of office equipment and environments, musculoskeletal problems among computer users are still common. Thus, attention has increasingly turned to other occupational risk factors, namely work organization factors, which may, in conjunction with physical risk factors, play a role in the etiology of musculoskeletal disorders.

Good Working Positions

To understand the best way to set up a computer workstation, it is helpful to understand the concept of neutral body positioning. This is a comfortable working posture in which your joints are naturally aligned. Working with the body in a neutral position reduces stress and strain on the muscles, tendons, and skeletal system and reduces your risk of developing a musculoskeletal disorder (MSD). The following are important considerations when attempting to maintain neutral body postures while working at the computer workstation:

- Hands, wrists, and forearms are straight, in-line and roughly parallel to the floor.
- Head is level, forward facing, and balanced. Generally, it is in-line with the torso.
- Shoulders are relaxed, and upper arms hang normally at the side of the body.
- Elbows stay in close to the body and are bent between 90 and 120 degrees.
- Feet are fully supported by the floor or a footrest may be used if the desk height is not adjustable.
- Back is fully supported with appropriate lumbar support when sitting vertical or leaning back slightly.
- Thighs and hips are supported and generally parallel to the floor.
- Knees are about the same height as the hips, with the feet slightly forward.

Regardless of how good your working posture is, working in the same posture or sitting still for prolonged periods is not healthy. You should change your working position frequently throughout the day in the following ways:

- Make small adjustments to your chair or backrest.
- Stretch your fingers, hands, arms, and torso.
- Stand up and walk around for a few minutes periodically.
- Perform some of your tasks in standing: computing, reading, phone, meetings.

These four reference postures are examples of body posture changes that all provide neutral positioning for the body.

Upright Sitting

The user's torso and neck are approximately vertical and in-line, the thighs are approximately horizontal, and the lower legs are vertical.

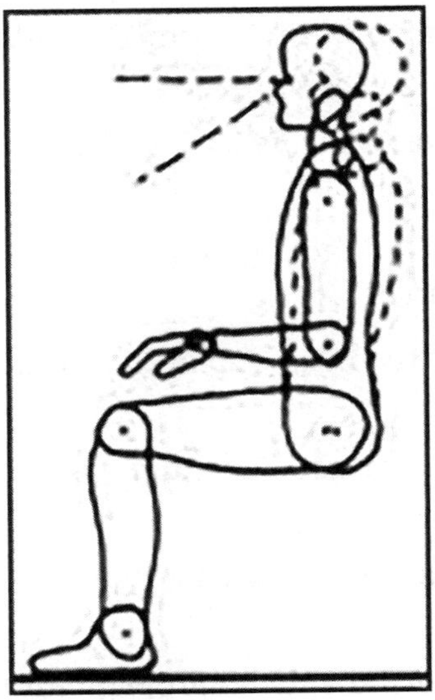

Figure 12.1. *Upright Sitting Posture*

Standing

The user's legs, torso, neck, and head are approximately in-line and vertical with feet slightly apart. The user may also elevate one foot on a rest while in this posture.

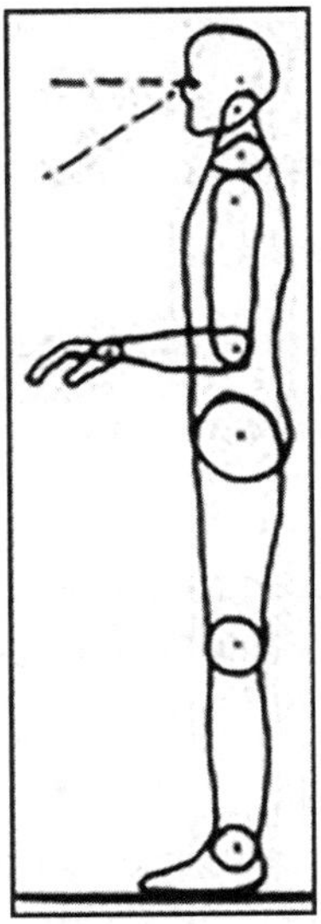

Figure 12.2. *Standing Posture*

Declined Sitting

The user's thighs are inclined with the buttocks higher than the knee, and the angle between the thighs and the torso is greater than 90 degrees. The torso is vertical or slightly reclined, and the legs are vertical. This position should not inhibit the ability to easily reach the keyboard or view the monitor.

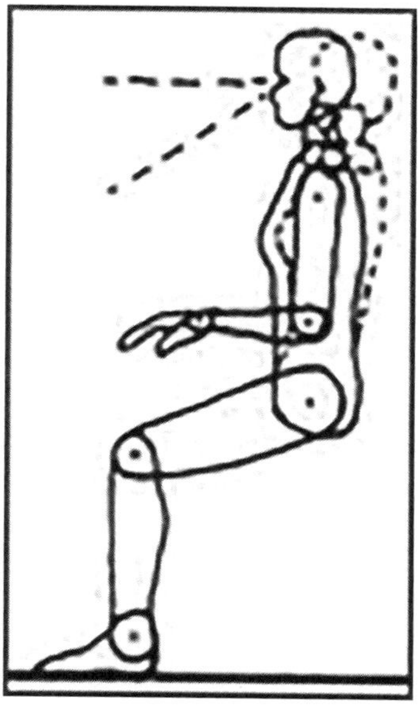

Figure 12.3. *Declined Sitting Posture*

Reclined Sitting

The user's torso and neck are straight and recline between 105 and 120 degrees from the thighs.

Selecting and Arranging Your Workstation Components

Appropriate placement of the components and accessories for the desktop computer workstation will allow you to work in neutral body positions, help you perform more efficiently, and work more comfortably and safe. A laptop workstation creates special challenges due to its computer design, size, and the variety of areas in which it is used.

The following sections explain how to select and arrange specific workstation components.

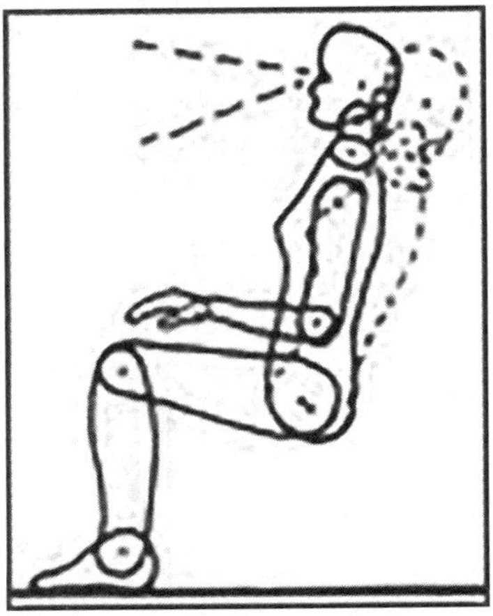

Figure 12.4. *Reclined Sitting Posture*

Chairs

A chair that is well-designed and appropriately adjusted is an essential element of a safe and productive computer workstation. A good chair provides the necessary support to the back, legs, buttocks, and arms, while reducing exposures to awkward postures, contact stress, and forceful exertions.

Desks

A well-designed and appropriately-adjusted desk will provide adequate clearance for your legs, allow proper placement of computer components and accessories, and minimize awkward postures and exertions.

Document Holders

Document holders keep printed materials needed during computer tasks close to the user and the monitor. Appropriate placement of the holder may reduce or eliminate risk factors, such as awkward head and neck postures, fatigue, headaches, and eye strain.

Keyboards

Proper selection and arrangement of the computer keyboard help reduce exposure to awkward postures, repetition, and contact stress.

Monitors

Choosing a suitable monitor and placing it in an appropriate position helps reduce exposure to forceful exertions, awkward postures, and overhead glare. This helps prevent possible health effects, such as excessive fatigue, eye strain, and neck and back pain.

Pointer / Mouse

In addition to the conventional mouse, there are trackballs, touchpads, fingertip joysticks, and pucks, to name a few. Selection and placement of a pointer/mouse is an important factor in creating a safe computer workstation.

Telephones

Telephones add to the convenience of a workstation; however, telephones have cords that can get tangled up and can cause the user to assume awkward postures.

Wrist or palm rests can also increase your comfort. Although opinions vary regarding the use of wrist/palm supports, proper use has been shown to reduce muscle activity and to facilitate neutral wrist angles.

Work Process and Recognition

Even when the design of the workstations is correct and environmental factors are at their best, users can face risks from task organization which can intensify the impact of other risk factors, such as repetition. Additionally, failing to recognize early warning signs could allow small problems to develop into serious injuries. Addressing task organization factors and medical awareness can help minimize the risk of developing musculoskeletal disorders (MSDs) and stop the progression to injury.

Prolonged Periods of Activity

Potential Hazard

Computer work, whether it is for a job or for fun, may appear to be a low effort activity when viewed from a total body perspective, but maintaining postures or performing highly repetitive tasks for extended periods can lead to problems in localized areas of the body. For example, using a mouse for a few minutes should not be a problem for most users, but performing this task for several uninterrupted hours can expose the small muscles and tendons of the hand to hundreds or even thousands of activations (repetitions). There may not be adequate time between activations for rest and recuperation, which can lead to localized fatigue, wear and tear, and injury. Likewise, maintaining static postures, such as viewing the monitor for a prolonged period of time without taking a break, can fatigue the muscles of the neck and shoulder that support the head.

Possible Solutions

Provide variation in tasks and workstations so there is time to recover from the effects of the activity. There are several ways to provide recovery time for overused muscles.

- Utilize an adjustable workstation so users can easily change their working postures. The use of easily adjustable furniture, for example, allows you to frequently change seated postures, which allows different muscle groups to provide support while others rest.
- Ensure that there is enough workspace so you can use each hand alternately to perform mouse tasks. This allows the tendons and muscles of the free hand to rest.
- Substitute keystrokes for mousing tasks, such as Ctrl+S to save, Ctrl+P to print. Especially if your job is highly mouse intensive.
- High repetition tasks or jobs that require long periods of static posture may require several, short rest breaks (micro breaks or rest pauses). During these breaks, users should be encouraged to stand, stretch, and move around. This provides rest and allows the muscles enough time to recover.
- Alternate tasks whenever possible, mixing noncomputer-related tasks into the workday. This encourages body movement and the use of different muscle groups.

Medical Awareness and Training

Potential Hazard

Employees who have not been adequately trained to recognize hazards or understand effective work practices designed to reduce these hazards are at a greater risk of harm. Without proper medical awareness, MSD signs and symptoms may go unnoticed and unaddressed. For example, users who do not understand the risk of bad body postures or techniques do not have the knowledge to actively participate in their own protection. Detection and reporting delays can result in more severe injury.

Possible Solutions

Computer users should take the time to obtain general ergonomics awareness training on the following issues:

- Factors related to specific computer components that may increase discomfort or risk of injury
- Being aware of discomfort (signs and symptoms)
- How to correctly use and adjust components and environmental factors

Chapter 13

Preventing Back Injury among Caregivers

Patient Handling and Musculoskeletal Disorders

Many nurses and nursing assistants suffer from work-related musculoskeletal disorders and pain. According to the most recent U.S. Bureau of Labor Statistics (BLS) data, workers in hospitals suffer injuries and illnesses at nearly twice the national average rate. Hospitals had an incidence rate of 6.8 nonfatal occupational injuries and illnesses per 100 full-time workers in 2011, compared with 3.5 per 100 in all U.S. industries combined. The incidence rate for injuries and illnesses resulting in days away from work, measured across all industries and occupations nationwide, was 1.2 per 100 full-time workers in 2011. The incidence rate for these injuries among nursing aides, orderlies, and attendants across the healthcare industry was nearly 4 times that, at 4.4 per 100 full-time workers. Nearly 50 percent of the reported

---

This chapter contains text excerpted from the following sources: Text beginning with the heading "Patient Handling and Musculoskeletal Disorders" is excerpted from "Safe Patient Handling Programs," Occupational Safety and Health Administration (OSHA), September 2013. Reviewed April 2019; Text under the heading "Back Injuries among Family Caregivers" is excerpted from "Accelerating Adoption of Assistive Technology to Reduce Physical Strain among Family Caregivers of the Chronically Disabled Elderly Living at Home. Appendix C. Helping to Reduce Caregiving Physical Strain: Guide for National Family Caregiver Support Programs," Office of the Assistant Secretary for Planning and Evaluation (ASPE), January 12, 2012. Reviewed April 2019.

injuries and illnesses among nurses and nursing support staff in 2011 were musculoskeletal disorders. Nursing assistants suffered more of these disorders in 2011 than any other occupation, while registered nurses ranked fifth.

Patient Handling Injuries Can Be Very Costly to the Healthcare System

According to one large national survey drawn from 53 healthcare systems with roughly 1,000 hospitals in all 50 states, patient handling injuries accounted for 25 percent of all workers' compensation claims for the healthcare industry in 2011. On average, a worker's compensation claim related to patient handling cost $15,600, and wage replacement accounted for the largest share of this cost ($12,000). In terms of wage replacement, patient handling injuries are among the most expensive type of hospital worker injuries.

In addition to these direct and highly visible costs, there are numerous indirect and less visible costs from patient handling injuries—difficult to measure, but with a very real impact on the healthcare system. These include employee turnover, training, overtime, incident investigation time, productivity, and morale. Patient safety, satisfaction, and recovery times may also be affected if workers are injured during patient handling and repositioning. These indirect costs can increase the total cost of patient handling injuries by two to four times.

Safe Patient Handling Programs

Safe patient handling can include permanent or portable lifts, transfer sheets and other equipment, training on equipment use and maintenance, implementation of a "minimal lift" policy that eliminates manual handling whenever possible, and/or a dedicated "lift team" that travels through the hospital moving patients with proper equipment. While the costs for instituting such programs can be significant, several studies have shown that the initial capital investment in safe patient handling policies, programs, and equipment can be recovered in fewer than five years.

Back Injuries among Family Caregivers

A major source of physical strain, such as back injuries, among family caregivers is lifting and transferring. Many nursing homes and hospitals have rules against manual lifting and provide mechanical lifting aids for caregiving staff to use. Family caregivers, however, are less likely to be aware of safe lifting techniques or to have access to devices, such as ceiling lifts. Safe handling guidelines state that 35 pounds is the most a person can safely lift. Whenever possible, equipment, such as a hoist or mechanical lift, should be used for a whole body lift of a non-weight-bearing person. Gait belts and slings can help position and provide back-up when assisting a partially weight-bearing person. They can also be used for maneuvering a non-weight-bearing person into a hoist sling.

Another source of physical strain is communication problems in caring for a person with dementia. Oftentimes, people with dementia become confused due to their inability to interpret signals from their bodies or from their surroundings. This contributes to resistance towards caregivers when they attempt to transfer them, which increases caregivers' risk for physical strain. Training on communicating with people with dementia can help address physical strain from caring for a person with dementia. Assistive technology (AT)/home modifications (HM) for cognitive impairment—such as activities/games, devices for memory and communication, additional lighting, labels, and signs—can also help in this area. Assistive technology includes any equipment or product that helps people with disabilities function better, and home modifications refer to changes to the home to make tasks easier, reduce accidents, and support independent living.

Homes that are in need of repairs or are not designed to meet the needs of older adults with functional impairments also contribute to increased physical strain. In addition, many family caregivers are themselves over the age of 60, which raises their risk of physical strain. Home repairs and modifications that may be needed range from removing clutter or repairing a handrail to major renovations, such as installing a wheelchair ramp, downstairs bathroom, or stair lift.

In addition to increasing safety for family caregivers, a wide range of AT/HM can assist older adults increase their functioning and independence. These range from complex technologies, such as telehealth and remote monitoring systems, to simple tools, such as grab bars and pillboxes. This can reduce the amount of help they need and ease the strain on family caregivers.

Assistive Technologies and Home Modifications to Reduce Caregiver Physical Strain

- Bathing/toileting aids (grab bars, raised toilet seats, shower benches)

- AT/HM for mobility (wheelchairs, walkers, canes, ramps, stair lifts)
- Transfer aids (lifting devices, hoists)
- Electronic systems for health record tracking, caregiving coordination, medication management, emergency response, monitoring
- Devices for dressing, food preparation (shoe horns, jar openers)
- Hearing and vision aids
- Medical supplies (incontinence supplies)
- Medication management aids (automated dispensers, pillboxes)
- Vehicle modifications/accessible car

Chapter 14

Compensatory Workplace Exercises for a Healthy Back

Musculoskeletal Exercises

Deep Breathing

While standing, or in an otherwise relaxed position:

- Place one hand on the abdomen and one on the chest.
- Inhale slowly through the nose.
- Hold for four seconds.
- Exhale slowly through the mouth.
- Repeat.

Cable Stretch

- While sitting with chin in, stomach in, shoulders relaxed, hands relaxed in lap, and feet flat on the floor, imagine a cable pulling your head upward.
- Hold for three seconds and relax.
- Repeat three times.

This chapter includes text excerpted from "Exercises and Stretches," Division of Occupational Health and Safety (DOHS), National Institutes of Health (NIH), February 1, 2001. Reviewed April 2019.

Side Bend: Neck Stretch

- Tilt head to 1 side (ear towards shoulder).
- Hold for 15 seconds.
- Relax.
- Repeat 3 times on each side.

Diagonal Neck Stretch

- Turn head slightly and then look down as if looking in your pocket.
- Hold for 15 seconds.
- Relax.
- Repeat 3 times on each side.

Shoulder Shrug

- Slowly bring shoulders up to the ears and hold for approximately 3 seconds.
- Rotate shoulders back and down.
- Repeat 10 times.

Executive Stretch

- While sitting, lock hands behind head.
- Bring your elbows back as far as possible.
- Inhale deeply while leaning back and stretching.
- Hold for 20 seconds.
- Exhale and relax.
- Repeat 1 time.

Foot Rotation

- While sitting, slowly rotate each foot from the ankle.
- Rotate three times in one direction, then three times in the opposite direction.

- Relax.
- Repeat one time.

Hand Shake

- While sitting, drop arms to the side.
- Shake hands downward gently.
- Repeat frequently.

Hand Massage

- Massage the inside and outside of the hand using the thumb and fingers.
- Repeat frequently (including before beginning work).

Finger Massage

- Massage fingers of each hand individually, slowly, and gently.
- Move toward nail gently.
- Massage space between fingers.
- Perform daily.

Wrist Stretch

- Hold arm straight out in front of you.
- Pull the hand backward with the other hand, then pull downward.
- Hold for 20 seconds.
- Relax.
- Repeat 3 times each.

Warming Up for Work

Just as an athlete prepares before playing a sport, you too should prepare before work to help prevent back injuries. These slow stretches help prevent back injuries and make your muscles more flexible. Hold each position for 20 seconds and repeat 3 times before work.

Back Exercises

It does not take much time to improve the strength and flexibility of your back. In just 10 minutes a day, you can perform a few exercises, which can prevent a lifetime of low back pain!

Partial Sit-Up

This exercise strengthens your stomach muscles:

- Lie on your back with both knees bent and your feet flat on the floor. Slowly raise your head and shoulders off the floor, keeping your hands across your chest.
- Work up to 30 repetitions.

Bridge

This exercise strengthens your low back:

- Lie on your back with both knees bent and your feet flat on the floor.
- With arms lying at your sides, tighten stomach muscles, squeeze the buttocks, and slowly raise your hips into the air. Hold for 5 seconds and then slowly bring the buttocks back to the floor.
- Repeat 20 times.

Wall Slide

This exercise strengthens your back and leg muscles:

- Stand with your back against a wall and your feet slightly apart.
- Slide into a half-sit. Hold as long as you can; slide back up.
- Repeat five times.

Aerobic Exercise

Aerobic exercise stretches and strengthens the muscles that support your low back, which, when combined with healthy eating, can also help you maintain your ideal weight. If you are overweight, the extra pounds add to the strain on your lower back. Aerobic exercise, such as walking, can help you lose weight.

Proper Rest

The best position for resting the back muscles is lying on your back on your living room floor with a pillow under your knees and a rolled up towel under your neck. You can also lie on your side in the fetal position—bend the knees to reduce strain on the lower back and put a pillow between your knees, and under your head and neck to keep them level.

Chapter 15

Ergonomic Tips for Driving

Driving Ergonomics

Surprisingly, many ergonomic risk factors (e.g., awkward postures, excessive force, and vibration) exist in relation to driving. Such risk factors become increasingly apparent during distance driving. Driving ergonomics has an overall goal of fitting the driver to their car so they can drive in a way that maximizes the natural ability of their body to move and respond to physical stress.

Driving puts an employee at greater risk for low back trouble than sitting and standing jobs/activities. Thus, the frequency of discomfort increases with the number of miles driven on an annual basis.

Commonly reported discomforts to include:

- Lower back pain
- Foot cramps
- Stiff neck
- Sore shoulders
- Finger cramps

This chapter includes text excerpted from "Driving Ergonomics," U.S. Department of Agriculture (USDA), February 25, 2016.

Causes of Driving Ergonomics

Causes of such discomfort often involve the following:

- The shape of the vehicle seat, as it may put pressure on selected parts of the legs, back, and buttocks. This contact can lead to pain or discomfort at pressure points and may affect blood flow to the legs and feet.
- Low-frequency whole-body vibration in moving cars and trucks, which can contribute to effects on the lower back and performance problems
- Poor driving conditions for which your body experiences up-and-down vibrations from the car traveling on uneven or bumpy road surfaces
    - The body moves sideways when you turn on corners.
    - Depending on how fast you accelerate or decelerate, you will feel a force on your body.

Tips to Improve Your Driving Habits

Tips to improve your driving habits start with reading the vehicle manual and understanding all the adjustments that you can do. Many vehicles allow for the following adjustments:

- Seat position
- Backrest angle
- Headrest position
- Steering wheel height and tilt
- Seat belt
- Mirrors

It is also important to do the following whether driving short or long distances:

- Take stretch breaks every three to four hours.
- Use a seat lumbar support.
- Adjust the seat and steering wheel to your comfort level.
- Get plenty of rest at night

The following driving practices should be avoided:

- Drive without taking a break.
- Rest arms on console or windowsill
- The obvious (e.g., writing, reading, eating, drinking, etc.)

Overall, it is important to recognize that poor seated postures are generally considered to contribute to work-related musculoskeletal disorders (WMSDs). Good posture is a key feature in the prevention of back pain during driving tasks. However, even good postures can result in discomfort. Thus, it is important to note that no single posture is ideal if maintained for long periods of time. Adopting a range of comfortable postures, and frequent changes of posture may help to delay the onset of discomfort in driving.

Chapter 16

Do Back Belts Really Work?

Back injuries account for nearly 20 percent of all injuries and illnesses in the workplace and cost the nation an estimated 20 to 50 billion dollars per year. The National Institute for Occupational Safety and Health (NIOSH) believes that the most effective way to prevent back injury is to implement an ergonomics program that focuses on redesigning the work environment and work tasks to reduce the hazards of lifting.

However, in response to the increasing human and economic costs of back injury, companies have implemented numerous other measures, either in conjunction with or in place of sound ergonomics programs. For instance, there has been a dramatic increase in the use of industrial back belts.

The decision to wear a back belt is a personal choice; however, the NIOSH believes that workers and employers should have the best available information to make that decision. This chapter outlines the current state of scientific knowledge on back belts and stresses the importance of an overall ergonomics program. Companies should not rely on back belts as a "cure all" for back injury, but they should begin to undertake prevention measures that reduce the risks of lifting tasks.

This chapter includes text excerpted from "Back Belts Do They Prevent Injury?" Centers for Disease Control and Prevention (CDC), June 6, 2014. Reviewed April 2019.

Do Back Belts Prevent Injury?

In recent years, there has been a dramatic increase in the number of workers who rely on back belts to prevent injury during lifting. Back belts, also called "back supports" or "abdominal belts," are currently worn by workers in numerous industries, including grocery store clerks, airline baggage handlers, and warehouse workers. As their use has risen, the NIOSH has increasingly been asked for advice on back belt selection. In response to these inquiries, the Institute decided to address a more fundamental question. Rather than ask "Which belt will best protect workers?" NIOSH researchers began with the question—"Do back belts protect workers?"

Employers relying on back belts to prevent injury should be aware of the lack of scientific evidence supporting their use.

A Lack of Scientific Support

After a review of the scientific literature, the NIOSH has concluded that, because of limitations of the studies that have analyzed workplace use of back belts, the results cannot be used to either support or refute the effectiveness of back belts in injury reduction. Although back belts are being bought and sold under the premise that they reduce the risk of back injury, there is insufficient scientific evidence that they actually deliver what is promised.

The Institute, therefore, does not recommend the use of back belts to prevent injuries among workers who have never been injured. If you or your workers are wearing back belts as protective equipment against back injury, you should be aware of the lack of scientific evidence supporting their use.

How Did the National Institute for Occupational Safety and Health Come to These Conclusions about Back Belts?

The NIOSH systematically reviewed published peer-reviewed scientific literature on back belts to determine if they actually reduce the risk of back injury. Because there were few studies on the association between workplace use of back belts and injuries, the NIOSH also reviewed studies of the relationship between back belt use and forces exerted on the spine during manual lifting. In other words, much of the existing research is based on theories of what causes back injury, rather than on the actual rates of workplace injury with and without back belt use.

Claims of Back Belts

- Reduce internal forces on the spine during forceful exertions of the back
- Increase intra-abdominal pressure (IAP), which may counter the forces on the spine
- Stiffen the spine, which may decrease forces on the spine
- Restrict bending motions (range of motion)
- Remind the wearer to lift properly
- Have reduced injuries in certain workplaces

While all of these claims have been put forth as support for the use of back belts, they remain unproven. There is currently inadequate scientific evidence or theory to suggest that back belts can reduce the risk of injury. Moreover, even if back belts produced the biomechanical effects listed above, there is no proven link to injury prevention.

The NIOSH searched the peer-reviewed literature for studies investigating these claims and evaluated the scientific evidence they produced. A summary of the findings is provided on the following pages.

Facts about the Back Belts

Reduce Forces on the Spine

Lifting may produce a variety of forces within the body that contribute to the pressure on the spine, termed "loading." Many of the studies the NIOSH reviewed sought to examine the impact of back belt use on loading. None of the studies provide sufficient data to indicate that industrial back belts significantly reduce loading during lifting. In fact, there is little evidence to suggest that these forces could be reduced with a back belt.

Increase Intra-Abdominal Pressure

While this theory remains controversial, some believe that if the pressure is increased within the abdomen, it will counterbalance the compressive force being exerted downward on the spine. The studies the NIOSH reviewed were inconclusive, and the relationship between IAP and spinal compression is not well understood. Therefore, even if a back belt increased IAP, there is, as yet, no evidence that it would reduce forces on the spine or decrease back injury.

Remind Workers to Lift Properly

At this point, there is little scientific evidence that back belts remind workers to avoid awkward postures and heavy loads.

Stiffen the Spine

Numerous ligaments, tendons, and other soft tissues surround the spine and help hold it in place. The theory is that if back belts increase this support, they would decrease the motion allowed between segments of the spine, and therefore, decrease damage to the discs in the lower back. There is no conclusive evidence that back belts increase the stiffness of the spine and no proven relationship between this stiffness and the reduction of injury.

Reduce Bending Motions

Loading on the spine increases when a person has to bend as far forward as possible. If the ability to bend this far forward could be restricted by a back belt, the risk of injury would possibly be decreased. It would appear that abdominal belts help restrict the range of motion during side to side bending and twisting. However, they do not have the same effect when the worker bends forward, as in many industrial lifting situations.

Reduce Injuries in Certain Workplaces

There have been anecdotal case reports of injury reduction in workplaces using back belts. However, many companies that have instituted back belt programs have also implemented training and ergonomic awareness programs. The reported injury reduction may be related to these or other factors. On the basis of available evidence, the potential effectiveness of back belts in reducing the occurrence of low back injuries remains unproven.

Why Is So Little Known about the Utility of Back Belts?

Back belts were initially used in medical settings. These belts, termed "orthoses," resemble the corsets worn by women in the nineteenth century and are typically used to provide additional back support during the rehabilitation of injuries. Subsequently, athletes began using leather belts for weight-lifting.

Only in recent years has the industrial back belt been widely used. While there are more than 70 types of industrial back belts, the typical abdominal support used in workplaces today is a lightweight, elastic belt worn around the lower back, sometimes held in place with suspenders.

Because of the recent emergence of back belt use in the workplace, there have been few published studies of the rate of injury among workers using the belts. These studies suffer from design flaws and have not produced sufficient support for or against the use of back belts. The NIOSH encourages efforts to more adequately determine the association between back belt use and the prevention of low back injury and is committed to supporting further research in this area.

Could Wearing a Back Belt Increase the Potential for Injury?

At this point, there are no definitive studies on either the beneficial or harmful effects of wearing back belts. Just as there is speculation that back belts may help, there is also concern that they may harm workers. As a result of the NIOSH review, the Institute is concerned with the potentially harmful effects associated with a false sense of security that may accompany back belt use.

There is some research showing that workers believe they can lift more when wearing a back belt. If workers falsely believe they are protected, they may subject themselves to even greater risk by lifting more weight than they would have without a belt.

How Can an Ergonomics Program Be Implemented?

A first step in implementing an ergonomics program would be to evaluate jobs that require frequent lifting, twisted or bent postures, or pushing or pulling.

Redesign these tasks so that the load is close to the body; the load is between shoulder and knuckle height; twisted lifts are eliminated; gravity moves the load when possible; slides, chutes, hoists, and hand trucks are used to move heavy loads; weight is reduced to the lowest feasible level.

What If I Still Decide to Use Back Belts?

The NIOSH believes that the decision to use back belts should be a voluntary decision by both employers and employees. Back belt use should not be a mandatory job requirement. If your workforce continues to wear back belts, you should remember the following points:

- There is a lack of scientific evidence that back belts work.
- Workers wearing back belts may attempt to lift more weight than they would have without a belt. A false sense of security may subject workers to a greater risk of injury.
- Workers and employers should redesign the work environment and work tasks to reduce lifting hazards, rather than rely solely on back belts to prevent injury.
- The research needed to adequately assess back belt effectiveness will take several years to complete. In the interim, workers should not assume that back belts are protective.

Chapter 17

When Wearing Backpacks, Are Kids Ergonomically Safe?

Backpack Overload in Children

Low back pain (LBP) unrelated to injury or other known cause is unusual in preteen children. However, a backpack overloaded with school books and supplies can strain the back and cause muscle fatigue. The American Academy of Orthopaedic Surgeons (AAOS) recommends that a child's backpack should weigh no more than 15 to 20 percent of the child's body weight.

Backpack Safety Tips

You may think it looks cool to sling your backpack onto one shoulder, but how cool will you look slumped over? If backpacks are not

---

This chapter contains text excerpted from the following sources: Text under the heading "Backpack Overload in Children" is excerpted from "Low Back Pain Fact Sheet," National Institute of Neurological Disorders and Stroke (NINDS), August 7, 2018; Text under the heading "Backpack Safety Tips" is excerpted from "Backpack Safety," girlshealth.gov, Office on Women's Health (OWH), May 28, 2014. Reviewed April 2019; Text under the heading "Preventing Strains and Sprains in Young Workers" is excerpted from "Young Retail Workers," Centers for Disease Control and Prevention (CDC), May 21, 2018.

used right, they can hurt your back, mess up your posture, and even make your hands tingle. And backpack troubles can be a greater risk for girls. That is because boys in your grade may be bigger than you, so their bodies suffer less pressure from the same amount of books.

Follow a few rules, and your backpack will be less of a pain in the neck—and back and shoulders!

- Make sure your loaded backpack does not weigh more than around 15 percent of what you weigh.
- Load the heaviest items closer to your back.
- If necessary, take some books out and carry them in your hands.
- Get a backpack with padded straps.
- Wear both straps to keep the weight even on both sides.
- Tighten the straps so the backpack is close to your body.
- Make sure the backpack does not hang down more than four inches below your waist.

You might want to get help from an adult to check on your backpack. And help yourself by clearing out any items you do not really need to carry. If wearing or carrying your backpack causes pain, stop using it for several days. If the pain does not get better, see a doctor.

Preventing Strains and Sprains in Young Workers

You overwork when you do more than your body can handle. For example, you can overwork by lifting things that are too heavy, doing the same motion over and over, using bad postures, or working too long without breaks.

Tips on Lifting/Carrying for Young Workers

You can make it easier on yourself when you pick up heavy or awkward things. If you consider this advice, you will be less likely to hurt your back.

- Can you get help from someone who knows more about the job? That person might know of tools or equipment you can use to help you lift or carry something heavy.
- Can you get someone to help you pick it up or carry it? That divides the weight between two people, making it easier and safer to lift.

- If the box or container seems too heavy or awkward for you, talk with your supervisor about other ways of doing that job, or ask about other jobs you could do that do not involve heavy lifting.
- If the task is making you feel overworked, talk with your supervisor about how to change the task to better suit your capabilities, or ask for a different task so that you can be productive without being fatigued.

How you position or move your body when you lift something can also make you more or less likely to be hurt. The suggestions below are in order, based on what studies have found.

Do the following when possible:

- Keep the item you are lifting close to your body.
- Avoid lifting off the floor and from overhead.
- Avoid twisting and bending while lifting.
- Keep your back straight and lift with your legs.

If your work requires a lot of strength and effort over long periods of time, consider the following tips:

- Pace yourself so that you avoid being sore the next day.
- Work on different jobs—some hard, some easy—that use different muscle groups.
- Ask for more rest breaks.
- Ask for help.

Chapter 18

Back Pain during Pregnancy

During pregnancy, a woman can expect some degree of discomfort in her back. Back pain is prevalent in almost 50 to 70 percent of all pregnant women and can be experienced at any point of the pregnancy. However, it occurs most commonly in the later stages of pregnancy. This pain may persist after delivery (postpartum)—but usually resolves after some months—and can sometimes be intense enough to disrupt daily activities and interfere with good night's sleep.

The types of back pain that occur during pregnancy are:

Lumbar or lower back pain generally occurs in the center of the back, at and above the waist. It is similar to the lower back pain experienced by a nonpregnant woman. Lumbar or lower back pain that radiates into the legs or feet is called "sciatica." Lower back pain during pregnancy may or may not be concurrent with sciatica.

Posterior pelvic pain is a deep pain felt below and at the side of the waistline and across the tailbone on either side. This kind of a pain in the back or pelvis can sometimes radiate down to the buttocks region and further down to the upper posterior portion of the thighs (the back of the thighs), but it does not extend below the knees. Posterior pelvic pain can sometimes be associated with pubic pain and morning stiffness.

Risk factors for back pain during pregnancy include obesity and a prior history of back pain.

Some of the potential causes of back pain or discomfort during pregnancy are:

Hormonal changes. Hormones released during pregnancy allow the softening and relaxation of ligaments attached to the pelvic bones and spine and loosen the joints in preparation for birth. These changes affect back support and cause pain while walking, climbing stairs, sitting for prolonged periods of time, rolling over in bed, getting out of a low chair or the tub, bending, and lifting.

Muscle separation. As the uterus expands during pregnancy, rectus abdominis muscles (two parallel sheets of muscles that run from the rib cage to the pubic bone) separate to create space for the fetus to grow. This can worsen the back pain or discomfort.

Center of gravity. An expectant mother's center of gravity shifts forward as a result of significant weight gain in the abdominal region. This postural change can trigger back pain.

Additional weight. As the fetus grows, the back is responsible for managing the additional weight, which can contribute to some amount of discomfort.

Posture or position. Poor posture while walking, sitting for prolonged periods of time, excessive standing, and inappropriate bending can escalate the back pain.

Increased stress. Stress increases muscle stiffness and pain, especially in weak areas, which contributes to pain.

Tips for Reducing Back Pain throughout the Pregnancy

- Avoid excessive weight gain. Gain a healthy amount of weight by maintaining a healthy diet.
- Maintain good posture. Stand straight with a high chest and relaxed shoulders and back.
- Avoid standing for long periods of time.
- Wear supportive footwear, and avoid high-heels. Move your feet while turning to avoid twisting your spine. Balance your weight on both sides when completing activities.

- Ensure that the chairs that you sit in provide good back support, and use a lumbar pillow for additional support.
- Elevate your feet while resting.
- When bending down, bend at your knees and try to keep your back straight (squat) as you pick things up.
- Avoid heavy lifting.
- Avoid sleeping on your back. Try to sleep on your side instead, with pillows tucked under your abdomen and between your knees for support.
- Avoid tight clothing. Wearing comfortable, loose garments may relieve back pressure to some extent.
- Include pregnancy-safe exercise in your daily routine. Pregnancy-safe exercises include swimming, relaxed walking, and pelvic tilts, and these exercises are designed to support and strengthen the abdomen and back.
- If the back pain seems to be related to stress, then prenatal yoga, meditation, and extra rest may be helpful.
- Use cold compresses (ice packs) and prenatal massage to relax and soothe an aching back.
- Get plenty of rest.

Contact a local chiropractor who specializes in pregnancy-related care, and learn how small adjustments can help ease the back pain. If the pain is unbearable, then contact your doctor. Do not take any pain-relief medication without prior approval from your doctor.

References

1. "Back Pain in Pregnancy," WebMD, August 4, 2018.
2. "Back Pain during Pregnancy," Mayoclinic, April 5, 2016.
3. "Types of Back Pain in Pregnancy," SPINE-health, May 28, 2008.

Chapter 19

Exercises for Low Back Pain

Pain is your body's way of warning you that something might be wrong, but that does not necessarily mean you should avoid exercise. In fact, depending on the type of pain you have, exercise could actually help.

Exercising with Acute Pain

If you experience a sharp pain in your muscles and/or joints, stop exercising and see your doctor. She or he will be able to say whether it is safe to exercise while experiencing acute pain and what activities might help. There may be simple stretching or strength training exercises, for instance, that you can do with a physical therapist or trainer to help with recovery. Your doctor might recommend that you reduce the intensity of your activity so you do not make the health issue worse, prolong the symptoms, or cause re-injury.

Warm up before exercising to get your body moving and ready for activity and to help reduce your risk of injury. For instance, you might do a few minutes of easy walking. Also, cool down after your workout

---

This chapter contains text excerpted from the following sources: Text in this chapter begins with excerpts from "Exercising with Pain," *Go4Life*, National Institutes of Health (NIH), July 8, 2016; Text under the heading "Flexibility Exercise for Lower Back" is excerpted from "Lower Back Exercise," *Go4Life*, National Institutes of Health (NIH), March 27, 2015. Reviewed April 2019; Text under the heading "Back Exercise" is excerpted from "Back Exercise 2," *Go4Life*, National Institutes of Health (NIH), January 23, 2009. Reviewed April 2019.

to help slow your heart rate and breathing back to normal, and to relax the muscles you just used.

Preventing Lower Back Pain

Exercise is an effective way to lower your risk for some pain. For example, research has shown that exercise combined with education can reduce the risk of lower back pain. The study looked at exercises such as strength-training activities targeting the back and abdominal muscles, stretching and spine range of motion exercises, and aerobic conditioning.

Flexibility Exercise for Lower Back

Targeted muscle: Lower back

Talk to your doctor: If you have had hip or back surgery, talk with your doctor before trying this stretch.

This exercise stretches the muscles of your lower back.

- Lie on your back with your legs together, knees bent, and feet flat on the floor. Try to keep both arms and shoulders flat on the floor throughout the stretch.
- Keeping knees bent and together, slowly lower both legs to one side as far as you comfortably can.
- Hold the position for 10 to 30 seconds.
- Bring legs back up slowly and repeat toward another side.
- Continue alternating sides for at least 3 to 5 times on each side.

Safety Measures

- Avoid "locking" your joints. Straighten your arms and legs when you stretch them, but do not hold them tightly in a straight position. Always keep them slightly bent while stretching.
- Always stretch with a smooth, steady movement. Do not jerk or bounce into the stretch; it may cause injury.
- A mild pulling feeling, while you are stretching, is normal. If you feel sharp or stabbing pain or joint pain, you are stretching too far. Reduce the stretch so it does not hurt.
- Always remember to breathe normally while holding a stretch.

- Always warm up before stretching exercises. Stretching your muscles before they are warmed up can result in injury. If you are doing only stretching exercises, warm up with a few minutes of easy walking first. If you are doing endurance or strength exercises, stretch after, not before.
- If you have had hip or back surgery, talk with your doctor before doing lower-back flexibility exercises.

Back Exercise

Targeted muscles: Back

What you need: Sturdy chair with armrests

Talk to your doctor: If you have had hip or back surgery, talk with your doctor before trying this stretch.

This exercise will help you do activities that require you to twist or turn to look behind you, such as backing out of a parking space or swinging a golf club.

- Sit up toward the front of a sturdy chair with armrests. Stay as straight as possible. Keep your feet flat on the floor and shoulder-width apart.
- Slowly twist to the left from your waist without moving your hips. Turn your head to the left. Lift your left hand and hold on to the left arm of the chair. Place your right hand on the outside of your left thigh. Twist farther, if possible.
- Hold the position for 10 to 30 seconds
- Slowly return to face forward
- Repeat on the right side
- Repeat at least 3 to 5 more times

As you progress, try lifting your left arm and resting it comfortably on the back of the chair. Hold on to the left armrest with your right arm. Repeat on right side.

Safety Measures

- Avoid "locking" your joints. Straighten your arms and legs when you stretch them, but do not hold them tightly in a straight position. Always keep them slightly bent while stretching.

- Always stretch with a smooth, steady movement. Do not jerk or bounce into the stretch; it may cause injury.
- A mild pulling feeling while you are stretching, is normal. If you feel sharp or stabbing pain or joint pain, you are stretching too far. Reduce the stretch so it does not hurt.
- Always remember to breathe normally while holding a stretch.
- Always warm up before stretching exercises. Stretching your muscles before they are warmed up can result in injury. If you are doing only stretching exercises, warm up with a few minutes of easy walking first. If you are doing endurance or strength exercises, stretch after, not before.
- If you have had hip or back surgery, talk with your doctor before doing lower-back flexibility exercises.

Chapter 20

Pilates Promotes Back Health

What Is Pilates?

Pilates is a fitness regimen for building flexibility, strength, endurance, and coordination. The emphasis is on improving core strength and fitness without adding muscle bulk. Pilates involves controlled movements done on a mat or with equipment. It improves physical and mental well-being, strengthens muscles, and tones the body, while also strengthening the torso and providing better posture and good health.

Pilates strongly emphasizes technique, and despite outward appearances, it is not as easy as doing crunches or other core-strengthening exercises. The moves look simple, but the execution requires precision and control. The exercises have names, such as "The 100," "The Elephant," and "The Swan," and are usually done in a specific order, one after the other.

The method was developed by Joseph H. Pilates, a German bodybuilder, gymnast, and physical trainer, who overcame childhood disease and fragility to become an accomplished athlete in various sports. Working as a nurse in Great Britain during World War I, he designed equipment and a system of exercises for rehabilitating immobilized soldiers and other patients. After immigrating to the United States in the 1920s, Pilates taught these exercises in a studio in New York.

What Are the Types of Pilates Exercises?

Pilates exercises can be generally categorized into two types:

The first requires primarily just a floor mat and a training routine and is designed to use body weight for resistance. Of the 500 exercises that were originally developed for Pilates, 34 are mat-based movements. In addition to the mat, these exercises utilize other traditional Pilates equipment—such as magic circles and hand weights or nonstandard gear, such as gym balls, stretch bands, and foam rollers.

The second type employs specialized equipment, such as "Reformer," "Cadillac," "Wunda Chair," "Spine Corrector," and "Ladder Barrel," which were designed by Pilates himself. This equipment uses a system of pulleys, springs, handles, and straps to provide resistance or support based on the requirements of the exercise.

Both kinds of exercises can be adapted for varying degrees of fitness and ability. If exercising on the mat turns out to be difficult for some people, the equipment offers alternative ways to exercise.

How Does Pilates Work?

Pilates can be practiced with a mat at home—possibly with the guidance of a home video—at a gymnasium or studio with special equipment or at a class with a trainer. Typically, classes last for 45 minutes to an hour. Pilates, which can be practiced for a few days per week along with aerobics, is considered a medium-intensity regimen, and though you will not necessarily work up a sweat, your muscles will get a thorough workout. Pilates focuses on concentration and breathing, as well as strengthening the core of the body, arms, and legs. It can also improve flexibility and joint mobility while strengthening the muscles and helping maintain a healthy body weight.

Who Can Do Pilates?

Pilates is suitable for people of all ages and fitness levels, from beginners to athletes. The equipment can be calibrated for support, to help beginners and people with health conditions, or for resistance in the case of athletes who want to challenge themselves. As with any exercise routine, it is a good idea to consult a healthcare professional if you have an injury or a medical condition before you begin working out.

What Are the Health Benefits of Pilates?

The benefits of Pilates can include improved posture, balance, muscle tone, joint mobility, and relief from stress and tension. Pilates has been shown to be particularly beneficial for athletes and dancers because it helps develop overall body strength and flexibility and reduces the risk of injury. While there is scientific evidence to support many of these benefits, there has not been enough rigorous scrutiny for definitive conclusions. More standardized research in this area is needed in order to verify the benefits scientifically.

What Are the Benefits of Pilates for People with Health Conditions?

Pilates has the advantage of being adaptable to a variety of individual needs. In many cases, it has been a useful addition to aerobics for people with heart disease, hypertension, and high cholesterol. For people with arthritis, it can be a beneficial strength-training program. Pilates may also be a good choice for lower back pain, helping to strengthen the muscles that support the back. Pregnant women who are already working out with Pilates should be able to continue, with their doctor's approval, as long as modifications are made to accommodate the pregnancy. It is important to understand that people with any medical condition should participate in a Pilates program only after consultation with a healthcare professional.

How Is Pilates Different from Yoga?

Pilates and yoga are different methods of exercises, but both offer similar benefits, such as improved posture, strength, balance, flexibility, and good breathing techniques. Although both systems promote physical and mental health, yoga tends to focus more on meditation and relaxation. Pilates makes use of equipment but yoga does not, and Pilates uses the flow of movement, while yoga features static poses.

How Should You Choose a Pilates Class?

Pilates classes are often taught in a studio with equipment or in open areas with mats, and they usually last for about an hour. Ideally, equipment-based Pilates should be taught on a one-to-one basis and mat exercises in small groups to ensure personal attention. If you are joining a group class for equipment training, make sure you gain sufficient familiarity with the equipment before attempting to use it on your own.

There are no legal requirements or qualifications needed to become a Pilates instructor. As a result, it is important to choose a teacher or class leader based on experience, recommendations, and personal rapport. Good instructors should have up to 450 hours of experience over a span of several years.

References

1. "A Guide to Pilates," NHS Choices, May 18, 2015.
2. "Pilates," The Nemours Foundation/KidsHealth®, February 2014.
3. Robinson, Kara Mayer. "Pilates," WebMD, 2017.

Part Three

Acute Injuries to the Back and Neck

Chapter 21

Neck Injuries

Chapter Contents

Section 21.1—Whiplash 140
Section 21.2—Cervical Fracture 141

Section 21.1

Whiplash

This section includes text excerpted from "Whiplash Information Page," National Institute of Neurological Disorders and Stroke (NINDS), March 27, 2019.

Whiplash—a soft tissue injury to the neck—is also called "neck sprain" or "neck strain." It is characterized by a collection of symptoms that occur following damage to the neck, usually because of sudden extension and flexion. The disorder commonly occurs as the result of an automobile accident and may include injury to intervertebral joints, discs, and ligaments; cervical muscles; and nerve roots.

Symptoms of Whiplash

Symptoms, such as neck pain, may be present directly after the injury or may be delayed for several days.

In addition to neck pain, other symptoms may include:

- Neck stiffness
- Injuries to the muscles and ligaments (myofascial injuries)
- Headache
- Dizziness
- Abnormal sensations, such as:
    - Burning or prickling (paresthesias)
    - Shoulder or back pain

In addition, some people experience cognitive, somatic, or psychological conditions—such as memory loss, concentration impairment, nervousness/irritability, sleep disturbances, fatigue, or depression.

Treatment for Whiplash

Treatment for individuals with whiplash may include:

- Pain medications
- Nonsteroidal anti-inflammatory drugs (NSAIDs)
- Antidepressants

- Muscle relaxants
- Cervical collar (usually worn for two to three weeks)

Range of motion exercises, physical therapy, and cervical traction may also be prescribed. Supplemental heat application may relieve muscle tension.

Prognosis for Whiplash

Generally, prognosis for individuals with whiplash is good. The neck and head pain clears within a few days or weeks. Most patients recover within three months after the injury; however, some may continue to have residual neck pain and headaches.

Section 21.2

Cervical Fracture

A cervical fracture, also known as a "broken neck," occurs due to a broken bone in any of the seven vertebrae of the neck (C1–C7). A cervical injury can have severe consequences on a person and may result in temporary or permanent paralysis from the neck down or even death. The majority of cervical fractures are seen in men between 15 and 24 years of age.

Classification

Cervical fractures are classified into two broad categories based on the nature of the fracture and region:

1. **Occipital-cervical spine injuries,** those that occur between the occiput and C2 vertebrae
2. **Subaxial cervical spine injuries,** those that occur between the C3–C7 vertebrae bones

Causes

A cervical fracture mostly occurs due to trauma to the head, or it can also result from any of the following:

- Diving in shallow water
- Falls from great heights
- Impact sports, such as football, ice hockey, rugby, and wrestling
- A severe blow to the head
- A severe and a sudden twist of the neck
- Vehicle accidents

Other risk factors include:

- Decreased muscle mass
- Osteoporosis, or thinning bones
- Diseases or conditions that weaken bones or result in bone or mineral loss, such as an abnormal menstrual cycle, postmenopause, tumors, or cysts

Even a slight twist of the neck during or after the trauma can cause the cervical bones to crack and cause irreversible and permanent damage to the spinal cord and neurologic structures, thereby resulting in a broken neck.

Symptoms

People with a cervical fracture may display or complain of the following symptoms:

- Bruising or swelling at the back of the neck
- Decreased range of motion (ROM) of the neck
- Radiating pain in the neck area
- Decreased feeling or muscle weakness of the arms and legs
- Pain in the neck area spreading to the shoulders, arms, and legs
- Tenderness and spasms
- Difficulty with breathing or an inability to take a deep breath

In case of a broken neck, the patient's neck has to be immobilized until medical examiners arrive and diagnose the patient.

Diagnosis

Patients that experienced trauma in the neck area should be suspected of a cervical fracture, and they should be evaluated immediately. Since the symptoms or physical findings can be atypical or the patient can complain about pain in other locations or downplay the severity of the neck injury, an X-ray of the cervical spine in its immobilized state is suggested to determine the presence of a cervical fracture. In case of a cervical fracture, the examiner may further suggest a magnetic resonance imaging (MRI) or a computerized tomography (CT) scan to determine the severity of the fracture.

Treatment

The treatment for cervical fractures can be categorized as:

1. Conservative or nonoperative
2. Surgical or operative

The type of treatment depends on the location and extent of the fracture. While nonoperative treatment methods—such as braces, traction, or a rigid cast—are suggested for a minor compression fracture, surgery or spinal fusion is recommended for an extensive fracture. Antibiotics, in case of an infection, and pain medication may also be prescribed during the recovery phase.

Recovery and Rehabilitation

A cervical brace is usually worn for 6 to 8 weeks, and traction is worn up to 12 weeks or until the bones heal. The patient's recovery also depends on other factors, such as their age, overall health, and associated injuries; hence, children and healthy people heal faster. Rehabilitation is suggested for patients with paralysis even though their necks have healed. Such rehabilitation can include support groups, psychotherapy, or occupational therapy.

Prevention

To reduce the chances of a cervical fracture:

- Do weight-bearing exercises to improve the bone and muscle strength.
- Wear all padding and safety equipment during combat sport activities, and follow proper tackling techniques.

- Wear seat belts while driving.
- Avoid diving in shallow waters.
- Avoid situations of physical harm, such as slippery or dark areas and physical bouts.

References

1. "Cervical Spine Fracture and Dislocations," University of Southern California, n.d.
2. "Cervical Fracture (Broken Neck)," OrthoInfo, n.d.
3. Quinn, Elizabeth. "Cervical Neck Fractures," Verywell Health, November 14, 2018.
4. "Neck Fracture," University of Virginia, n.d.

Chapter 22

Fractures of the Thoracic and Lumbar Spine

The spinal column consists of several small bones that are stacked on top of each other. There are flat and round-shaped discs in between these bones, which act as shock-absorbers. This allows the spine to bend and adjust, according to the movements. The spine consists of four segments: the coccygeal, lumbar, thoracic, and cervical. The coccyx, also known as the "tailbone," is a small triangular bone. It comprises 3 to 4 coccygeal vertebrae. The lumbar spine consists of 5 vertebrae and carries most of the body weight. The thoracic spine consists of 12 vertebrae and starts from the chest and extends up to rib cage.

Spinal fractures mostly occur in the thoracic (middle) and lumbar (lower) regions of the back. A fracture in the spinal column is a very serious injury, and it requires immediate attention and treatments in order to prevent further damage. The symptoms of a thoracic and lumbar fracture include the following:

- Back pain that ranges from moderate to severe, and gets worse when moving
- Experience of tingling, numbness, weakness, or bowel/bladder dysfunction

---

Causes

These fractures are often due to high-energy trauma, such as a car crash, falling off of a building, a sports accident, violent actions, a gunshot, etc. Men are four times more likely to experience these kinds of fractures when compared to women. Depending upon the severity, spinal fractures can be prone to a spinal cord injury (SCI).

People who have osteoporosis (low bone density), tumors, or any other underlying conditions that weaken the bone are more likely to have spinal fractures, even when caused by low-impact activities, such as lifting small weights or twisting their body. These fractures might not show symptoms or cause discomfort until a bone breaks.

Emergency Procedure

There are certain things to do and things to avoid when a person experiences a spinal fracture. If a fracture is suspected, do not move the patient as it may cause further damage to the spinal column. It may also be difficult to locate and categorize the fracture right after the accident. Call 911 immediately after the injury, and wait for the emergency medical service (EMS) workers. The EMS workers will check for vital signs, such as breathing and heartbeat, and will temporarily immobilize the patient and transport the patient to a hospital.

The Doctor's Examination

When the patient arrives at the hospital, a doctor will examine them from head to toe to check for bruising, swelling, or any other signs of injury to the head, chest, abdomen, pelvis, spine, and legs. This may include neurological tests, in which the doctor checks the patient's ability to move, sense, and feel the position of all limbs. Imaging tests—such as X-ray, computed tomography (CT) scans, and magnetic resonance imaging (MRI) scans—of various areas, including the thoracic and lumbar spine, will be conducted. Once all the required tests are done, the doctor categorizes the fracture and plans further appropriate treatment for the patient.

Types of Spinal Fractures

There are three different types of spinal fractures, and they depend upon the pattern of injury as determined by the doctors.

- Flexion fractures

- Extension fracture
- Rotation fractures

Flexion Fractures

There are two types of flexion fractures.

- **Compression fracture:** This type of fracture occurs when the front part of the vertebra breaks and loses height, while the rear does not. This fracture is usually stable, as the bone stays in place and induces impact without dislocating its position. The compression fracture rarely pertains to neurological problems. The chances of this kind of fracture are higher for patients with osteoporosis.
- **Axial-burst fracture:** When the vertebra loses height on both the front and back sides, it results in axial-burst fracture. This kind of fracture occurs when an individual falls from a distant height and lands on their feet. This fracture has more severity than the compression fracture, as it is often associated with other problems, especially long-term neurological damage.

Extension Fracture

This type of fracture (the flexion/distraction/change fracture) occurs when the vertebra is pulled apart. It is also referred to as a "seat belt injury," in which the lower part of the body is stabilized by a seat belt and the upper part of the body is thrust forward, which pulls apart and displaces the bone.

Rotation Fractures

- **Transverse process fracture:** This type of fracture is caused by extreme sideways (lateral) bending or rotation of the spinal column. This fracture does not greatly affect stability.
- **Fracture dislocation:** A very serious and unstable injury that involves bone and/or soft tissue, in which a vertebra moves off an adjacent one. The fracture dislocation is a result of the bone enduring a high-impact trauma. This type of fracture may lead to nerve damage in older patients.

Treatments

The main goal of spinal fracture treatment is to help the bones return to their functionality before the SCI, while preventing further damage.

The treatment plan depends upon the following:

- Type of fracture
- Other injuries accompanying the spinal fracture

Treatment may be nonsurgical or surgical, depending upon the severity of the fracture.

Nonsurgical Treatment

Doctors treat minor spinal fractures without surgery. The time period and precautions taken for the nonsurgical treatment varies depending upon the type of fracture.

- **Flexion fracture pattern:** Most burst fractures and some compression fractures do not require surgical treatment and can be treated by nonsurgical treatment methods. Patients with this fracture pattern are supposed to wear hyper-extension braces for 6 to 12 weeks and participate in physical exercises to repair the bones and to prevent postfracture complications.
- **Extension fracture pattern:** When treating this type of fracture, a doctor will closely monitor a patient as they wear a brace or cast for 12 weeks.
- **Rotation fracture pattern:** If the patient has a rotation fracture pattern, she or he needs to wear a thoracolumbar corset and follow an aerobic walking program.

Surgical Treatment

When the spinal fracture is unstable and severe, surgical treatment is done in order to restore the bone's proper position, relieve pressure, and allow early movement of the limbs. Depending on the fracture pattern, the doctor may perform the surgery in the front (anterior), side (lateral), or back (posterior)—or a combination of all the three. The surgical treatment includes fixation of metal plates and screws and/or spinal fusion.

Treatment Follow-Up

Regardless of the treatment received by the patient, rehabilitation is necessary for the injury to heal. Rehabilitation includes exercises to facilitate limb movements and relieve pain. If unexpected pain or swelling is felt in the spinal cord and/or the surrounding areas, consult your doctor immediately.

References

1. "Spinal Trauma/Fractures," Midwest Orthopaedics at Rush, April 26, 2012.
2. "Fractures of the Thoracic and Lumbar Spine," Midwest Orthopaedics at Rush, September 11, 2015.
3. "Fractures, Sprains and Strains," Shoreline Orthopaedics, February 17, 2015.
4. "Thoracic Compression Fractures," The University of Maryland Medical Center (UMMC), February 1, 2001.

Chapter 23

Osteoporosis and Fractures

Osteoporosis is a disease in which bones are weakened and have a higher chance of breaking. Bone strength has two main features:

- Bone mass or amount of bone
- Bone quality

You may think that osteoporosis is a natural and unavoidable part of aging. However, medical experts now believe that osteoporosis is largely preventable. Furthermore, if you already have osteoporosis, you can take steps to prevent or slow further progress of the disease and reduce your risk of future fractures. Even though osteoporosis was once viewed as a disease of old age, it is now recognized as a disease that can stem from less-than-optimal bone growth during childhood and adolescence, as well as from bone loss later in life.

In addition to the financial costs, osteoporosis takes a toll in terms of reduced quality of life (QOL) for many people who suffer fractures. It can also affect the lives of your family members and friends who serve as your caregivers.

This chapter includes text excerpted from "Osteoporosis," National Institute of Arthritis and Musculoskeletal and Skin Diseases (NIAMS), February 28, 2016.

Osteoporosis is the major underlying cause of fractures in postmenopausal women and the elderly. Fractures can occur in any bone, but happen most often in bones of the:

- Hip
- Spine
- Wrist

Of all fractures, hip fractures have the most serious impact. Most hip fractures require hospitalization and surgery; some hip-fracture patients require nursing home placement. Vertebral fractures also can have serious consequences, including chronic back pain and disability. They have also been linked to increased mortality in older people.

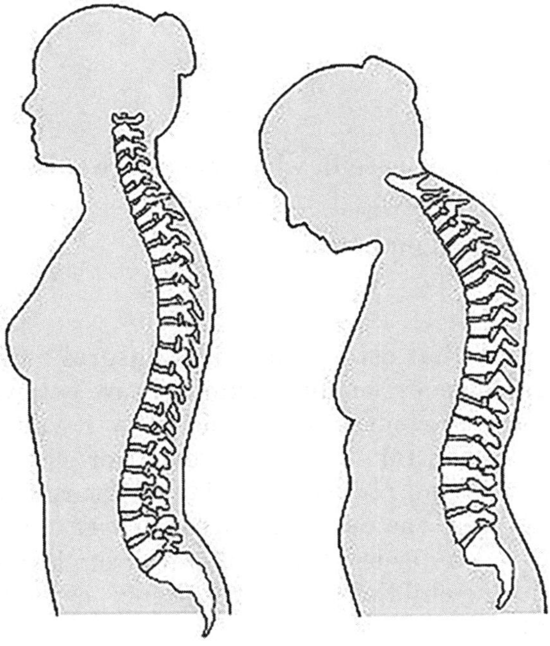

Figure 23.1. *Normal Vertebrae versus Vertebrae with Osteoporosis* (Source: "Osteoporosis," Office on Women's Health (OWH), U.S. Department of Health and Human Services (HHS).)

Some children and adolescents develop osteoporosis that has no known cause, known as "idiopathic juvenile osteoporosis" (IJO). Young people who have this rare form of osteoporosis usually recover within two to four years. The basic treatment strategy may include:

- Protecting the spine and other bones from fracture until recovery occurs
- Recommending calcium and vitamin D supplements
- Prescribing certain medications used to treat adults with osteoporosis, especially in severe cases

Symptoms of Osteoporosis

Osteoporosis is often called a "silent disease" because it usually progresses without any symptoms until a fracture occurs or one or more vertebrae (bones in the spine) collapse. Collapsed vertebrae may first be felt or seen when a person develops severe back pain; loss of height; or spine malformations, such as a stooped or hunched posture. Bones affected by osteoporosis may become so fragile that fractures occur spontaneously or as the result of:

- Minor bumps
- Falls
- Normal stresses and strains, such as bending, lifting, or even coughing

Causes of Osteoporosis

Osteoporosis affects women and men of all races and ethnic groups. Osteoporosis can strike at any age, although the risk for developing the disease increases as you get older. Osteoporosis:

- Is most common in non-Hispanic White women and Asian women
- African American and Hispanic women have a lower risk of developing osteoporosis, but they are still at significant risk.
- For Native American women, the data is not clear.
- Among men, osteoporosis is more common in non-Hispanic Whites and Asians than in men of other ethnic or racial groups.

Factors that are linked to the development of osteoporosis or contribute to an individual's likelihood of developing the disease are called "risk factors." Many people with osteoporosis have several risk factors for the disease, but others who develop osteoporosis have no identified risk factors. There are some risk factors that you cannot change, and others that you can or may be able to change.

Risk Factors for Osteoporosis

Risk Factors You Can or May Be Able to Change

Hormone changes. Low levels of estrogen from amenorrhea, the abnormal absence of menstrual periods, is the most common reason premenopausal women have changes in estrogen levels. Missed or irregular periods can be caused by various factors, including:

- Hormonal disorders
- Extreme levels of physical activity combined with restricted calorie intake. For example, in female marathon runners, ballet dancers, and women who spend a great deal of time and energy working out at the gym

Low estrogen levels in women after menopause and low testosterone levels in men also increase the risk of osteoporosis. Lower-than-normal estrogen levels in men may also play a role. Low testosterone and estrogen levels are often a cause of osteoporosis in men being treated with certain medications for prostate cancer.

Diet. From childhood into old age, a diet low in calcium and vitamin D can increase your risk of osteoporosis and fractures. Excessive dieting or inadequate caloric intake can also be bad for bone health. People who are very thin and do not have much body fat to cushion falls have an increased risk of fracture.

Certain medical conditions. In addition to sex hormone problems and eating disorders, other medical conditions can increase the risk of osteoporosis, including:

- Genetic disorders
- Endocrine diseases
- Gastrointestinal diseases and conditions
- Blood diseases
- Rheumatic disorders
- Anorexia nervosa
- Late onset of puberty and early menopause

Medications. Long-term use of certain medications linked with osteoporosis include:

- Anticoagulants (heparin)

- Anticonvulsants (some)
- Aromatase inhibitors
- Cyclosporine A and tacrolimus
- Cancer chemotherapy drugs
- Glucocorticoids (and adrenocorticotropic hormone (ACTH))
- Gonadotropin-releasing hormone agonists
- Lithium
- Methotrexate
- Proton pump inhibitors
- Selective serotonin reuptake inhibitors (SSRIs)
- Thyroxine

An inactive lifestyle or extended bed rest. Low levels of physical activity and prolonged periods of inactivity can contribute to an increased rate of bone loss. These lifestyles also leave you in poor physical condition, which can increase your risk of falling and breaking a bone.

- **Excessive use of alcohol**. Chronic heavy drinking is a significant risk factor for osteoporosis.
- **Smoking**. Most studies indicate that smoking is a risk factor for osteoporosis and fracture, although the exact reasons for the harmful effects of tobacco use on bone health are unclear.

Risk Factors You Cannot Change

Sex. Your chances of developing osteoporosis are greater if you are a woman. Women have lower peak bone mass and smaller bones than men. They also lose bone more rapidly than men in middle age because of the dramatic reduction in estrogen levels that occurs with menopause.

Age. The older you are, the greater your risk of osteoporosis. Bone loss builds up over time, and your bones become weaker as you age.

Body size. Slender, thin-boned women are at greater risk, as are, surprisingly, taller women.

Race. White and Asian women are at highest risk. African American and Hispanic women have a lower but significant risk. Among men, Whites are at higher risk than others. These differences in risk can be explained in part, although not entirely. by differences in peak bone mass among these groups.

Family history. Susceptibility to osteoporosis and fractures appears to be, in part, hereditary. People whose parents have a history of fractures also tend to have reduced bone mass and an increased risk for fractures.

You may have a higher risk for a hip fracture, independent of your bone density, if you have:

- An existing spine fracture
- A mother who fractured her hip
- More risk factors

Treatment of Osteoporosis

The primary goal in treating people with osteoporosis is preventing fractures. A comprehensive treatment program includes:

- Proper nutrition
- Lifestyle changes
- Exercise
- Prevention of falls that may result in fractures
- Medications
- Alternative therapies

If you take medication to prevent or treat osteoporosis, it is still essential that you obtain the recommended amounts of calcium and vitamin D. Exercising and maintaining other aspects of a healthy lifestyle are also important.

For people with osteoporosis resulting from another condition, the best approach is to identify and treat the underlying cause. If you are taking a medication that causes bone loss, your doctor may be able to reduce the dose of that medication or switch you to another medication that is effective but not harmful to your bones. If you have a disease that requires long-term glucocorticoid therapy, such as rheumatoid arthritis or lupus, you can also take certain medications approved for the prevention or treatment of osteoporosis associated with aging or menopause.

Nutrition

A healthy, balanced diet that includes:

- Plenty of fruits and vegetables
- Enough calories
- Adequate calcium, vitamin D, and vitamin K is essential for minimizing bone loss and maintaining overall health. Calcium and vitamin D are especially important for bone health.

Calcium

Calcium is the most important nutrient for preventing osteoporosis and for reaching peak bone mass. For healthy postmenopausal women who are not consuming enough calcium (1,200 mg per day) in their diet, calcium and vitamin D supplements help to preserve bone mass and prevent hip fracture. Calcium is also needed for the proper function of:

- The heart
- Muscles
- Nerves
- Blood clotting

We take in calcium from our diet and lose it from the body mainly through urine, feces, and sweat. The body depends on dietary calcium to build healthy new bone and avoid excessive loss of calcium from bone to meet other needs. The Institute of Medicine of the National Academy of Sciences recommends specific amounts of dietary calcium and vitamin D for various stages of life. Men and women up to 50 years of age need 1,000 milligrams of calcium per day, and the recommendation increases to 1,200 milligrams for women older than 50 years of age and for men older than 70 years of age.

Many people in the United States consume much less than the recommended amount of calcium in their diets. Good sources of calcium include:

- Low-fat dairy products
- Dark green leafy vegetables, such as bok choy, collards, and turnip greens
- Broccoli

- Sardines and salmon with bones
- Soybeans, tofu, and other soy products
- Calcium-fortified foods, such as orange juice, cereals, and breads

If you have trouble getting enough calcium in your diet, you may need to take a calcium supplement, such as calcium carbonate, calcium phosphate, or calcium citrate. If you are between the ages of 19 and 50, your daily calcium intake should not exceed 2,500 milligrams because too much calcium can cause problems, such as kidney stones. (After the age of 50, intakes should not exceed 2,000 milligrams per day.) Calcium coming from food sources provides better protection from kidney stones. Anyone who has had a kidney stone should increase their dietary calcium and decrease the amount from supplements, as well as increase fluid intake.

Vitamin D

Vitamin D is required for proper absorption of calcium from the intestine. It is made in the skin after exposure to sunlight. Only a few

Table 23.1. Recommended Calcium and Vitamin D Intakes

Life-Stage Group	Calcium mg/day	Vitamin D (IU/day)
Infants 0 to 6 months	200	400
Infants 6 to 12 months	260	400
1 to 3 years old	700	600
4 to 8 years old	1,000	600
9 to 13 years old	1,300	600
14 to 18 years old	1,300	600
19 to 30 years old	1,000	600
31 to 50 years old	1,000	600
51 to 70 years old males	1,000	600
51 to 70 years old females	1,200	600
>70 years old	1,200	800
14 to 18 years old, pregnant/lactating	1,300	600
19 to 50 years old, pregnant/lactating	1,000	600

Definitions: mg = milligrams; IU = International Units
(Source: Food and Nutrition Board (FNB), Institute of Medicine (IOM), National Academy of Sciences (NAS), 2010.)

foods naturally contain significant amounts of vitamin D, including fatty fish and fish oils. Foods fortified with vitamin D, such as milk and cereals, are a major dietary source of vitamin D. Although many people obtain enough vitamin D naturally, studies show that vitamin D production decreases in older adults, in people who are housebound, and during the winter—especially in northern latitudes.

If you are at risk for vitamin D deficiency, you can take multivitamins or calcium supplements that contain vitamin D to meet the recommended daily intake of 600 International Units (IU) for men and women up to the age of 70 and 800 IU for people over 70 years of age. Doses of more than 2,000 IU per day are not advised unless under the supervision of a doctor. Larger doses can be given initially to people who are deficient as a way to replenish stores of vitamin D.

Lifestyle

In addition to a healthy diet, a healthy lifestyle is important for optimizing bone health. You should:

- Avoid smoking and second-hand smoke.
- Drink alcohol in moderation (no more than one drink per day is a good general guideline).
- Talk to your doctor about medications you are taking. Some prescription medications can cause bone loss or increase your risk of falling and breaking a bone.

Exercise

Exercise is an important part of an osteoporosis treatment program. The evidence suggests that the most beneficial physical activities for bone health include strength training or resistance training. Physical activity can:

- Build and maintain bone throughout adulthood
- Help maintain or even modestly increase bone density in adulthood
- Reduce your risk of falling by increasing muscle mass and strength and improving coordination and balance
- Help older people improve function and delay loss of independence

Although exercise is beneficial for people with osteoporosis, it should not put any sudden or excessive strain on your bones. If you have osteoporosis, you should avoid high-impact exercise. To help ensure against fractures, a physical therapist or rehabilitation medicine specialist can:

- Recommend specific exercises to strengthen and support your back
- Teach you safe ways of moving and carrying out daily activities
- Recommend an exercise program that is tailored to your circumstances

Other trained exercise specialists, such as exercise physiologists, may also be able to help you develop a safe and effective exercise program.

Fall Prevention

Fall prevention is a critical concern for men and women with osteoporosis. Falls increase your likelihood of fracturing a bone in the hip, wrist, spine, or other parts of the skeleton. Fractures can affect your quality of life and lead to loss of independence and even premature death. A host of factors can contribute to your risk of falling.

Falls can be caused by:

- Impaired vision or balance
- Loss of muscle mass
- Chronic or short-term illnesses that impair your mental or physical functioning
- Use of four or more prescription medications
- Side effects of certain medications, such as:
    - Sedatives or tranquilizers
    - Sleeping pills
    - Antidepressants
    - Anticonvulsants
    - Muscle relaxants
    - Heart medicines
    - Blood pressure pills

- Diuretics
- Drinking alcoholic beverages

If you have osteoporosis, it is important to be aware of any physical changes you may be experiencing that affect your balance or gait and to discuss these changes with your doctor or other healthcare providers. It is also important to have regular checkups and tell your doctor if you have had problems with falling.

The force or impact of a fall (how hard you land) plays a major role in determining whether you will break a bone. Catching yourself so that you land on your hands or grabbing onto an object as you fall can prevent a hip fracture. You may break your wrist or arm instead, but the consequences are not as serious as if you break your hip. Studies have shown that wearing a specially designed garment that contains hip padding may reduce hip fractures resulting from falls in frail, elderly people living in nursing homes or residential care facilities, but use of the garments by residents is often low.

Falls can also be caused by factors in your environment that create unsafe conditions. Some tips to help eliminate the environmental factors that lead to falls include:

Outdoors and Away from Home

- Use a cane or walker for added stability.
- Wear shoes that give good support and have thin nonslip soles. Avoid wearing slippers and athletic shoes with deep treads.
- Walk on grass when sidewalks are slippery; in winter, sprinkle salt or kitty litter on slippery sidewalks.
- Be careful on highly polished floors that are slick and dangerous, especially when wet, and walk on plastic or carpet runners when possible.
- Stop at curbs and check their height before stepping up or down.

Indoors

- Keep rooms free of clutter, especially on floors.
- Keep floor surfaces smooth but not slippery.
- Wear shoes that give good support and have thin nonslip soles. Avoid wearing slippers and athletic shoes with deep treads.

- Be sure carpets and area rugs have skid-proof backing or are tacked to the floor. Use double-stick tape to keep rugs from slipping.
- Be sure stairwells are well lit and that stairs have handrails.
- Install grab bars on bathroom walls near tub, shower, and toilet.
- Use a rubber bath mat or slip-proof seat in the shower or tub.
- Improve the lighting in your home. Use a nightlight or flashlight if you get up at night.
- Use step ladders that are stable and have a handrail.
- Install ceiling fixtures or lamps that can be turned on by a switch near the room's entrance.
- If you live alone (or spend large amounts of time alone), consider purchasing a cordless phone; you will not have to rush to answer the phone when it rings, and you can call for help if you do fall.
- Consider having a personal emergency-response system; you can use it to call for help if you fall.

Medications

Your doctor may prescribe medications that have been shown to slow or stop bone loss or build new bone, increase bone density, and reduce fracture risk. The U.S. Food and Drug Administration (FDA) has approved several medications for prevention or treatment of osteoporosis, based on their ability to reduce fractures.

- **Bisphosphonates**: Several bisphosphonates are approved for the prevention or treatment of osteoporosis. These medications reduce the activity of cells that cause bone loss.
- **Parathyroid hormone**: A form of human parathyroid hormone (PTH) is approved for postmenopausal women and men with osteoporosis who are at high risk for having a fracture. Use of the drug for more than two years is not recommended.
- **RANK ligand (RANKL) inhibitor**: A RANK ligand (RANKL) inhibitor is approved for postmenopausal women with osteoporosis who are at high risk for fracture.
- **Estrogen agonists/antagonists**: An estrogen agonist/ antagonist (also called a "selective estrogen receptor modulator"

or "SERM") is approved for the prevention and treatment of osteoporosis in postmenopausal women. SERMs are not estrogens, but they have estrogen-like effects on some tissues and estrogen-blocking effects on other tissues.

- **Calcitonin**: Calcitonin is approved for the treatment of osteoporosis in women who are at least 5 years beyond menopause. Calcitonin is a hormone involved in calcium regulation and bone metabolism.
- **Estrogen and hormone therapy**: Estrogen and combined estrogen and progestin (hormone therapy) are approved for the prevention of postmenopausal osteoporosis, as well as the treatment of moderate to severe hot flashes and vaginal dryness that may accompany menopause. Estrogen without an added progestin is recommended only for women who have had a hysterectomy (surgery to remove the uterus) because estrogen increases the risk of developing cancer of the uterine lining and progestin reduces that risk.

Results of the National Institutes of Health (NIH)-sponsored Women's Health Initiative, a large, long-term study of disease prevention strategies in postmenopausal women, suggest that, in most women, the harmful effects of long-term use of hormone therapy are likely to outweigh the disease prevention benefits.

The FDA has recommended that women use hormone therapy at the lowest dose and for the shortest time, and carefully consider and discuss with their doctor other approved osteoporosis treatments.

Alternative Therapies

Isoflavones are naturally occurring compounds found in soybeans. Because they are structurally similar to estrogen, researchers have thought that they may hold promise as an alternative to estrogen therapy to protect postmenopausal women from osteoporosis. Several studies have explored the effects of soy isoflavones on bone health, but results have been mixed, ranging from a modest impact to no effect. Most of these studies had various limitations, including their short duration and small sample size, making it difficult to fully evaluate the impact of these compounds on bone health. Moreover, reports from NIH-supported clinical trials have failed to demonstrate a bone-sparing effect of soy isoflavones.

Who Treats Osteoporosis

Medical specialists who treat osteoporosis include:

- Family physicians
- Internists
- Endocrinologists
- Geriatricians
- Gynecologists
- Orthopedic surgeons
- Rheumatologists
- Physiatrists (doctors specializing in physical medicine and rehabilitation)

Physical and occupational therapists and nurses may also participate in the care of people with osteoporosis.

Living with Osteoporosis

Many of the things you do to prevent osteoporosis also help you to manage it. To help keep your bones strong and slow down bone loss, you can:

- Diet
- Exercise
- Lead a healthy lifestyle
- Prevent falls

Diet

A healthy diet with enough calcium and vitamin D helps make your bones strong. Many people get less than half the calcium they need. Good sources of calcium are:

- Low-fat milk, yogurt, and cheese
- Foods with added calcium, such as orange juice, cereals, and breads

Vitamin D is also needed for strong bones. You may need to take vitamin D pills.

Exercise

Exercise helps your bones grow stronger. The best exercises for healthy bones are strength building and weight bearing, such as:

- Walking
- Hiking
- Jogging
- Climbing stairs
- Lifting weights
- Playing tennis
- Dancing

Healthy Lifestyle

Smoking is bad for bones, as well as the heart and lungs. Also, people who drink a lot of alcohol are more prone to bone loss and broken bones due to poor diet and risk of falling.

Preventing Falls

Men and women with osteoporosis need to take care not to fall down. Falls can break bones. Some reasons people fall are:

- Poor vision
- Poor balance
- Certain diseases that affect how you walk
- Some types of medicine, such as sleeping pills

Some tips to help prevent falls outdoors are:

- Use a cane or walker.
- Wear rubber-soled shoes so you do not slip.
- Walk on grass when sidewalks are slippery.
- In winter, put salt or kitty litter on icy sidewalks.

Some ways to help prevent falls indoors are:

- Keep rooms free of clutter, especially on floors.
- Use plastic or carpet runners on slippery floors.

- Wear low-heeled shoes that provide good support.
- Do not walk in socks, stockings, or slippers.
- Be sure carpets and area rugs have skid-proof backs or are tacked to the floor.
- Be sure stairs are well lit and have rails on both sides.
- Put grab bars on bathroom walls near tub, shower, and toilet.
- Use a rubber bath mat in the shower or tub.
- Keep a flashlight next to your bed.
- Use a sturdy step stool with a handrail and wide steps.
- Add more lights in rooms.
- Keep a cordless phone to keep with you so that you do not have to rush to the phone when it rings, and if you fall, you can call for help.

Emotional Impacts of Osteoporosis

- If you are nervous about the risk of breaking a bone when you go out to crowded places, such as malls, movie theaters, or museums, try going at less crowded times. Take breaks and sit down when you feel tired.
- If you have been feeling symptoms of depression, such as loss of appetite, hopelessness, feeling useless and helpless, or having thoughts of suicide, for more than two weeks, consult a doctor, social worker, or therapist. Medications and counseling are available to fight depression.
- If you are feeling self-conscious about changes in your appearance, such as the curvature (kyphosis) that occurs in the upper spine after multiple vertebral fractures, look for styles of clothing that minimize figure changes.

Functional and Physical Aspects of Osteoporosis

- If you have trouble working, doing chores around the house, or other routine activities, such as grocery shopping, try breaking them into short segments. Get up from sitting every half hour or so to ease muscle strain and reposition your skeleton. Also, be aware of your posture, and avoid bending and twisting at the same time.

- Look for ways to modify sports and leisure activities that you enjoy to protect your bones, or cultivate new forms of physical activity that put less stress on your skeleton.
- If you experience pain after a fracture, try pain-relief strategies, such as hot and cold compresses, biofeedback, and other relaxation strategies. Avoid long periods of inactivity or bed rest, which will worsen osteoporosis. Consult your healthcare professional about the use of analgesics, such as acetaminophen.
- For chronic (long-term) back pain or tiredness caused by fractures in the spine, consult a physical therapist or rehabilitation specialist for exercises to strengthen the back muscles, which may minimize or relieve pain. You will need to continue these exercises faithfully to maintain their benefits.

Social Aspects of Osteoporosis

- Support groups, friends, and family members can help you manage the social challenges and limitations resulting from osteoporosis.
- Do not be afraid to ask others for help in dealing with the effects of osteoporosis on your life. For example, you may need to ask a family member, friend, or neighbor to help you bring groceries into your house or apartment. Find ways to give to others who help you so that you do not feel forced to choose between feeling that you are taking too much help and not taking any help at all.
- Remember that it is normal to want and need help from others, as well as to help other people. You can work to keep relationships balanced so that no one does most of the talking over a long period of time, and keep in mind that we all help others throughout life. Friends and family are probably happy to help you, just as you feel good when you help others.
- Concern about experiencing or causing fractures can affect intimate relations between significant others when one or both individuals have osteoporosis. Although these topics can be difficult to discuss, couples can look for ways to achieve intimacy without increasing fracture risk. Most physical therapists have been trained to address this issue and can offer advice.

Prevention of Osteoporosis

Preventing osteoporosis is a lifelong endeavor. To reach optimal peak bone mass and minimize loss of bone as you get older, there are several factors you should consider. Addressing all of these factors is the best way to optimize bone health throughout life.

Screening for Osteoporosis

Prevention also includes screening for osteoporosis. The U.S. Preventive Services Task Force (USPSTF), an independent panel of experts in primary care and prevention, recommends screening for osteoporosis for:

- All women 65 years of age and older
- Women under the age of 65 who are at high risk for fractures

You should also ask your doctor about osteoporosis if you:

- Are over 50 years of age and have broken a bone
- Have lost height or your posture has become stooped or hunched
- Experience sudden back pain
- Have a chronic disease or eating disorder known to increase the risk of osteoporosis
- Are taking one or more medications known to cause bone loss
- Have multiple risk factors for osteoporosis and osteoporosis-related fractures

Consider talking to your doctor about being evaluated for osteoporosis if:

- You are a man or woman over the age of 50 or a postmenopausal woman and you break a bone
- You are a woman 65 years of age or older
- You are a woman younger than 65 years of age and at high risk for fractures
- You have lost height, developed a stooped or hunched posture, or experienced sudden back pain with no apparent cause
- You have been taking glucocorticoid medications, such as prednisone, cortisone, or dexamethasone, for two months or longer or are taking other medications known to cause bone loss

- You have a chronic illness or are taking a medication that is known to cause bone loss
- You have anorexia nervosa or a history of this eating disorder
- You are a premenopausal woman, not pregnant, and your menstrual periods have stopped, are irregular, or never started when you reached puberty

Overall Nutrition

A healthy, balanced diet that includes lots of fruits and vegetables and enough calories is also important for lifelong bone health. If you take in adequate amounts of calcium and vitamin D throughout your life, you are more likely to have optimal skeletal mass early in life and are less likely to lose bone later in life.

Calcium

Taking the recommended amount of calcium over a lifetime is thought to play an important role in the development of osteoporosis. Many published studies show that low calcium intakes are associated with:

- Low bone mass
- Rapid bone loss
- High fracture rates

National surveys suggest that the average calcium intake of individuals is far below the levels recommended for optimal bone health.

The body's demand for calcium is greater in:

- Childhood and adolescence, when the skeleton is growing rapidly
- Women during pregnancy and breastfeeding
- Postmenopausal women and older men. Increased calcium requirements in older people may be related to vitamin D deficiencies that reduce intestinal absorption of calcium.

Also, as you age, your body becomes less efficient at absorbing calcium and other nutrients. Older adults are also more likely to have chronic medical problems and to use medications that may impair calcium absorption.

Adolescence is the most critical period for building bone mass that helps protect against osteoporosis later in life. Yet, studies show that among children between the ages of 9 and 19 in the United States, few meet the recommended levels. Therefore, it is especially important for parents, other caregivers, and pediatricians to talk to children and young teens about developing bone-healthy habits, including eating calcium-rich foods and getting enough exercise.

Vitamin D

Vitamin D plays an important role in calcium absorption and bone health. It is made in the skin after exposure to sunlight and can also be obtained through the diet. Although many people are able to obtain enough vitamin D naturally, vitamin D production decreases if you:

- Are older
- Are housebound
- Do not get enough sun
- Have a chronic neurological or gastrointestinal disease

If you are at risk for vitamin D deficiency, your doctor may recommend vitamin D supplements. Calcium and vitamin D supplements may help slow bone loss and prevent hip fracture.

Exercise

Similar to muscle, bone is living tissue that responds to exercise by becoming stronger. There is good evidence that physical activity early in life contributes to higher peak bone mass. The best exercise for building and maintaining bone mass is weight-bearing exercise—exercise that you do on your feet and that forces you to work against gravity. Weight-bearing exercises include:

- Jogging
- Aerobics
- Hiking
- Walking
- Stair climbing

- Gardening
- Weight training
- Tennis
- Dancing

High-impact exercises may provide the most benefit. Bicycling and swimming are not weight-bearing exercises, but they have other health benefits. Exercise machines that provide some degree of weight-bearing exercise include:

- Treadmills
- Stair-climbing machines
- Ski machines
- Exercise bicycles

Strength training to build and maintain muscle mass and exercises that help with coordination and balance are also important. Later in life, the benefits of exercise for building and maintaining bone mass are not nearly as great, but staying active and doing weight-bearing exercise is still important.

A properly designed exercise program that builds muscles and improves balance and coordination provides other benefits for older people, including helping to prevent falls and maintaining overall health and independence. Experts recommend 30 minutes or more of moderate physical activity on most (preferably all) days of the week, including a mix of weight-bearing exercises, strength training (2 or 3 times a week), and balance training.

Smoking

Smoking is bad for your bones and for your heart and lungs. Women who smoke have lower levels of estrogen when compared to nonsmokers and frequently go through menopause earlier.

Alcohol

People who drink heavily are more prone to bone loss and fractures because of poor nutrition and harmful effects on calcium balance and hormonal factors. Drinking too much also increases the risk of falling, which is likely to increase fracture risk.

Medications

The long-term use of glucocorticoids can lead to a loss of bone density and fractures. Other forms of drug therapy that can cause bone loss include:

- Long-term treatment with certain antiseizure drugs and barbiturates
- Some drugs used to treat endometriosis
- Excessive use of aluminum-containing antacids
- Certain cancer treatments and excessive thyroid hormone

It is important to discuss the use of these drugs with your doctor and not to stop or alter your medication dose on your own.

Chapter 24

Understanding Spinal Cord Injury

Spinal cord injury (SCI) is usually associated with what is commonly called a "broken neck" or "broken back." Generally speaking, SCI is damage to the spinal nerves, the body's central and most important nerve bundle, as a result of trauma to the backbone.

Most cases of SCI take place when trauma breaks and squeezes the vertebrae or the bones of the back. This, in turn, damages the axons—the long nerve cell "wires" that pass through vertebrae, carrying signals between the brain and the rest of the body. The axons might be crushed or completely severed by this damage. Someone with an injury to only a few axons might be able to recover completely from their injury. On the other hand, a person with damage to all axons will most likely be paralyzed in the areas below the injury.

An SCI is described by its level, type, and severity. The level of injury for a person with an SCI is the lowest point on the spinal cord below which sensory feeling and motor movement diminish or disappear.

The level is denoted by the letter and number name of the vertebra at the injury site (such as C3, T2, or L4).

- There are 7 cervical vertebrae (C1 through C7), which are in the neck.

This chapter includes text excerpted from "Spinal Cord Injury (SCI): Condition Information," *Eunice Kennedy Shriver* National Institute of Child Health and Human Development (NICHD), December 2016.

- There are 12 thoracic vertebrae (T1 through T12), which are located in the upper back. There are 5 lumbar vertebrae (L1 through L5), which are found in the lower back.
- Below those are 5 sacral vertebrae, which are fused to form the sacrum. Finally, there are 4 vertebrae of the coccyx or tailbone.

There are two broad types of SCI, each comprising a number of different levels:

- Tetraplegia (formerly called "quadriplegia") generally describes the condition of a person with an SCI that is at a level anywhere from the C1 vertebra down to the T1. These individuals can experience a loss of sensation, function, or movement in their head, neck, shoulders, arms, hands, upper chest, pelvic organs, and legs.
- Paraplegia is the general term describing the condition of people who have lost feeling in or are not able to move the lower parts of their bodies. The body parts that may be affected are the chest, stomach, hips, legs, and feet. The state of an individual with an SCI level from the T2 vertebra to the S5 can usually be called "paraplegic."

In addition, there are two degrees of SCI severity:

- A complete injury is a situation when the injury is so severe that almost all feeling (sensory function) and all ability to control movement (motor function) are lost below the area of the SCI.
- Incomplete injury occurs when there is some sensory or motor function below the damaged area on the spine. There are many degrees of incomplete injury.

The closer the spinal injury is to the skull, the more extensive is the curtailment of the body's ability to move and feel. If the lesion is low on the spine, say, in the sacral area, it is likely that there will be a lack of feeling and movement in the thighs and lower parts of the legs, the feet, most of the external genital organs, and the anal area. But the person will be able to breathe freely and move his head, neck, arms, and hands. By contrast, someone with a broken neck may be almost completely incapacitated, even to the extent of requiring breathing assistance.

What Are the Symptoms of Spinal Cord Injury?

According to the American Association of Neurological Surgeons (AANS), there are many different symptoms or signs of an SCI. Some of the more common signs of SCI include:

- Extreme pain or pressure in the neck, head, or back
- Tingling or loss of sensation in the hand, fingers, feet, or toes
- Partial or complete loss of control over any part of the body
- Urinary or bowel urgency, incontinence, or retention
- A difficulty with balance and walking
- Abnormal band-like sensations in the thorax—pain, pressure
- Impaired breathing after injury
- Unusual lumps on the head or spine

How Many People Are Affected by Spinal Cord Injury?

According to the National Spinal Cord Injury Statistical Center (NSCISC), annually there are about 12,000 new cases of SCIs in the United States, which amounts to about 40 cases per million people. The last studies of the incidence of SCIs were conducted in the 1990s, however, and so it is not known whether incidence has changed in recent years. In 2010, about a quarter of a million people in the United States were living with an SCI.

The majority of SCIs occur in young to middle-aged adults. From 1973 to 1979, the average age at injury was 28.7 years of age, and most injuries occurred between the ages of 16 and 30. However, demographic changes since the mid-1970s have resulted in an increase of 9 years in the median age of the U.S. population. Similarly, the average age for an SCI has increased over time. From 2005 to 2010, the average was 40 years of age.

Who Is at Risk for Spinal Cord Injury?

SCIs are typically the result of accidents and, therefore, can happen to anyone.

Factors that increase the risk of SCI:

- Driving or riding in a car. Using a seatbelt can reduce the possibility of an SCI by 60 percent; using a seatbelt plus having a functioning airbag can cut the odds of this injury by 80 percent.

- Being male. 80 percent of SCI patients are male.
- Operating machinery without using safety equipment
- Improper or unsafe use of a ladder, which can result in a fall from the ladder
- Using drugs or alcohol while driving, operating machinery, or playing sports
- Having arthritis, osteoporosis, or another bone or joint disorder

What Do Cause Spinal Cord Injury and How Does It Affect Your Body?

SCIs result from damage to the vertebrae, ligaments, or discs of the spinal column or to the spinal cord itself.

A traumatic SCI may stem from a sudden blow to the spine that fractures, dislocates, crushes, or compresses one or more vertebrae. Car crashes are the leading cause of SCIs among people younger than 65 years of age. Falls cause most SCIs in persons 65 years of age and older.

Since 2005, an SCI has been caused by:

- Car crashes (40.4%)
- Falls (27.9%)
- Violence, including gunshot wounds (15%)
- Other/unknown (8.5%)
- Sport-related accidents (8%)

What Does Happen in Your Body When Your Spinal Cord Is Injured?

When an SCI occurs, the spinal cord starts to swell at the damaged area, cutting off the vital blood supply to the nerve tissue and starving it of oxygen. This sets off a cascade of devastation that affects the entire body, causing the injured spinal tissue to die, be stripped of its insulation, and be further damaged by a massive response of the immune system.

- **Blood flow.** The sluggish blood flow at the injury site begins to reduce the flow of blood in adjacent areas, which soon affects all areas of the body. The body begins to lose the ability to self-regulate, leading to drastic drops in blood pressure and heart rate.

- **Flood of neurotransmitters.** The SCI leads to an excessive release of neurotransmitters or biochemicals that let nerve cells communicate with each other. These chemicals, especially glutamate, overexcite nerve cells, killing them through a process known as "excitotoxicity." The process also kills the vital oligodendrocytes that surround and protect the spinal axons with the myelin insulation that allows the spinal nerves to transmit information to and from the brain.
- **Invasion of immune cells.** An army of cells of the immune system speeds to the damaged area of the spine. While they help by preventing infection and cleaning up dead cellular debris, they also promote inflammation. These immune cells stimulate the release of certain cytokines that, in high concentrations, can be toxic to nerve cells, especially those needed to maintain the myelin sheath around axons.
- **An onslaught of free radicals.** The inflammation caused by cells in the immune system unleashes waves of free radicals, which are highly reactive forms of oxygen molecules. These free radicals react destructively with many types of cellular molecules, severely damaging healthy nerve cells in the process.
- **Nerve cell self-destruction.** A normally natural process of programmed cell death, known as "apoptosis," goes out of control at the injury site. The reasons are not known. Days or weeks after the injury, oligodendrocytes die from no apparent cause, reducing the integrity of the spinal cord.

Additional damage usually occurs over the days or weeks following the initial injury because of bleeding, swelling, inflammation, and accumulation of fluid in and around the spinal cord.

How Is Spinal Cord Injury Diagnosed?

SCIs are not always immediately recognizable. The following injuries should be assessed for possible damage to the spinal cord:

- Head injuries, particularly those with trauma to the face
- Pelvic fractures

- Penetrating injuries in the area of the spine
- Injuries from falling from heights

If any of these injuries occur together with any of the symptoms mentioned above (acute head, neck, or back pain; decline of feeling in the extremities; loss of control over part of the body; urinary or bowel problems; walking difficulty; pain or pressure bands in the chest area; difficulty breathing; and head or spine lumps), then an SCI may be implicated.

A person suspected of having an SCI must be carefully transported—to prevent further injury, the spine should be kept immobile—to an emergency room or trauma center. A doctor will question the person to determine the nature of the accident, and the medical staff may test the patient for sensory function and movement. If the injured person complains of neck pain, is not fully awake, or has obvious signs of weakness or neurological injury, diagnostic tests will be performed.

These tests may include:

- **A computed tomography (CT) scan.** This approach uses computers to form a series of cross-sectional images that may show the location and extent of the damage and reveal problems, such as blood clots (hematomas).
- **A magnetic resonance imaging (MRI) scan.** An MRI machine takes a picture of the injured area using a strong magnetic field and radio waves. A computer creates an image of the spine to reveal herniated discs and other abnormalities.
- **A myelogram.** This is an X-ray of the spine taken after a dye is injected.
- **Somatosensory evoked potential (SSEP) testing or magnetic stimulation.** Performing these tests may show if nerve signals can pass through the spinal cord.
- **Spine X-rays.** These may show fractures or damage to the bones of the spine.

On about the third day after the injury, doctors give patients a complete neurological examination to diagnose the severity of the injury and predict the likely extent of recovery. This involves testing the patient's muscle strength and ability to sense light touch and a pinprick. Doctors use the standard American Spinal Injury Association (ASIA) Impairment Scale for this diagnosis. X-rays, MRIs, or more advanced imaging techniques are also used to visualize the entire length of the spine.

The ASIA Impairment Scale has five classification levels (A to E), ranging from complete loss of neural function in the affected area to completely normal.

- **A: The impairment is complete.** There is no motor or sensory function left below the level of injury.
- **B: The impairment is incomplete.** Sensory function, but not motor function, is preserved below the neurologic level (the first normal level above the level of injury), and some sensation is preserved in the sacral segments S4 and S5.
- **C: The impairment is incomplete.** Motor function is preserved below the neurologic level, but more than half of the key muscles below the neurologic level have a muscle grade less than 3 (i.e., they are not strong enough to move against gravity).
- **D: The impairment is incomplete.** Motor function is preserved below the neurologic level, and at least half of the key muscles below the neurologic level have a muscle grade of 3 or more (i.e., the joints can be moved against gravity).
- **E: The patient's functions are normal.** All motor and sensory functions are unhindered.

To illustrate, a person classified as C-level on the ASIA scale functions better than a person at the B level. Time was, a patient might have been labeled a C4 quadriplegic. However, using the ASIA scale, the classification might be C4 ASIA A tetraplegic. Regarding muscle-strength grades, zero is the lowest, corresponding to the complete absence of muscle movement. Five is the highest, representing full, normal strength.

What Are the Treatments for Spinal Cord Injury?

Unfortunately, there are at present no known ways to reverse damage to the spinal cord. However, researchers are continually working on new treatments, including prostheses and medications, which may promote the regeneration of nerve cells or improve the function of the nerves that remain after an SCI.

SCI treatment currently focuses on preventing further injury and empowering people with an SCI to return to an active and productive life.

At the Scene of the Incident

Quick medical attention is critical to minimizing the effects of head, neck, or back trauma. Therefore, treatment for an SCI often begins at the scene of the injury.

Emergency personnel typically:

- Immobilize the spine as gently and quickly as possible by using a rigid neck collar and a rigid carrying board
- Use the carrying board to transport the patient to the hospital

In the Emergency Room

Once the patient is at the hospital, healthcare providers focus on:

- Maintaining the person's ability to breathe
- Immobilizing the neck to prevent further spinal cord damage

Healthcare providers also may treat an acute injury with:

- **Surgery.** Doctors may use surgery to remove fluid or tissue that presses on the spinal cord (decompression laminectomy); remove bone fragments, disc fragments, or foreign objects; fuse broken spinal bones; or place spinal braces.
- **Traction.** This technique stabilizes the spine and brings it into proper alignment.
- **Methylprednisolone (Medrol).** If this steroid medication is administered within hours of injury, some patients experience improvement. It appears to work by reducing damage to nerve cells and decreasing inflammation near the site of injury.
- **Experimental treatments.** Scientists are pursuing research on how to halt cell death, control inflammation, and promote the repair or regeneration of nerves.

People with an SCI may benefit from rehabilitation, including:

- Physical therapy geared toward muscle strengthening, communication, and mobility
- Use of assistive devices, such as wheelchairs, walkers, and leg braces
- Use of adaptive devices for communication
- Occupational therapy focused on fine motor skills

- Techniques for self-grooming and bladder and bowel management
- Coping strategies for dealing with spasticity and pain
- Vocational therapy to help people get back to work with the use of assistive devices, if needed
- Recreational therapy, such as sports and social activities
- Improved strategies for exercise and healthy diets (obesity and diabetes are potential risk factors for persons with an SCI)
- Functional electrical stimulation for assistance with restoration of neuromuscular function, sensory function, or autonomic function (e.g., bladder, bowel, or respiratory function)

What Conditions Are Associated with Spinal Cord Injury?

An SCI is associated with many secondary conditions that have significant impacts on medical rehabilitation management, long-term outcome, and quality of life (QOL).

- Secondary conditions associated with SCIs include:
  - Breathing problems
  - Bowel and bladder problems, including overactive bladder and incontinence
  - Heart problems
  - Pressure sores
  - Sexual function problems
  - Pain
  - Blood clots
  - Impaired muscle coordination (or spasticity)
  - Pneumonia
  - Autonomic dysreflexia (or hyperreflexia), which causes a potentially lethal increase in blood pressure
  - Increased likelihood of certain cancers, including bladder cancer

How Does Spinal Cord Injury Affect Children?

While the number of cases of SCI in children and adolescents is not high relative to other age groups, their medical outcomes may be more negatively affected by an SCI. Few studies performed to date have examined SCI in children and adolescents, and many questions remain unanswered. Some of these questions include how having an SCI affects the growth and development of children and adolescents. For example, as young people grow, their bones and bodies grow with them; however, this growth may be altered in children and adolescents with an SCI. In addition, because the trunk support system is less developed in a child when compared to an adult, a child with an SCI may have more frequent secondary conditions (e.g., respiratory and bowel/bladder problems). Also, children and adolescents may have a higher risk for a secondary skeletal condition because of skeletal immaturity.

How Do People Adjust to Living with Spinal Cord Injury?

Paralysis can completely change a person's life. It can be depressing, frightening, and daunting at first to consider how to reengage with previous activities and relationships, such as those involving family, employment, friendships, and recreation/exercise. Even so, a patient with an SCI can develop strong motivation and a good support system for recovery and enjoy a fulfilling and happy life.

While the *Eunice Kennedy Shriver* National Institute of Child Health and Human Development (NICHD) conducts studies to examine various aspects of SCI outcomes and QOL for those affected by SCIs and their families, the manner of adjustment is not currently a focus of their research on SCIs. However, many other organizations and agencies do focus solely on adjustment and provide information for patients and their families.

After an SCI, many of the body's functions may change dramatically. The following issues may arise:

- Bone loss
- Obesity
- Muscle atrophy
- Pressure ulcers
- Bladder/bowel disorders

- Cardiovascular problems
- Changes in sexual and reproductive functions
- Pain
- Depression and adjustment to illness

In recent decades, individuals with an SCI have been gaining longer life spans, and the importance of understanding the impact of aging on the above issues has become increasingly evident.

Is There a Cure for Spinal Cord Injury?

There is no known cure for the loss of nerve tissue associated with an SCI. However, depending on the extent of damage to the spinal tissue, partial or almost complete recovery may occur for some people from one week to six months after an injury. Other people may experience small improvements for up to one year or even longer.

The major developments in the treatment of SCI have been in the areas of rehabilitation and improvement in the QOL. Even though an SCI may disrupt one's life, those who have experienced this injury can be taught how to use mechanical and technological devices to provide more independence in terms of mobility, working, interacting with their families, and recreation. Additional help can be provided to help people with SCIs manage emotional and sexual issues.

Research is ongoing to treat the various symptoms and problems associated with SCI and to develop therapies that promote the regeneration of nerves. The National Institute of Neurological Disorders and Stroke (NINDS) supports research to help people with SCI, as do other institutions, including the NICHD. This includes research on the four principles of spinal cord repair:

- Protecting surviving nerve cells from further damage
- Replacing damaged nerve cells
- Stimulating the regrowth of axons and targeting their connections appropriately
- Retraining neural circuits to restore body functions

Part Four

Chronic Disorders Associated with Back and Neck Pain

Chapter 25

Skeletal Deformities of Spine

Chapter Contents

Section 25.1—Kyphosis 188
Section 25.2—Lordosis.. 192
Section 25.3—Scoliosis.. 196

Section 25.1

Kyphosis

“Kyphosis,” © 2019 Omnigraphics.
Reviewed April 2019.

Kyphosis, also known as “roundback” or “hunchback,” is a spinal disorder in which the upper back is rounded because of an excessive outward curve of the thoracic spine (the part of the spine near the chest area). The normal thoracic spine is supposed to be curved at any angle between 20 and 40 degrees. This natural curvature is highly essential in balancing one’s body weight and standing upright. But, when the curve goes beyond 40 or 45 degrees it is called “kyphosis.” This disorder leads to a slouching posture, and it may occur at any age.

Types

The different types of kyphosis are:

- **Postural kyphosis:** This occurs because of an abnormal development of the spine during the adolescent stage. It can be a result of slouching or poor posture.
- **Scheuermann kyphosis:** This is named after Danish surgeon Holger Scheuermann who first identified the condition. It occurs due to structural deformity in which some of the consecutive vertebrae take a more triangular shape rather than a rectangular shape and results in a rounded spine. As with postural kyphosis, it also occurs in adolescent stages. But, it is more severe than postural kyphosis.
- **Congenital kyphosis:** This is a birth defect that occurs when the spine does not develop properly within the womb. As the child grows, the condition may worsen. The only way to treat congenital kyphosis is spinal surgery.

Causes

The spine is made up of small rectangular bones called “vertebrae” that are stacked on each other. This structure provides support to the spine and makes it flexible. Kyphosis occurs when the vertebrae in the thoracic region bends and becomes wedge-shaped. This can happen due to:

- Poor posture

- Injuries and fractures
- Disc degeneration
- Birth defects
- Developmental issues
- Aging

Certain diseases and infections can also lead to kyphosis. They include:

- Osteoporosis
- Spondylolisthesis
- Polio
- Paget disease
- Spina bifida
- Muscular dystrophy
- Neurofibromatosis
- Tumors
- Tuberculosis
- Cancer

Symptoms

The primary symptom of kyphosis is the bowing or bending of the thoracic spine, resulting in a hunchback. But, in mild cases, the bend may not be noticeable. Other signs and symptoms of kyphosis include:

- Back pain
- Back stiffness
- Tight hamstrings
- Fatigue

These symptoms may vary from person to person, and as the bend becomes more severe, it may lead to serious complications, such as:

- Shortness or difficulty in breathing

- Loss of sensation
- Numbness or tingling in the arms and legs

Diagnosis

When a person is suspected to have kyphosis, a proper diagnosis should be made in order to determine the appropriate treatment plan. The diagnosis includes the following stages.

Medical History

The diagnosis usually begins with the analysis of the patient's medical history, which includes:

- Family history
- Time of onset of curvature in the back
- Presence and severity of pain
- Bowel or bladder dysfunction
- Details about any previous surgery

Physical Examination

During the physical examination, the doctor makes the patient lie on a flat surface and examines the spine. The doctor may then ask the patient to do some stretches in order to assess the range of motion and curvature of the back. The doctor may also perform neurological examinations to check the sensation, reflexes, and muscle strength.

Additional Tests

Depending on the results of the medical history analysis and physical examination, the doctor may recommend a few additional tests for further clarity of the disorder. These tests include:

- **X-rays:** Doctors may recommend taking X-rays from different angles to identify the deformities in the vertebrae.
- **Computed tomography (CT) scan:** These scans may be recommended if the doctor wants a clearer image of the deformities in the vertebrae.

- **Magnetic resonance imaging (MRI) scan:** These scans may be used to detect infections and tumors in the spine.
- **Nerve tests:** These special tests are done to check if any nerves are being pinched or irritated due to the bending of the spine.
- **Pulmonary function tests:** If the curve is severe, pulmonary function tests may be recommended in order to determine if breathing is restricted due to reduced chest space.

Treatments

The treatment for kyphosis generally focuses on preventing the spine from bending further and restoring the normal posture wherever possible. The treatment procedure depends upon the type and severity of the condition.

Nonsurgical Treatments

Nonsurgical treatment is often recommended for patients with postural or Scheuermann kyphosis. It includes:

- **Physical therapy:** Physical therapy and exercises can relieve pressure on the spine, strengthen the back muscles, and significantly improve posture. Certain exercises can be helpful in correcting the misalignment of the spine and stretching tight hamstrings.
- **Medications:** Doctors recommend nonsteroidal anti-inflammatory drugs (NSAIDs), such as aspirin and ibuprofen, to relieve the pain and discomfort. Bone-strengthening medicines may also be recommended to avoid additional spine fractures.
- **Bracings:** Back bracings are recommended for young children and adolescents with Scheuermann kyphosis. These braces are to be worn until the child or adolescent attains full growth and reaches skeletal maturity.

Surgical Treatment

Surgical treatment is generally recommended for people with congenital kyphosis. Rarely, it may also be recommended for severe conditions of postural or Scheuermann kyphosis that does not respond to nonsurgical treatments. The surgical procedures may vary, depending on the cause and severity of the disorder. Spinal fusion is the most common surgical procedure for kyphosis. During the procedure, the curved part of the vertebrae is realigned, and small pieces of bones (grafts) are placed and fused in the empty spaces. Other surgical procedures include inserting metal rods and plates in the spine region to keep the vertebrae aligned.

However, there are certain complications associated with spinal surgery, such as impairment, subsequent pain, etc. Hence, it is important to discuss the complications with your doctor before undergoing spinal surgery.

References

1. Kandola, Aaron. "What to Know about Kyphosis," Medical News Today, January 2, 2019.
2. "Kyphosis (Roundback) of the Spine," OrthoInfo, August 2016.
3. "Kyphosis," Mayo Clinic, May 23, 2018.
4. "Kyphosis," MedlinePlus, National Institutes of Health (NIH), April 1, 2019.
5. "Adult Kyphosis," University of Maryland, February 1, 2001.

Section 25.2

Lordosis

Lordosis, also known as "hyperlordosis" or "swayback," is a condition in which the lumbar spine (region above the buttocks) is bent inwards. Normally, the spine has curves, such as scoliotic (side curves), lordotic (back curves), and kyphotic (front curves), that work as a shock-absorber during stress, bend and adjust themselves, and support the weight of the head. However, too much bending of the spinal curves is a disorder.

Lordosis can affect people of any age group. It occurs in the lower region of the spine, and it sometimes may occur in the neck (cervical lordosis). People with lordosis may seem to appear swayback, in which the buttocks is prominent.

Lordosis leads to excess pressure in the spine, which may result in pain and/or discomfort. This condition, if left untreated for a long time, becomes fatal and may affect your ability to move. This condition may last for years or it may be lifelong, depending upon the severity.

Causes

Certain conditions/diseases may affect the integrity of the spine and lead to lordosis. Some of these conditions/diseases may include:

- **Obesity.** Some overweight people tend to lean backward for balance. This may result in lordosis.
- **Osteoporosis** is a condition in which density of the bones is low. This condition weakens the vertebrae, and the spine loses its integrity.
- **Spondylolisthesis** occurs when vertebrae slip to one side of the body due to a defect in the spine.
- **Discitis** is an inflammation that has developed between the intervertebral discs in the spine.
- **Achondroplasia** is an inherited bone growth disorder that causes short-limbed dwarfism.

Symptoms

The most common symptom of lordosis is muscle pain. The extreme curving of the spine pulls the muscles in different directions, causing the muscle to spasm or stretch. If you have cervical lordosis, pain may extend to your neck, shoulder, and upper back.

You can check yourselves at home for lordosis by lying on a flat surface. Check the amount of space between your back and the surface; you may have lordosis if space is large. From a side-view while standing, you may notice a visible C-like arch in which the abdomen and buttocks stick out; this may also point to a lordosis diagnosis.

Check with your doctor if you are experiencing any of the following symptoms:

- Weakness

- Numbness
- Weak bladder control
- Difficulties in controlling muscle
- Tingling

These symptoms may be signs of a trapped nerve and need immediate treatment.

Diagnosis

Lordosis is diagnosed by physical, neurological, and radiological examinations.

Physical Examination

The doctor will do a complete physical examination in order to find out whether the condition of lordosis requires treatment or not. The physical examination forms a baseline in which the doctor can observe the patient's progress throughout the treatment. The most common physical examination may include palpation (sensing abnormalities by the feel of touch) and observing the patient's range of motion after asking them to perform movements of extension, flexion, spinal rotation, and lateral bending.

Neurological Examination

The neurological examination includes an assessment of the lordosis and when the patient experienced the symptoms for the first time. This examination helps to check for the presence of nerve damage.

Radiographic Evaluation

X-rays of the anterior, posterior, and lateral are taken while the patient is standing and revealing the entire spine. Magnetic resonance imaging (MRI) is required if the doctor suspects any additional damage to the spinal cord.

Treatment

The treatment for lordosis may be conventional or surgical, depending upon the degree and rigidity of the curve. The conventional treatments include:

- **Physical therapy**, to build flexibility, strength, and to increase the range of motion while performing various exercises
- **Braces**, to control the progress of the curving
- Weight reduction
- Anti-inflammatory and analgesic medications may be prescribed.

Surgical treatment may be considered if the lordosis involves nerves, severe bending, or if the conventional treatment is not effective to provide relief.

The surgical procedure and approach are decided by a spine surgeon and based upon the radiographic images, the patient's medical history, and their symptoms.

Recovery

It is important to follow the physical therapist's and/or physician's instructions, despite the type of treatment a patient gets.

If the patient undergoes surgery, medications and instructions are provided prior to the discharge from the hospital. The patient has to visit the surgeon on a regular basis to continue their care.

References

1. "Swayback (Lordosis)," Cedars-Sinai, August 1, 2004.
2. "Lordosis," Boston Children's Hospital, February 1, 2001.
3. "What Causes Lordosis?" Healthline, September 6, 2016.

Section 25.3

Scoliosis

This section includes text excerpted from "Scoliosis in Children and Adolescents," National Institute of Arthritis and Musculoskeletal and Skin Diseases (NIAMS), December 30, 2015. Reviewed April 2019.

Scoliosis is a disorder in which there is a sideways curve of the spine. Curves are often S-shaped or C-shaped. In most people, there is no known cause for this curve. Curves frequently follow patterns that have been studied in previous patients (see figure 25.1).

People with milder curves may just need to visit their doctor for regular check-ups. Some people who have scoliosis require treatment.

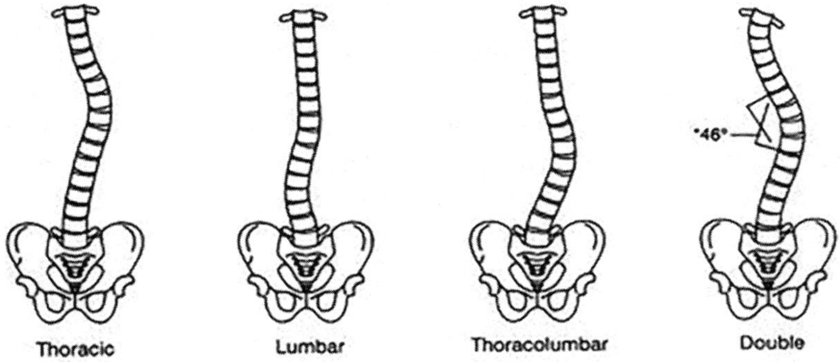

Figure 25.1. *Curved Patterns of the Spine*

Who Gets Scoliosis

People of all ages can have scoliosis. The most common type is caused by unknown factors and typically occurs in children between the ages of 10 and 12 and in their early teens. Girls are more likely than boys to have scoliosis. You are more likely to have scoliosis if your parent, brother, or sister have it.

Symptoms of Scoliosis

Scoliosis is a disorder in which there is a sideways curve of the spine. Signs of scoliosis can include:

- Uneven shoulders

- Head that is not centered
- Sides of the body are not level with each other
- One side of the rib cage is higher than the other when bending forward

Causes of Scoliosis

In most cases, the cause of scoliosis is unknown. Causes of curves are classified as:

- **Nonstructural (functional) scoliosis.** A structurally normal spine that temporarily appears curved. It is caused by a condition such as a difference in leg length, muscle spasms, or appendicitis. Doctors treat this type of scoliosis by correcting the underlying problem.
- **Structural scoliosis.** A curve that can be caused by disease, birth defect, injury, infection, tumors, connective tissue disorders, or unknown factors.

Diagnosis of Scoliosis

Your doctor may do the following to diagnosis you with scoliosis:

- **Medical history** to look for medical problems that might be causing your spine to curve.
- **Physical examination** to look at your back, chest, pelvis, legs, feet, and skin.
- **X-rays** to measure the curve of the spine. This information is used to determine how to treat scoliosis.

Treatment of Scoliosis

Your doctor may recommend the following treatments:

- **Observation.** If the curve is mild and your skeleton is still growing, your doctor will re-examine you every few months.
- **Bracing.** If the curve is moderate and you are still growing, your doctor may recommend a brace to keep the curve from getting any worse. Braces must be selected for the specific curve problem and fitted to each patient. Braces must be worn every day for the full number of hours prescribed by the doctor.

- **Surgery.** If you are still growing and have a severe curve that is getting worse, your doctor may suggest surgery. This often involves fusing together two or more bones in the spine. The doctor may also put in a metal rod or other device to help keep the spine straight after surgery. You should seek the advice of at least two experts and ask about the benefits and risks of the surgery.

The following treatments have not been shown to keep curves from getting worse in scoliosis:

- Chiropractic treatment
- Electrical stimulation
- Nutritional supplements

Living with Scoliosis

Exercise programs have not been shown to keep scoliosis from getting worse. But, it is important for all people, including those with scoliosis, to exercise and remain physically fit. Weight-bearing exercise, such as walking, running, soccer, and gymnastics, helps keep bones strong. For both boys and girls, exercising and playing sports can improve their sense of well-being.

Chapter 26

Inflammatory Joint Disease of the Spine

Chapter Contents

Section 26.1—Arthritis 200

Section 26.2—Ankylosing Spondylitis 203

Section 26.1

Arthritis

This section includes text excerpted from "Arthritis," National Institute of Arthritis and Musculoskeletal and Skin Diseases (NIAMS), April 30, 2017.

"Arthritis" literally means joint inflammation. Although joint inflammation is a symptom or sign rather than a specific diagnosis, the term "arthritis" is often used to refer to any disorder that affects the joints. Joints are places where two bones meet, such as your elbow or knee.

There are different types of arthritis. In some diseases in which arthritis occurs, other organs, such as your eyes, heart, or skin, can also be affected.

Fortunately, current treatments allow most people with arthritis to lead active and productive lives.

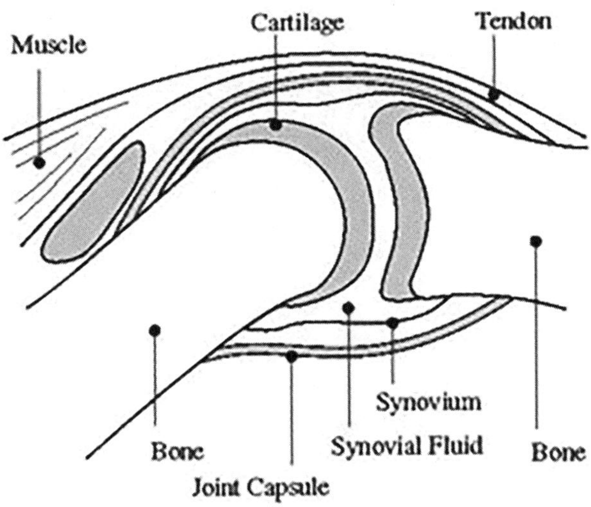

Figure 26.1. *Normal Joints*

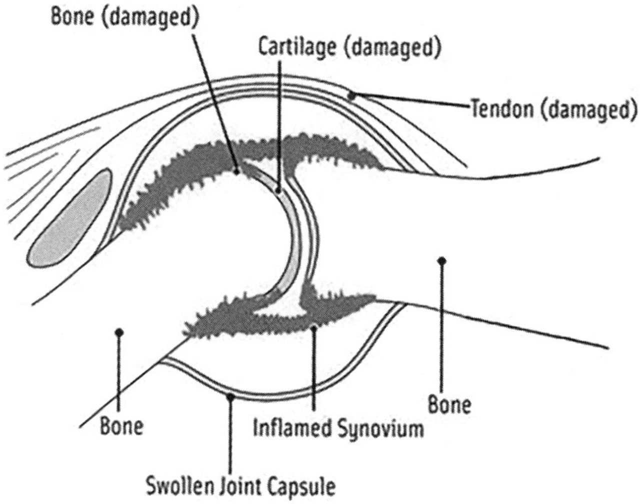

Figure 26.2. *Joints Affected by Rheumatoid Arthritis* (Source: National Center for Biotechnology Information (NCBI).)

What Are the Types of Arthritis?

There are several types of arthritis. Common ones include:

- **Ankylosing spondylitis** is arthritis that affects the spine. It often involves redness, heat, swelling, and pain in the spine or in the joint where the bottom of the spine joins the pelvic bone.
- **Gout** is caused by crystals that build up in the joints. It usually affects the big toe, but many other joints may be affected.
- **Juvenile arthritis** is the term used to describe arthritis in children. Arthritis is caused by inflammation of the joints.
- **Osteoarthritis** usually comes with age and most often affects the fingers, knees, and hips. Sometimes, osteoarthritis follows a joint injury. For example, you might have badly injured your knee when you were young, and you develop arthritis in your knee joint years later.
- **Psoriatic arthritis** can occur in people who have psoriasis (scaly red and white skin patches). It affects the skin, joints, and areas where tissues attach to the bone.

- **Reactive arthritis** is pain or swelling in a joint that is caused by an infection in your body. You may also have red, swollen eyes and a swollen urinary tract.
- **Rheumatoid arthritis** happens when the body's own defense system does not work properly. It affects joints and bones (often of the hands and feet), and it may also affect internal organs and systems. You may feel sick or tired, and you may have a fever.

Arthritis is seen with other conditions. These include:

- **Lupus** happens when the body's defense system harms the joints, heart, skin, kidneys, and other organs.
- **Infection** that gets into a joint and destroys the cushion between the bones.

What Are the Symptoms of Arthritis?

Symptoms of arthritis can include:

- Pain, redness, heat, and swelling in your joints
- Trouble moving around
- Fever
- Weight loss
- Breathing problems
- Rash or itch

These symptoms may also be signs of other illnesses.

What Causes Arthritis

There are probably many genes that make people more likely to have arthritis. Research has found some of these genes.

If you have the gene linked with arthritis, something in your environment—such as a virus or injury—may trigger the condition.

Is There a Test for Arthritis?

To diagnosis you with arthritis or another rheumatic disease, your doctor may:

- Ask you about your medical history

- Give you a physical exam
- Take samples for a laboratory test
- Take X-rays

How Is Arthritis Treated?

There are many treatments that can help relieve pain and help you live with arthritis. You should talk to your doctor about the best treatments for you, which can include:

- Medications to relieve pain, slow the condition, and prevent further damage
- Surgery to repair joint damage or relieve pain

Who Treats Arthritis

Doctors who diagnose and treat arthritis and other rheumatic disease include:

- A general practitioner, such as your family doctor
- A rheumatologist, who treats arthritis and other diseases of the bones, joints, and muscles

Section 26.2

Ankylosing Spondylitis

This section includes text excerpted from "Ankylosing Spondylitis," National Institute of Arthritis and Musculoskeletal and Skin Diseases (NIAMS), June 30, 2016.

Ankylosing spondylitis (AS) is a type of arthritis that affects the joints in the spine. Its name comes from the Greek words "ankylos," meaning stiffening of a joint, and "spondylo," meaning vertebrae (small bones in the backbone).

Ankylosing spondylitis belongs to a group of disorders that are associated with swelling of the joints and spine. Although these disorders have similarities, they also have features that distinguish them from one another. The hallmark of ankylosing spondylitis is swelling of the joint where the bottom vertebra of the spine (sacrum) joins the pelvic bone (ilium).

In some people, ankylosing spondylitis can also affect the shoulders, ribs, hips, knees, and feet. It can also affect areas where the tendons and ligaments attach to the bones. It is possible that it can affect other organs, such as the eyes, bowel, and—more rarely—the heart and lungs.

Many people with ankylosing spondylitis have mild episodes of back pain that come and go. But others have severe, ongoing pain with loss of flexibility in the spine. In the most severe cases, long-term swelling causes two or more bones of the spine to fuse. If the rib cage is affected, you may have trouble taking a deep breath.

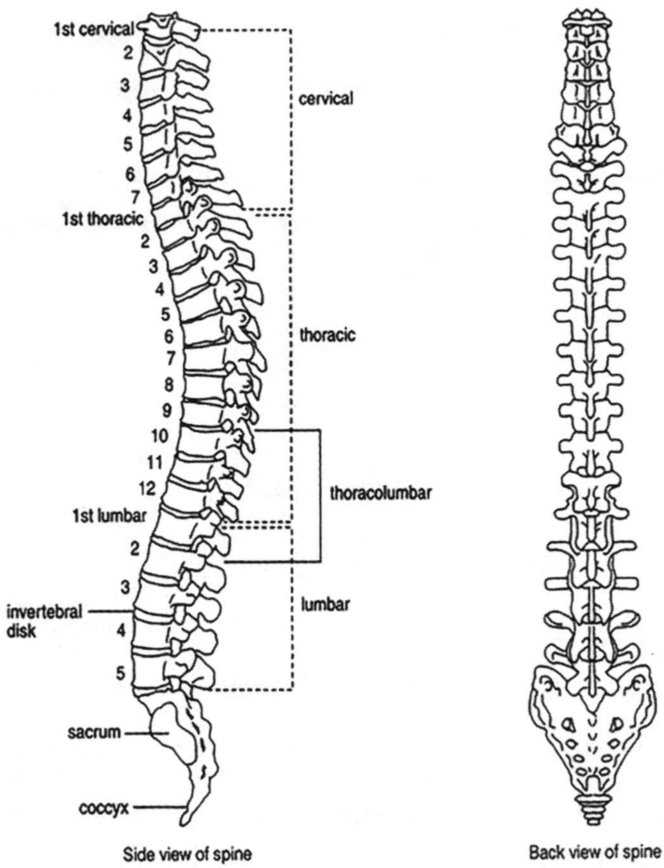

Figure 26.3. *Side and Back Views of the Spine*

Who Gets Ankylosing Spondylitis

Ankylosing spondylitis typically begins when you are a teenager or young adult. Once you develop the disease, it will affect you for the rest of your life. Men are more likely to develop ankylosing spondylitis than women.

The main gene associated with ankylosing spondylitis is called "*HLA-B27*." If you have ankylosing spondylitis, then you probably have this gene. However, this does not mean you will get the disease if you have the gene; fewer than 1 of 20 people with *HLA-B27* gets ankylosing spondylitis. Scientists recently discovered two more genes (*IL23R* and *ERAP1*) that, along with *HLA-B27*, increase your risk for ankylosing spondylitis.

Diagnosis of Ankylosing Spondylitis

Your doctor will give you a physical exam and ask you about your medical history in order to diagnose you with ankylosing spondylitis. Bone/joint scans and lab tests may help confirm a diagnosis.

Medical History

Your doctor will probably ask you the following questions during a medical history:

- How long have you had pain?
- Where is the pain in your back or neck? Are other joints affected?
- Is back pain better with exercise and worse after inactivity, such as when you first get up in the morning?
- Do you have other problems, such as eye problems or fatigue?
- Does anyone in your family have back problems or arthritis?
- Have you recently suffered from an upset stomach or diarrhea?
- Do you have any skin rashes, such as psoriasis?

Physical Exam

During the physical exam, your doctor will look for symptoms of ankylosing spondylitis. These include pain in the spine, pelvis, joint between the pelvis and spine, heels, or chest. Your doctor may ask you to move and bend in different directions. This is to check the flexibility of your spine. You will also be asked to breathe deeply. This is to check for rib stiffness caused by continued swelling of the joints where the ribs attach to the spine.

Bone and Joint Scans

Your doctor may confirm you have ankylosing spondylitis by taking pictures of your spine and of the joint between your spine and pelvic bone. Pictures are taken using X-rays or magnetic resonance imaging (MRI), which uses magnets and radio waves (not radiation). However, you may have the disease for years before changes show on X-rays. MRI may allow for earlier diagnosis because it can show damage to soft tissues and bone before it can be seen on an X-ray. Both tests may also be used to see if the disease worsens.

Lab Tests

Your blood may be tested for the *HLA-B27* gene, which is present in most people with ankylosing spondylitis. The test is less useful if you are African American or from some Mediterranean countries, since you are less likely to have the gene even if you do have ankylosing spondylitis. The gene is also found in many people who do not have ankylosing spondylitis and will never get it. Still, having the gene is one more indicator you have ankylosing spondylitis when you also have symptoms and X-ray evidence of the disease.

Treatment for Ankylosing Spondylitis

There is no cure for ankylosing spondylitis, but some treatments that relieve symptoms may possibly prevent the disease from getting worse. In most cases, treatment involves a combination of medication, exercise, and self-help measures. In some cases, surgery may be used to repair some of the joint damage caused by the disease.

You should work with your doctor to find the safest and most effective medications for you, which will likely include one or more of the following:

Nonsteroidal Anti-Inflammatory Drugs

Nonsteroidal anti-inflammatory drugs (NSAIDs) relieve pain and inflammation and are commonly used to treat ankylosing spondylitis. Examples include aspirin, ibuprofen, and naproxen.

Some NSAIDs are available over-the-counter (OTC), but others are available only with a prescription.

NSAIDs can have side effects, and some people seem to respond better to one NSAID than another. You should see your doctor on a regular basis if you take NSAIDs over a long period of time.

Corticosteroids

These strong inflammation-fighting drugs are similar to the cortisone made by your body. If NSAIDs alone do not control your joint swelling, your doctor may inject corticosteroids directly into the affected joints to bring quick, but temporary, relief. Injections may be given to the hip joint, knee joint, or joint between the spine and pelvic bone. Injections are not given in the spine.

Disease-Modifying Antirheumatic Drugs

Disease-modifying antirheumatic drugs (DMARDs) work in different ways. The most common DMARDs for ankylosing spondylitis are sulfasalazine and methotrexate.

Biologic Agents

These medications block proteins involved in your body's inflammatory response. Several biologics are approved by the U.S. Food and Drug Administration (FDA) for treating ankylosing spondylitis. These drugs are either injected or given intravenously (IV) and are often effective for ankylosing spondylitis when other treatments are not.

Surgery

Total joint replacement may be an option if ankylosing spondylitis causes severe joint damage that makes it difficult to do your daily activities. Your surgeon will remove the damaged joint and replace it with a human-made one made of metals, plastics, and/or ceramic materials. The most commonly replaced joints are the knee and hip.

There is also surgery to straighten the spine, if it has fused into a curved-forward position. This is generally considered a high-risk procedure, and it is only done in very rare cases. A surgeon who is highly experienced in the procedure will cut through the spine so that it can be placed into a straighter up/down position. Hardware may be needed to hold the spine in its new position while it heals.

Who Treats Ankylosing Spondylitis

The diagnosis of ankylosing spondylitis is often made by a rheumatologist, a doctor trained to diagnose and treat arthritis. However, because ankylosing spondylitis can affect different parts of your body, you may need to see several different types of doctors for treatment, including:

- **Ophthalmologist**, who treats eye diseases
- **Gastroenterologist,** who treats bowel diseases
- **Physiatrist**, a medical doctor who specializes in physical medicine and rehabilitation
- **Physical therapist** or rehabilitation specialist, who supervises stretching and exercise programs

You and your doctors may find it helpful to select one doctor to manage the overall treatment plan.

Prognosis of Ankylosing Spondylitis

The course of ankylosing spondylitis varies from person to person. Some people will have only mild episodes of back pain that come and go, while others will have chronic, severe back pain. In almost all cases, there are short-term, painful episodes and remissions, or periods of time when the pain lessens.

Swelling can cause stiffness in the spine and the joint between the spine and pelvic bone. Over time, bony outgrowths can develop that cause the small bones in the spine to grow together, or fuse. Fusion can also stiffen the rib cage, which would make it difficult to take a deep breath.

Ankylosing spondylitis is more likely to affect your ability to function if you have had the disease for at least 20 years, a physically demanding job, other health problems, or smoked. You will tend to have less severe limitations from the disease if you have a higher level of education and a history of ankylosing spondylitis in the family.

You are more likely to have severe joint damage if you got the disease at an earlier age, are a man, or a current smoker. A genetic marker called "DRB1*0801" seems to protect against severe spine damage.

Living with Ankylosing Spondylitis

Exercise

Besides seeing your doctor regularly and following your treatment plan, staying active is probably the best thing you can do for ankylosing spondylitis. Regular exercise can help relieve pain, improve posture, and maintain flexibility. Before beginning an exercise program, speak with your doctor or physical therapist about designing a program that is right for you. Some helpful exercises include:

- Strengthening exercises, performed with weights or done by tightening muscles without moving the joints, build the muscles around your painful joints to better support them. Exercises that do not require joint movement can be done even when your joints are painful and inflamed.
- You should gently straighten and bend your joints as far as they will comfortably go. This will improve movement flexibility and reduce stiffness in the painful joint. If the spine is painful and/or inflamed, exercises to stretch and extend the back can be helpful in preventing long-term disability.
- You may find it helpful to exercise in water

Diet

A healthy diet is good for everyone, and it may be very helpful if you have ankylosing spondylitis. There is no specific diet for people with ankylosing spondylitis, but keeping a healthy weight is important. It reduces stress on painful joints. Omega-3 fatty acids, found in cold water fish (such as tuna and salmon), flax seeds, and walnuts, might reduce disease activity. This is still being studied.

Posture

Another important thing you can do for yourself is to practice good posture. A good test for posture is to check yourself in a mirror. First, stand with a full-length mirror to your side and, if possible, turn your head to look at your profile. Next, imagine you have dropped a weighted string from the top of your head to the soles of your feet. Where does the string fall? If your posture is good, it should pass through your earlobe, the front of your shoulder, the center of your hip, behind your kneecap, and in front of your ankle bone. If you are not standing that way already, practice holding your body that way in front of a mirror until you know how it feels. Practicing good posture can help you avoid some of the complications that can occur with ankylosing spondylitis.

Chapter 27

Osteoarthritis: Degenerative Spinal Joint Disease

Osteoarthritis (OA) is the most common type of arthritis and is seen especially among older people. It is sometimes called "degenerative joint disease."

People with OA usually have joint pain and stiffness. The most commonly affected joints are in the hands (ends of the fingers and thumbs), neck, lower back, knees, and hips. Unlike some other forms of arthritis, OA does not affect the skin, lungs, eyes, or blood vessels. It can also occur in only one joint or can affect a joint on one side of the body much more severely.

Osteoarthritis affects each person differently. For some people, OA is relatively mild and interferes little with day-to-day life. For others, it causes significant pain and disability. Joint damage usually develops gradually over years, although it could worsen quickly in some people.

Who Gets Osteoarthritis

Osteoarthritis becomes more common with age. However, younger people can also develop it, usually as the result of a joint injury, an abnormal joint structure, or a genetic defect in joint cartilage.

This chapter contains text excerpted from the following sources: Text in this chapter begins with excerpts from "Osteoarthritis," National Institute of Arthritis and Musculoskeletal and Skin Diseases (NIAMS), May 30, 2016; Text under the heading "Living with Osteoarthritis" is excerpted from "Osteoarthritis (OA)," Centers for Disease Control and Prevention (CDC), January 10, 2019.

Before the age of 45, more men than women have OA. After the age of 45, it is more common in women. It is also more likely to occur in people who are overweight and in those with jobs that stress particular joints.

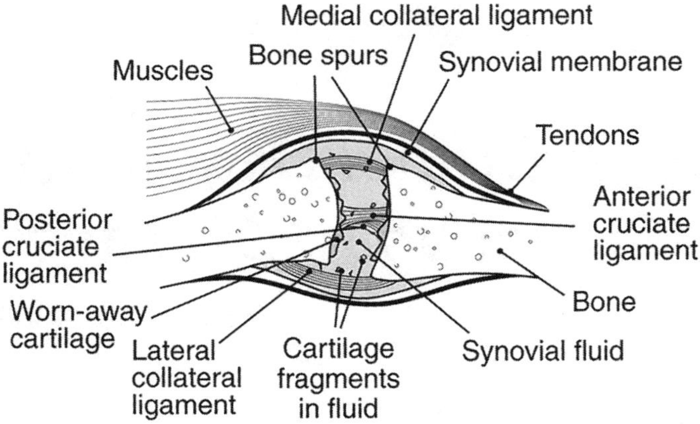

Figure 27.1. *Joint with Severe Osteoarthritis*

Symptoms of Osteoarthritis

Early in the disease, your joints may ache after physical work or exercise. Later on, joint pain may become more persistent. You may also experience joint stiffness, especially when you first wake up in the morning or have been in one position for a long time.

Joints often affected by OA include:

- **Hands**: If your mother or grandmother has or had OA in their hands, you are at an increased risk of having it too. Women are more likely than men to have OA in the hands. For most women, it develops after menopause.
- **Knees**: Stiffness, swelling, and pain in the knees can make it hard to walk, climb, and get in and out of chairs and bathtubs. OA in the knees can lead to disability.
- **Hips**: You might feel pain and stiffness in the hip joint or in the groin, inner thigh, buttocks, or even in the knees. Moving and bending may be limited, making daily activities—such as dressing and putting on shoes—a challenge.
- **Spine**: You may feel stiffness and pain in the neck or lower back. In some cases, arthritis-related changes in the spine can

cause pressure on the nerves where they exit the spinal column, resulting in weakness, tingling, or numbness of the arms and legs. In severe cases, this can even affect bladder and bowel function.

Causes of Osteoarthritis

Osteoarthritis usually happens gradually over time. Some things that might make it more likely include:

- Being overweight
- Getting older
- Joint injury
- Joints that are not properly formed
- A genetic defect in joint cartilage

Tests for Osteoarthritis

Although there is no single test for OA, your doctor may do the following to diagnosis you with the condition:

- **Medical history** to learn about your symptoms, any other medical problems you and your close family members have, and about any medications you are taking.
- **Physical exam** to check your general health, reflexes, and problem joints.
- Take pictures of your joint.
  - **X-rays** can show things such as cartilage loss, bone damage, and bone spurs. Early damage may not show on X-rays.
  - **Magnetic resonance imaging (MRI)** can show damage to connective tissues.
- **Blood tests** to rule out other causes for symptoms.
- **Joint fluid samples** to look for other causes of joint pain, such as infection or gout.

Treatment of Osteoarthritis

Treatment for OA can include medications or surgery to reduce pain and improve functioning.

- **Medications** commonly used in treating OA include:
  - Over-the-counter (OTC) pain relievers, such as acetaminophen.
  - Nonsteroidal anti-inflammatory drugs (NSAIDs) to treat pain and inflammation. Ibuprofen and naproxen sodium are available OTC, whereas other NSAIDs are available by prescription only.
  - Creams, rubs, or sprays that are applied to the skin over sore joints to relieve pain
  - Other prescription pain relievers are sometimes prescribed when OTC medications do not work or a person may not be able to take NSAIDs.
  - Corticosteroids are strong inflammation-fighting drugs that can be injected into the joint to temporarily relieve pain. This type of treatment is usually not recommended for more than two to four treatments per year. These types of drugs are not typically given by mouth to treat OA, unless treating inflammatory flares.
  - Hyaluronic acid substitutes (viscosupplements) are injected into the knee to replace a normal component of the joint involved in lubrication and nutrition.
- **Surgery** may be a factor after considering a variety of factors, including your age, occupation, level of disability, pain intensity, and the degree to which arthritis interferes with your lifestyle. Surgeries can include one or more of the following:
  - **Arthroscopic debridement**—removal of loose pieces of bone and cartilage from the joint
  - **Osteotomy**—repositioning of bones
  - **Joint resurfacing**—smoothing out bones
  - **Prostheses** are artificial joints that replace affected joints. The artificial joints can be made from metals, high-density plastic, or ceramic material. Artificial joints can last 10 to 15 years or longer. In some cases, your surgeon may replace only the damaged part of the knee joint, leaving undamaged parts of the joint in place.
- **Transcutaneous electrical nerve stimulation (TENS)** directs mild electric pulses to nerve endings that lie beneath

the skin in the painful area. It seems to work by blocking pain messages to the brain and by changing pain perception.

- **Alternative therapies** for OA can include:
  - **Massage** can increase blood flow and bring warmth to a stressed area. However, arthritis-stressed joints are sensitive, so the therapist must be familiar with the problems of the disease.
  - **Acupuncture** uses thin needles to relieve pain and restore health. Scientists think the needles stimulate the release of natural, pain-relieving chemicals produced by the nervous system.

Who Treats Osteoarthritis

Treating OA requires a team effort involving you and several types of healthcare professionals. These may include:

- **Primary care doctors**, such as a family physician or internal medicine specialist, who coordinates care between the different health providers and treats other problems as they arise
- **Rheumatologists**, who specialize in arthritis and other diseases of the bones, joints, and muscles
- **Orthopedists**, who specialize in treatment and surgery for bone and joint diseases
- **Physical therapists**, who help improve joint function
- **Occupational therapists**, who teach ways to protect joints, minimize pain, perform activities of daily living, and conserve energy
- **Dietitians**, who teach about good diets and maintaining a healthy weight
- **Nurse educators**, who help you understand your condition and help start treatment plans
- **Physiatrists** (rehabilitation specialists), who supervise exercise programs
- **Licensed acupuncture therapists**, who reduce pain and improve physical functioning by inserting fine needles into the skin at specific points on the body

- **Psychologists** or social workers, who help with social challenges caused by medical conditions
- **Chiropractors**, who focus treatment on the relationship between the body's structure, mainly the spine, and its functioning
- **Massage therapists**, who press, rub, and otherwise manipulate the muscles and other soft tissues of the body

Living with Osteoarthritis

- **Learn self-management skills**. Join a self-management education class, which helps people with arthritis and other chronic conditions—including OA—understand how arthritis affects their lives and increase their confidence in controlling their symptoms and living well.
- **Get physically active**. Experts recommend that adults engage in 150 minutes per week of at least moderate physical activity. Every minute of activity counts, and any activity is better than none. Moderate, low impact activities recommended include walking, swimming, or biking. Regular physical activity can also reduce the risk of developing other chronic diseases such as heart disease, stroke, and diabetes.
    - **Go to effective physical activity programs**. For people who worry that physical activity may make OA worse or are unsure how to exercise safely, participation in physical activity programs can help reduce pain and disability related to arthritis and improve mood and the ability to move. Classes take place at local Ys, parks, and community centers. These classes can help people with OA feel better.
- **Talk to your doctor**. You can play an active role in controlling your arthritis by attending regular appointments with your healthcare provider and following your recommended treatment plan. This is especially important if you also have other chronic conditions, such as diabetes or heart disease.
- **Lose weight**. For people who are overweight or obese, losing weight reduces pressure on joints, particularly weight-bearing joints, such as the hips and knees. Reaching or maintaining a healthy weight can relieve pain, improve function, and slow the progression of OA.

- **Protect your joints**. Joint injuries can cause or worsen arthritis. Choose activities that are easy on the joints, such as walking, bicycling, and swimming. These low-impact activities have a low risk of injury and do not twist or put too much stress on the joints.

Chapter 28

Intervertebral Disc Disease

Intervertebral disc disease (IVDD) is a common condition characterized by the breakdown (degeneration) of one or more of the discs that separate the bones of the spine, causing pain in the back or neck and frequently in the legs and arms. The intervertebral discs provide cushioning between vertebrae and absorb pressure put on the spine.

While the discs in the lower region of the spine are most often affected in intervertebral disc disease, any part of the spine can have disc degeneration. Depending on the location of the affected disc or discs, intervertebral disc disease can cause periodic or chronic pain in the back or neck. Pain is often worse when sitting, bending, twisting, or lifting objects.

Degenerated discs are prone to outpouching (herniation); the protruding disc can press against one of the spinal nerves that run from the spinal cord to the rest of the body. This pressure causes pain, weakness, and numbness in the back and legs. Herniated discs often cause nerve pain called "sciatica" that travels along the sciatic nerve, which runs from the lower back down the length of each leg.

This chapter contains text excerpted from the following sources: Text in this chapter begins with excerpts from "Intervertebral Disc Disease," Genetics Home Reference (GHR), National Institutes of Health (NIH), October 2016; Text under the heading "How Might Intervertebral Disc Disease Be Treated?" is excerpted from "Intervertebral Disc Disease," Genetic and Rare Diseases Information Center (GARD), National Center for Advancing Translational Sciences (NCATS), March 12, 2012. Reviewed April 2019.

As a disc degenerates, small bony outgrowths (bone spurs) may form at the edges of the affected vertebrae. These bone spurs may pinch (compress) the spinal nerves, leading to weakness or numbness in the arms or legs. If the bone spurs compress the spinal cord, affected individuals can develop problems with walking and bladder and bowel control. Over time, a degenerating disc may break down completely and leave no space between vertebrae, which can result in impaired movement, pain, and nerve damage.

Causes

Intervertebral disc disease results from a combination of genetic and environmental factors. Some of these factors have been identified, but many remain unknown. Researchers have identified variations in several genes that may influence the risk of developing intervertebral disc disease. The most commonly associated genes provide instructions for producing proteins called "collagens." Collagens are a family of proteins that strengthen and support connective tissues, such as skin, bone, cartilage, tendons, and ligaments. Collagens form a network of fibers that create structure and stability within the intervertebral discs. Specific variations in several collagen genes seem to affect the risk of developing intervertebral disc disease by impairing the ability of collagens to interact with each other, decreasing the stability of the disc and leading to its degeneration.

Normal variations in genes related to the body's immune function are also associated with an increased risk of developing intervertebral disc disease. These genes play a role in triggering an immune response when the body detects a foreign invader, such as a virus. It is thought that these gene variants can lead to an immune response that results in inflammation and water loss (dehydration) of the discs, which causes their degeneration.

Variants in genes that play roles in the development and maintenance of the intervertebral discs and have also been found to be associated with intervertebral disc disease. The associated variants can lead to disc degeneration and herniation. Researchers are working to identify and confirm other genetic changes associated with an increased risk of intervertebral disc disease.

Nongenetic factors that contribute to the risk of intervertebral disc disease are also being studied. These factors include aging, smoking, obesity, chronic inflammation, and driving for long periods of time (for example, as a long-haul trucker or taxi driver).

Frequency

Intervertebral disc disease is estimated to affect about five percent of the population in developed countries each year. Most individuals experience disc degeneration as they age; however, the severity of the degeneration and the pain associated with it varies.

How Might Intervertebral Disc Disease Be Treated?

In the absence of red flags, the initial approach to treatment is typically conservative and includes physical therapy and pain medications. In 90 percent of affected individuals, acute attacks of sciatica usually improve within 4 to 6 weeks without surgical intervention. In cases where surgical intervention is necessary, surgical procedures may include discectomy or spinal fusion.

Chapter 29

Slipped (Herniated) Disc

Discs are small, cushion-like structures that support the vertebral bodies of the spine. The discs look similar to a jelly donut as they have a soft center layer called a "nucleus," which is surrounded by a tough exterior called the "annulus." Located between the vertebral bones, the discs act as shock absorbers and minimize the impact of motion on the spine. The annulus pulls the vertebrae bones together against the resistance of the gel-filled nucleus. The nucleus acts like a ball bearing allowing the vertebral bodies to roll over the incompressible gel. Disc herniation occurs when the tough external surface of the disc ruptures, pushing out the soft layer from the center. The condition is also termed as a "slipped disc," "ruptured disc," or "disc prolapse." Although the disc herniation can occur in any part of the spine, it is more common in the lower back (lumbar spine) and neck (cervical spine). If the herniation is large enough, the disc tissue may press and irritate the surrounding spinal nerves, causing discomfort, pain, and numbness in the arms and legs.

Causes

Disc herniation usually occurs due to the degeneration of disc structure. Various factors may contribute to disc degeneration, and the most common risk factors are:

- Injury
- Improper lifting of heavy objects

- Applying sudden force or pressure on the spine
- Excess body weight
- Sudden bending
- Aging
- Smoking

The worst location for the disc herniation to occur is the lower back, especially in the region between the fourth and fifth lumbar vertebrae. This region bears the entire weight of the upper body, and it is more prone to herniation.

Certain people are considered to be so vulnerable to disc degeneration problems that even a small force applied on the spine can cause disc herniation. Aging is one of the factors that can weaken the tissues, resulting in quick disc degeneration. However, some researchers show that family history also plays a vital role in determining the rate of disc degeneration.

Symptoms

Most people experience no symptoms from a herniated disc, as long as the disc does not press on any nerve. The symptoms are evident only when the disc tissue becomes large enough to compress or irritate the spinal nerves nearby. Moreover, the symptoms may vary depending on the exact location of where herniation occurs and the size of the herniation. Since disc herniations predominantly occur either in the lower back or the neck region, the common signs and symptoms of these two conditions are discussed below.

Lower Back (Lumbar Spine)

Sciatica is the most common symptom of a herniated disc in the lower back. This symptom refers to the radiating pain that occurs when the herniated disc directly compresses the sciatic nerve, the longest and largest nerve in the human body that originates from the nerve roots in the spinal cord. The pain caused by sciatica begins in the lower back and radiates all the way down to the foot. The discomfort can be felt everywhere along the pathway of the nerve. The pain is aggravated by coughing, sneezing, and prolonged sitting or standing. Aging, obesity, and diabetes are some of the risk factors that worsen the symptoms of sciatica. The complications include:

- Leg weakness

- Numbness or a tingling sensation in the legs
- Loss of bladder control

Although mild sciatica can heal on its own with time, it is best to consult with a doctor if the person experiences severe pain or numbness in the legs. The condition is often treated with medications or physical therapies. Surgery is recommended only in critical cases.

Neck (Cervical Spine)

The symptoms of a herniated disc in the neck region include:

- Mild to severe pain in the neck, shoulder blades, and arms
- Weakness in the arms
- Numbness or tingling sensation in the arms

Diagnosis

The diagnosis of a herniated disc is done by a neurosurgeon and is based on the symptoms explained above. The diagnostic process generally includes a physical examination, neurological tests, and imaging tests.

Physical Examination

The doctor goes through the complete medical history of the patient before conducting a physical examination. During the physical examination, the patient will lie on a flat surface and move her or his arms and legs in different directions to determine the range of motion and tenderness of the back.

Neurological Tests

The neurological tests are performed to assess:

- Reflexes
- Strength of the muscles
- Ability to walk
- Sensitivity to touch

Imaging Tests

- **X-rays:** In general, disc herniations cannot be detected directly from X-rays. But X-rays can be helpful in ruling out other potential causes of pain, such as injuries, fractures, infections, tumors, a misalignment of the spine, etc.
- **Computed tomography (CT) scans:** In a CT scan, X-rays of the spine are taken from several directions and then combined to create cross-sectional images of the spine. It is helpful to analyze various aspects of the spine, such as its size, shape, and structures around it.
- **Magnetic resonance imaging (MRI):** Using MRI scans, three-dimensional images of the spine can be created. These images can be helpful in determining the exact position of the herniated disc and affected nerves.
- **Myelogram:** In this procedure, a dye is injected into the spinal fluid, and X-rays are taken. These special X-rays can reveal the pressure exerted by the herniations on the spinal nerves.
- **Electromyogram (EMG):** This test measures the electrical impulses along the nerves and precisely determines which nerves are affected by the disc herniation.

Treatment

The treatment for disc herniation can either be surgical or nonsurgical. Depending on the severity of the condition, the treatment procedure varies.

Nonsurgical Treatment

Fortunately, most of the herniated disc conditions do not require a surgical treatment. Conservative and nonsurgical procedures can cure the disorder in its initial stages. A doctor may recommend bed rest and avoiding heavy activities for few days or weeks. This can reduce the inflammation of the spinal nerve and relieve the pain. Other nonsurgical treatments include:

- **Medications:** Over-the-counter (OTC) medications and narcotics can be helpful in reducing the pain. Doctors may also prescribe anticonvulsants for radiating nerve pain and muscle relaxers for muscle spasms.

- **Physical therapy:** A physical therapist may recommend a few exercises that can reduce the pain associated with a herniated disc. Heat therapy, cold therapy, ultrasound therapy, electrotherapy, wearing back/cervical braces, etc. can be helpful in treating various symptoms of disc herniation.
- **Complementary and alternative medicine (CAM):** Chiropractic adjustment, massage, yoga, and acupuncture are some of the alternative treatment methods that may ease the chronic pain associated with disc herniation.

Surgical Treatment

Surgical treatment is considered only if the conservative treatment methods are ineffective or if the patient experiences critical conditions, such as:

- Aggravated back pain that limits daily activities
- Loss of bowel and bladder control
- An inability to stand or walk properly

A normal surgical procedure involves removal of the protruding portion of the disc. In some rare cases, the entire disc may be removed and replaced with an artificial disc. After surgery, it is important to rest enough before resuming normal activities.

References

1. Shiel, William C. "Herniated Disc (Disc Herniation of the Spine)," MedicineNet, March 16, 2018.
2. Newman, Tim. "Causes and Treatment of a Herniated Disk," Medical News Today, August 21, 2018.
3. "Herniated disk," Mayo Clinic, March 6, 2018.
4. "Herniated Disc," American Association of Neurological Surgeons (AANS), July 1, 2010.
5. "Herniated Disk," OrthoInfo, October 2, 2007.
6. "Sciatica," Mayo Clinic, May 30, 2018.
7. Shiel, William C. "Sciatica," MedicineNet, March 6, 2019.

Chapter 30

Spinal Stenosis

What Is Spinal Stenosis?

Spinal stenosis is a narrowing of spaces in the spine (backbone) that results in pressure on the spinal cord and/or nerve roots. This disorder involves the narrowing of one or more of three areas of the spine:

- The canal in the center of the column of bones (vertebral or spinal column), through which the spinal cord and nerve roots run
- The canals at the base or roots of nerves branching out from the spinal cord
- The openings between vertebrae (bones of the spine), through which nerves leave the spine and go to other parts of the body

The spine is a column of 26 bones that extend in a line from the base of the skull to the pelvis.

24 of the bones are vertebrae. The bones of the spine include (see figure 30.1):

- 7 cervical vertebrae in the neck
- 12 thoracic vertebrae at the back wall of the chest
- 5 lumbar vertebrae at the inward curve (small) of the lower back

---

This chapter includes text excerpted from "Spinal Stenosis," National Institute of Arthritis and Musculoskeletal and Skin Diseases (NIAMS), August 30, 2016.

- The sacrum, composed of 5 fused vertebrae between the hip bones
- The coccyx, composed of 3 to 5 fused bones at the lower tip of the vertebral column

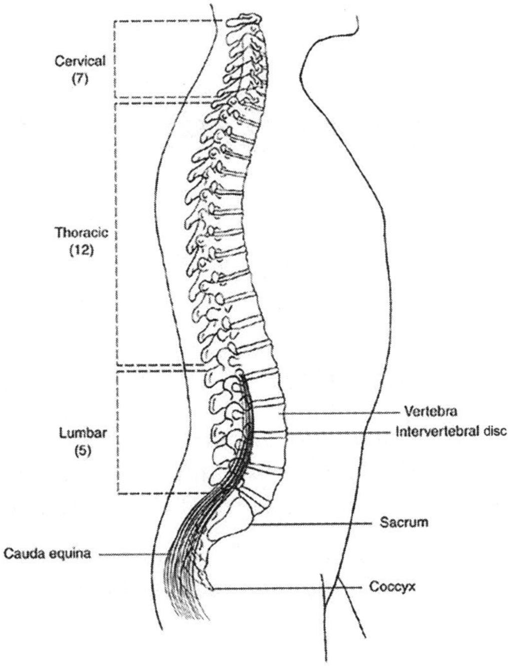

Figure 30.1. *Side View of Spine*

The vertebrae link to each other and have shock-absorbing intervertebral discs that lie between them to cushion them.

The vertebral column provides the main support for the upper body, allowing you to stand upright or bend and twist. It also protects the spinal cord from injury.

What Structures of the Spine Are Involved in Stenosis?

The following structures of the spine are the ones most involved in spinal stenosis (see figures 30.1, 30.2, and 30.3):

- **Facet joints.** Joints located on the back of the main part of the vertebra. They are formed by a portion of one vertebra and the vertebra above it. They connect the vertebrae to each other and permit backward motion.

- **Ligaments.** Elastic bands of tissue that support the spine by preventing the vertebrae from slipping out of line as the spine moves.
- **Spinal cord/nerve roots.** A major part of the central nervous system (CNS) that extends from the base of the brain down to the lower back and is encased by the vertebral column. It consists of nerve cells and bundles of nerves. The cord connects the brain to all parts of the body via 31 pairs of nerves that branch out from the cord and leave the spine between vertebrae.
- **Synovium.** A thin membrane that produces fluid to lubricate the facet joints, allowing them to move easily.
- **Vertebral arch.** A circle of bone around the canal through which the spinal cord passes. It is composed of a floor at the back of the vertebra, walls (the pedicles), and a ceiling where two laminae join.
- **Cauda equina.** A sack of nerve roots that continues from the lumbar region, where the spinal cord ends and continues down to provide neurologic function to the lower part of the body. It resembles a "horse's tail" (cauda equina in Latin).

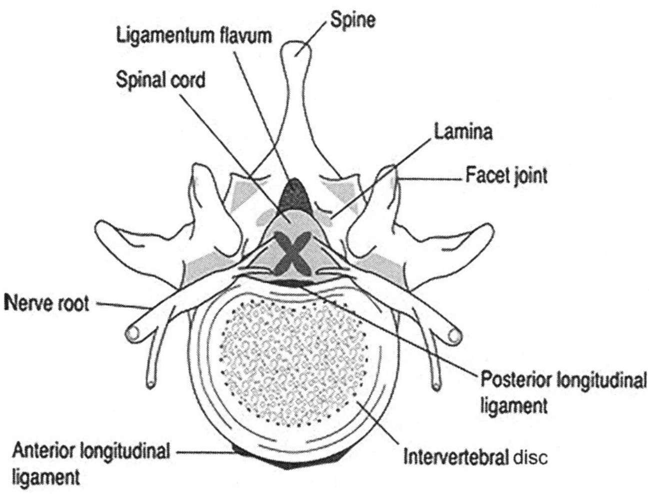

Figure 30.2. *Structures of the Spine*

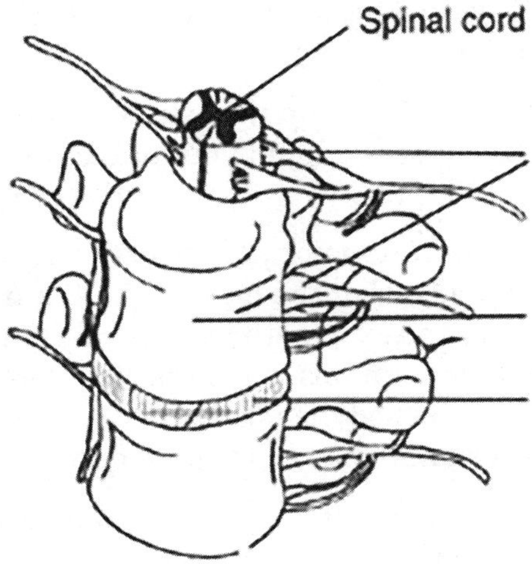

Figure 30.3. *Section of the Spine*

Who Gets Spinal Stenosis

This disorder is most common in men and women over 50 years of age. However, it may occur in younger people who are born with a narrowing of the spinal canal or who suffer an injury to the spine.

Symptoms of Spinal Stenosis

The space within the spinal canal may narrow without producing any symptoms. The neck or back may or may not hurt. However, if narrowing places pressure on the spinal cord, cauda equina, or nerve roots, there may be a slow onset and progression of symptoms. In the arms and legs, people may have:

- Numbness
- Weakness
- Cramping, or general pain
- Pain radiating down the leg (sciatica)

Sitting or flexing the lower back should relieve symptoms. The flexed position "opens up" the spinal column, enlarging the spaces between vertebrae at the back of the spine. Flexing exercises are often advised, along with stretching and strengthening exercises.

People with more severe stenosis, such as with cauda equine syndrome, may have problems with:

- Bowel function
- Bladder function
- Sexual function
- Pain, weakness, or loss of feeling in one or both legs
- Foot disorders

Causes of Spinal Stenosis

The normal vertebral canal (see figure 30.4) provides enough room for the spinal cord and cauda equina. Narrowing of the canal, which occurs in spinal stenosis, may be inherited or acquired.

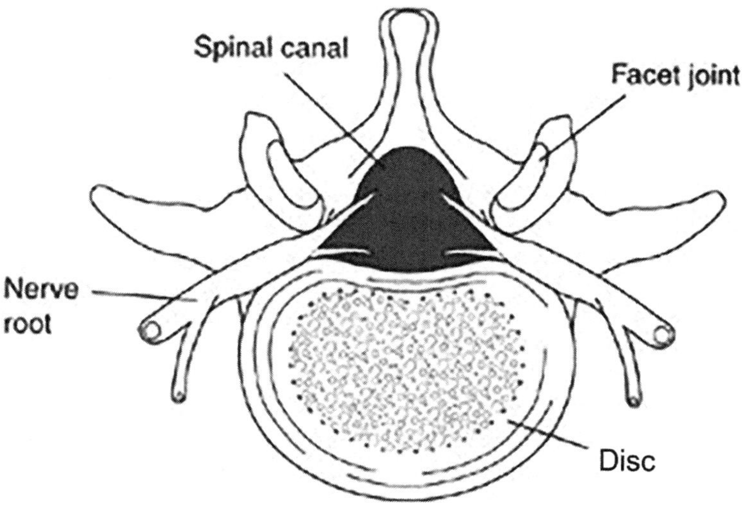

Figure 30.4. *Normal Vertebra (Cross Section)*

Inherited Conditions

Some people inherit a small spinal canal (see figure 30.5) or have a curvature of the spine (scoliosis) that produces pressure on nerves and soft tissue and compresses or stretches ligaments.

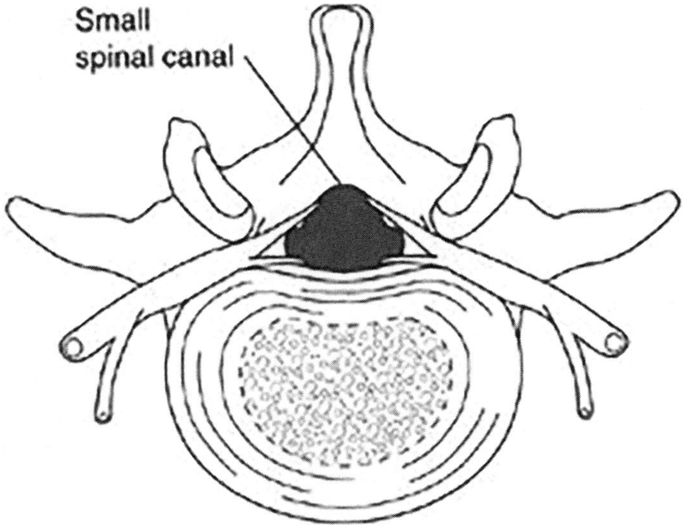

Figure 30.5. *Small Spinal Canal*

In an inherited condition called "achondroplasia," defective bone formation results in changes that reduce the diameter (distance across) of the spinal canal.

Aging

Spinal stenosis most often results from a gradual, degenerative aging process. Either structural changes or inflammation can begin the process. As people age, the ligaments of the spine may thicken and calcify (harden from deposits of calcium salts). Bones and joints may also enlarge. When the surfaces of the bone begin to project out from the body, these projections are called "osteophytes" (bone spurs).

When the health of one part of the spine fails, it usually places increased stress on other parts of the spine. For example, a herniated (bulging) disc may place pressure on the spinal cord or nerve root (see figure 30.6).

When a segment of the spine becomes too mobile, the capsules (enclosing membranes) of the facet joints thicken in an effort to stabilize the segment, and bone spurs may occur. This decreases the space available for nerve roots leaving the spinal cord.

Spondylolisthesis, a condition in which one vertebra slips forward on another, may result from a degenerative condition or an accident, or, very rarely, may be present at birth. Poor alignment of the spinal column when a vertebra slips forward onto the one below it can place pressure on the spinal cord or nerve roots at that place.

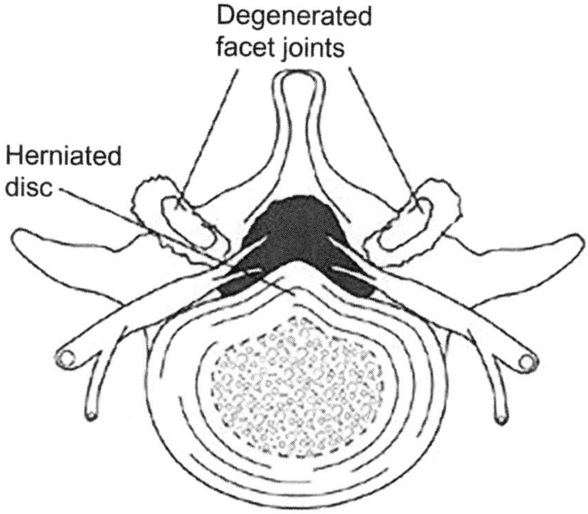

Figure 30.6. *Herniated Disc*

Arthritis

Aging, along with arthritis, is the most common cause of spinal stenosis. Two forms of arthritis that may affect the spine are osteoarthritis (OA) and rheumatoid arthritis (RA).

- **Osteoarthritis.** OA is the most common form of arthritis and is more likely to occur in middle-aged and older people. It is a chronic, degenerative process that may involve multiple joints of the body. It wears away the surface cartilage layer of joints and is often accompanied by overgrowth of bone, a formation of bone spurs, and impaired function. If the degenerative process of OA affects the facet joint and the disc, the condition is sometimes referred to as "spondylosis." With this condition, a person may have disc degeneration and an enlargement or overgrowth of bone that narrows the central and nerve root canals.
- **Rheumatoid arthritis.** RA usually affects people at an earlier age than OA does and causes inflammation and enlargement of the soft tissues (the synovium) of the joints. Although not a common cause of spinal stenosis, damage to ligaments, bones, and joints that begins as synovitis (inflammation of the synovial membrane that lines the inside of the joint) has a severe and

disrupting effect on joint function. The portions of the vertebral column with the greatest mobility (for example, the neck area) are often the ones most affected in people with RA.

Other Acquired Conditions

The following conditions that are not related to aging or degenerative disease are causes of acquired spinal stenosis:

- Tumors of the spine are abnormal growths of soft tissue that may affect the spinal canal directly by inflammation or by the growth of tissue into the canal. Tissue growth may lead to bone resorption (bone loss due to overactivity of certain bone cells) or displacement of the bone.
- Trauma (accidents) may either dislocate the spine and the spinal canal or cause burst fractures that produce fragments of bone that penetrate the canal.
- Paget disease of bone is a chronic (long-term) disorder that typically results in enlarged and abnormal bones. Excessive bone breakdown and formation cause thick and fragile bone. As a result, bone pain, arthritis, noticeable bone structure changes, and fractures can occur. The disease can affect any bone of the body but is often found in the spine. The blood supply that feeds healthy nerve tissue may be diverted to the area of the involved bone. Also, structural problems of the involved vertebrae can cause narrowing of the spinal canal, producing a variety of neurological symptoms. Other developmental conditions may also result in spinal stenosis.
- Ossification of the posterior longitudinal ligament occurs when calcium deposits form on the ligament that runs up and down behind the spine and inside the spinal canal (see figure 30.7). These deposits turn the fibrous tissue of the ligament into the bone. (Ossification means "forming bone.") These deposits may press on the nerves in the spinal canal.

Diagnosis of Spinal Stenosis

A doctor may use a variety of approaches to diagnose spinal stenosis and rule out other conditions.

- **Medical history.** You tell your doctor details about symptoms and about any injury, condition, or general health problem that might be causing the symptoms.

- **Physical examination.** The doctor:
  - Examines you to determine the extent of limitation of movement
  - Checks for pain or symptoms when you hyperextend the spine (bend backwards)
  - Checks for normal neurologic function (for instance, sensation, muscle strength, and reflexes) in the arms and legs

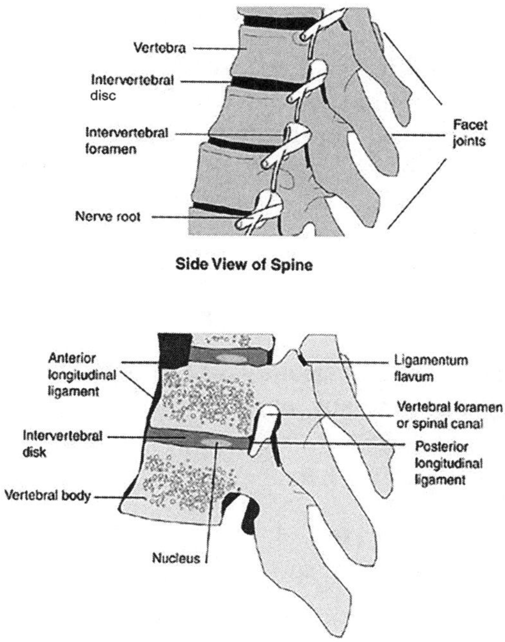

Figure 30.7. *Side View of Spine and Its Cross Section*

- **X-ray.** An X-ray beam is passed through the back to produce a two-dimensional picture. An X-ray may be done before other tests to look for signs of an injury, tumor, or inherited problem. This test can show the structure of the vertebrae and the outlines of joints, and it can detect calcification.
- **Magnetic resonance imaging (MRI).** Energy from a powerful magnet (rather than X-rays) produces signals that are detected by a scanner and analyzed by the computer. This produces a series of cross-sectional images ("slices") and/

or a three-dimensional view of parts of the back. An MRI is particularly sensitive for detecting damage or disease of soft tissues, such as the discs between vertebrae or ligaments. It shows the spinal cord, nerve roots, and surrounding spaces, as well as enlargement, degeneration, or tumors.

- **Computerized axial tomography (CAT) scan.** X-rays are passed through the back at different angles, detected by a scanner, and analyzed by a computer. This produces a series of cross-sectional images and/or three-dimensional views of the parts of the back. The scan shows the shape and size of the spinal canal, its contents, and the structures surrounding it.
- **Myelogram.** A liquid dye that X-rays cannot penetrate is injected into the spinal column. The dye circulates around the spinal cord and spinal nerves, which appear as white objects against the bone on an X-ray film. A myelogram can show pressure on the spinal cord or nerves from herniated discs, bone spurs, or tumors.

Treatment of Spinal Stenosis

Treatment of spinal stenosis may consist of nonsurgical treatments, alternative therapies, and surgery.

Nonsurgical Treatments

In the absence of severe or progressive nerve involvement, a doctor may prescribe one or more of the following conservative treatments:

- Nonsteroidal anti-inflammatory drugs (NSAIDs), such as aspirin, naproxen, ibuprofen, or indomethacin, to reduce inflammation and relieve pain. The longer a person uses NSAIDs, the more likely he or she is to have side effects, ranging from mild to serious. Side effects of NSAIDs include stomach problems; skin rashes; high blood pressure; fluid retention; and liver, kidney, and heart problems. Many other drugs cannot be taken when a patient is being treated with NSAIDs because NSAIDs alter the way the body uses or eliminates these other drugs. Check with your healthcare provider or pharmacist before you take NSAIDs. NSAIDs should only be used at the lowest dose possible for the shortest time needed.
- Analgesics, such as acetaminophen, to relieve pain

- Corticosteroid injections into the outermost of the membranes covering the spinal cord and nerve roots to reduce inflammation and treat acute pain that radiates to the hips or down a leg.
- Anesthetic injections, known as "nerve blocks," near the affected nerve to temporarily relieve pain.
- Restricted activity (varies depending on the extent of nerve involvement).
- Prescribed exercises and/or physical therapy to maintain motion of the spine, strengthen abdominal and back muscles, and build endurance, all of which help stabilize the spine. You may be encouraged to try slowly progressive aerobic activity, such as swimming or using exercise bicycles.
- A lumbar brace or corset to provide some support and help you regain mobility. This approach is sometimes used for people with weak abdominal muscles or older patients with degeneration at several levels of the spine.

Alternative Therapies

Alternative (or complementary) therapies are diverse medical and healthcare systems, practices, and products that are not presently considered to be part of conventional medicine. Some examples of these therapies that can treat spinal stenosis include:

- **Chiropractic treatment.** This treatment is based on the philosophy that restricted movement in the spine reduces proper function and may cause pain. Chiropractors may manipulate (adjust) the spine to restore normal spinal movement. They may also employ traction, a pulling force, to help increase space between the vertebrae and reduce pressure on affected nerves. Some people report that they benefit from chiropractic care. Research thus far has shown that chiropractic treatment is about as effective as conventional, nonsurgical treatments for acute back pain.
- **Acupuncture.** This treatment involves stimulating certain places on the skin by a variety of techniques, in most cases by manipulating thin, solid, metallic needles that penetrate the skin. Research has shown that low back pain is one area in which acupuncture has benefited some people.

More research is needed before the effectiveness of these or other possible alternative therapies can be definitively stated. Healthcare providers may suggest these therapies in addition to more conventional treatments.

Surgery

In many cases, the conditions causing spinal stenosis cannot be permanently altered by nonsurgical treatment, even though these measures may relieve pain for a period of time. To find out how much nonsurgical treatment will help, a doctor may recommend such treatment first. However, surgery might be considered right away if you have numbness or weakness that interferes with walking, impaired bowel or bladder function, or other neurological involvement.

The decision to have surgery depends on:

- The effectiveness of nonsurgical treatments
- The extent of your pain
- Other diseases that you may have
- Your physical condition
- Your preferences

The purpose of surgery is to:

- Relieve pressure on the spinal cord or nerves
- Restore and maintain alignment and strength of the spine

This can be done by removing, trimming, or adjusting diseased parts that are causing the pressure or loss of alignment.

The most common surgery is called "decompressive laminectomy," performed for the removal of the lamina (roof) of one or more vertebrae to create more space for the nerves. A surgeon may perform a laminectomy with or without fusing vertebrae or removing part of a disc. She or he may use various devices to enhance fusion and strengthen unstable segments of the spine.

If you have spinal stenosis caused by spinal trauma or achondroplasia, you may need surgery at a young age. When a person with achondroplasia needs surgery, laminectomy (removal of the roof) without fusion is usually effective.

Major Risks of Surgery

All surgery, particularly when involving general anesthesia and older patients, carries risks. The most common complications of surgery for spinal stenosis are:

- A tear in the membrane covering the spinal cord at the site of the operation
- Infection
- A blood clot that forms in the veins

These conditions can be treated but may prolong recovery.

Long-Term Outcomes of Surgical Treatment

Removal of the obstruction that has caused the symptoms usually gives a person some relief; most people have less leg pain and are able to walk better after surgery. However, if nerves were badly damaged before surgery, there may be some remaining pain or numbness or no improvement. Also, the degenerative process will likely continue, and pain or limitation of activity may reappear after surgery.

Who Treats Spinal Stenosis

Doctors who can provide nonsurgical treatment of spinal stenosis may be:

- Internists
- General practitioners
- Rheumatologists, who treat arthritis and related disorders
- Neurologists, who treat nerve diseases
- Orthopedic surgeons
- Neurosurgeons

Orthopedic surgeons and neurosurgeons also perform spinal surgery if you need it. Allied health professionals, such as physical therapists, may also help treat patients.

Chapter 31

Radiculopathy

Chapter Contents

Section 31.1—Pinched Nerve (Compressed Nerve).................. 244
Section 31.2—Cauda Equina Syndrome.................................... 245

Section 31.1

Pinched Nerve (Compressed Nerve)

This section includes text excerpted from "Pinched Nerve Information Page," National Institute of Neurological Disorders and Stroke (NINDS), March 27, 2019.

The term "pinched nerve" is a colloquial term and not a true medical term. It is used to describe one type of damage or injury to a nerve or set of nerves. The injury may result from compression, constriction, or stretching.

Symptoms

Symptoms include numbness, "pins and needles" or burning sensations, and pain radiating outward from the injured area. One of the most common examples of a single compressed nerve is the feeling of a foot or hand "falling asleep." A "pinched nerve" frequently is associated with pain in the neck or lower back. This type of pain can be caused by inflammation or pressure on the nerve root as it exits the spine. If the pain is severe or lasts a long time, you may need to have further evaluation from your physician.

Several problems can lead to similar symptoms of numbness, pain, and tingling in the hands or feet but without pain in the neck or back. These can include peripheral neuropathy, carpal tunnel syndrome, and tennis elbow. The extent of such injuries may vary from minor, temporary damage to a more permanent condition. Early diagnosis is important to prevent further damage or complications. Pinched nerve is a common cause of on-the-job injury.

Treatment

The most frequently recommended treatment for pinched nerve is rest for the affected area. Nonsteroidal anti-inflammatory drugs (NSAIDs) or corticosteroids may be recommended to help alleviate pain. Physical therapy is often useful, and splints or collars may be used to relieve symptoms. Depending on the cause and severity of the pinched nerve, surgery may be needed.

Prognosis

With treatment, most people recover from the pinched nerve. However, in some cases, the damage is irreversible.

Section 31.2

Cauda Equina Syndrome

This section includes text excerpted from "Cauda Equina Syndrome," Genetic and Rare Diseases Information Center (GARD), National Center for Advancing Translational Sciences (NCATS), March 6, 2018.

What Is Cauda Equina Syndrome?

Cauda equina syndrome (CES) refers to a group of symptoms that occur when nerves in the cauda equina (a collection of nerve roots that spread out from the bottom of the spinal cord) become compressed or damaged. These nerves roots connect the central nervous system and peripheral nervous system. CES can lead to pain, numbness, and weakness in the lower back, pelvic area and legs; "foot drop"; problems with bowel or bladder control; sexual dysfunction; and even paralysis. CES is considered a medical emergency and requires hospitalization. Therefore, people with unexplained onset of symptoms should seek medical attention as soon as possible and consult with a neurologist or neurosurgeon.

What Causes Cauda Equina Syndrome

Cauda equina syndrome is most commonly caused by a herniated disc in the lumbar spine. Other causes of CES may include a birth abnormality (such as spina bifida), spinal infection or tumor, trauma or injury to the lower back, spinal stenosis, a spinal arteriovenous malformation, and complications after spinal surgery.

How Is Cauda Equina Syndrome Diagnosed?

Cauda equina syndrome can be difficult to diagnose since symptoms vary, and they may mimic other conditions. Tests that may be used to diagnose CES include magnetic resonance imaging (MRI), a computed tomography (CT) scan, and myelogram (a special type of X-ray of the spinal canal).

What Is the Treatment for Cauda Equina Syndrome?

Treatment usually targets the underlying cause of CES (removing the cause of nerve pressure) and most often involves urgent surgery to prevent permanent neurologic impairment. How well a person recovers from CES often depends on the underlying cause and how promptly they are treated. Symptoms are more likely to improve or go away if the cause is identified quickly and treatment begins right away. Some people have significant improvement of symptoms and quality of life after treatment. However, others may have permanent neurologic impairment, chronic pain, and/or mental-health problems due to the impact of symptoms on social life and relationships.

Chapter 32

Spina Bifida and Tethered Spinal Cord Syndrome

Chapter Contents

Section 32.1—Spina Bifida 248
Section 32.2—Living with Spina Bifida at Different Ages 254
Section 32.3—Tethered Spinal Cord Syndrome 271

Section 32.1

Spina Bifida

This section contains text excerpted from the following sources: Text in this section begins with excerpts from "Spina Bifida," Centers for Disease Control and Prevention (CDC), September 13, 2018; Text beginning with the heading "Are There Disorders or Conditions Associated with Spina Bifida?" is excerpted from "Are There Disorders or Conditions Associated with Spina Bifida?" *Eunice Kennedy Shriver* National Institute of Child Health and Human Development (NICHD), December 2016.

Spina bifida is a condition that affects the spine and is usually apparent at birth. It is a type of neural tube defect (NTD).

Spina bifida can happen anywhere along the spine if the neural tube does not close all the way. When the neural tube does not close all the way, the backbone that protects the spinal cord does not form and close as it should. This often results in damage to the spinal cord and nerves.

Spina bifida might cause physical and intellectual disabilities that range from mild to severe. The severity depends on:

- The size and location of the opening in the spine
- Whether part of the spinal cord and nerves are affected

Types of Spina Bifida

The three most common types of spina bifida are:

Myelomeningocele

When people talk about spina bifida, most often they are referring to myelomeningocele. Myelomeningocele is the most serious type of spina bifida. With this condition, a sac of fluid comes through an opening in the fetus's back. Part of the spinal cord and nerves are in this sac and are damaged. This type of spina bifida causes moderate to severe disabilities, such as problems affecting how the person goes to the bathroom, loss of feeling in the person's legs or feet, and not being able to move the legs.

Meningocele

Another type of spina bifida is meningocele. With meningocele, a sac of fluid comes through an opening in the fetus's back. But, the spinal cord is not in this sac. There is usually little or no nerve damage. This type of spina bifida can cause minor disabilities.

Spina Bifida Occulta

Spina bifida occulta is the mildest type of spina bifida. It is sometimes called "hidden spina bifida." With it, there is a small gap in the spine, but no opening or sac on the back. The spinal cord and the nerves usually are normal. Many times, spina bifida occulta is not discovered until late childhood or adulthood. This type of spina bifida usually does not cause any disabilities.

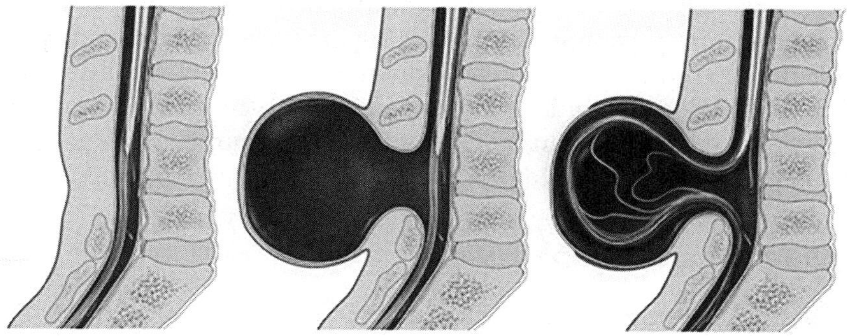

Figure 32.1. *Types of Spina Bifida*

Causes and Prevention of Spina Bifida

We do not know all of the causes of spina bifida. The role that genetics and the environment play in causing spina bifida needs to be studied further.

However, we do know that there are ways for women to reduce the risk of having a baby with spina bifida both before and during her pregnancy.

If you are pregnant or could get pregnant, use the following tips to help prevent your baby from having spina bifida:

- Take 400 micrograms (mcg) of folic acid every day. If you have already had a pregnancy affected by spina bifida, you may need to take a higher dose of folic acid before pregnancy and during early pregnancy. Talk to your doctor to discuss what is best for you.

- Talk to your doctor or pharmacist about any prescription and over-the-counter (OTC) drugs, vitamins, and dietary or herbal supplements you are taking.
- If you have a medical condition—such as diabetes or obesity—be sure it is under control before you become pregnant.
- Avoid overheating your body, as what might happen if you use a hot tub or sauna.
- Treat any fever you have right away with Tylenol® (or store brand acetaminophen).

Spina bifida happens in the first few weeks of pregnancy, often before a woman knows she is pregnant. Although folic acid is not a guarantee that a woman will have a healthy pregnancy, taking folic acid can help reduce a woman's risk of having a pregnancy affected by spina bifida. Because half of all pregnancies in the United States are unplanned, it is important that all women who can become pregnant take 400 mcg of folic acid daily.

Diagnosis of Spina Bifida

Spina bifida can be diagnosed during pregnancy or after the baby is born. Spina bifida occulta might not be diagnosed until late childhood or adulthood, or it might never be diagnosed.

During Pregnancy

During pregnancy, there are screening tests (prenatal tests) to check for spina bifida and other birth defects. Talk with your doctor about any questions or concerns you have about this prenatal testing.

- **Alpha-fetoprotein (AFP)**, a protein the fetus produces. This is a simple blood test that measures how much AFP has passed into the mother's bloodstream from the fetus. A high level of AFP might mean that the fetus has spina bifida. An AFP test might be part of a test called the "triple screen" that looks for neural tube defects and other issues.
- **Ultrasound.** An ultrasound is a type of picture of the fetus. In some cases, the doctor can see if the fetus has spina bifida or find other reasons that there might be a high level of AFP. Frequently, spina bifida can be seen with this test.

- **Amniocentesis.** For this test, the doctor takes a small sample of the amniotic fluid surrounding the fetus in the womb. Higher-than-average levels of AFP in the fluid might mean that the fetus has spina bifida.

After the Baby Is Born

In some cases, spina bifida might not be diagnosed until after the baby is born.

Sometimes, there is a hairy patch of skin or a dimple on the baby's back that is first seen after the baby is born. A doctor can use an image scan, such as an X-ray, magnetic resonance imaging (MRI), or computed tomography (CT) scan, to get a clearer view of the baby's spine and the bones in the back.

Sometimes, spina bifida is not diagnosed until after the baby is born because the mother did not receive prenatal care, or an ultrasound did not show clear pictures of the affected part of the spine.

Are There Disorders or Conditions Associated with Spina Bifida?

Health issues are different for each person with spina bifida. Open spina bifida (myelomeningocele)—in which the spinal cord is exposed—tends to cause more severe problems.

Hydrocephalus

Many infants born with spina bifida get extra fluid in and around the brain, a condition called "hydrocephalus," or "water on the brain." The extra fluid can cause swelling of the head, which may lead to brain injury.

Chiari II Malformation

The brains of most children with open spina bifida are positioned abnormally. The lower part of the brain rests farther down than normal, partially in the upper spinal canal. The cerebrospinal fluid can get blocked and cause hydrocephalus. While most affected children have no other symptoms, a few may have upper body weakness and trouble breathing and swallowing.

Tethered Spinal Cord

Typically, the bottom of the spinal cord floats freely in the spinal canal, but for many people with spina bifida, the spinal cord is attached to the spinal canal. Thus, the spinal cord stretches as a person grows, and this stretching can cause spinal nerve damage. The person might have back pain, scoliosis, weakness in the legs and feet, bladder or bowel control problems, and other issues.

Paralysis and Mobility Limitations

People with spina bifida high on the back (near the head, for instance) might not be able to move their legs. People with spina bifida low on the back (near the hips, for example) might have some leg mobility and be able to walk unassisted or with crutches, braces, or walkers.

Lack of Bladder and Bowel Control

People with spina bifida often cannot control their bladder and bowel movements. They also can develop urinary tract infections (UTIs).

Latex Allergy

Many people with spina bifida—possibly three-quarters of those with the condition—are allergic to latex, or natural rubber. While researchers still do not entirely understand why the rate in those with spina bifida is so high, some experts believe such an allergy can be caused by frequent exposure to latex, which is common for people with spina bifida who have shunts and have had many surgeries.

Learning Disabilities

While at least 80 percent of children with open spina bifida do not have learning deficiencies, some do have learning problems.

Other Conditions

Some people with open spina bifida have additional physical and psychological conditions, including digestive, vision, sexual, social, and emotional problems; obesity; and depression.

What Are the Treatments for Spina Bifida and Related Conditions?

Open Spina Bifida

An infant with open spina bifida can have surgery to close the hole in the back before birth or within the first few days after birth.

Hydrocephalus

If an infant with spina bifida has hydrocephalus, a surgeon can implant a shunt—a small hollow tube to drain the extra fluid and relieve pressure on the brain. The shunt may need to be replaced during childhood.

Tethered Spinal Cord

For a child with this condition, in which the spinal cord is attached to the spinal canal and stretches as the child grows, surgery can separate the spinal cord from surrounding tissue, allowing the child to regain her or his usual level of functioning.

Paralysis and Mobility Limitations

People with spina bifida use different ways to get around, according to their needs. They may be able to walk without assistance, or they may use braces, crutches, walkers, or wheelchairs.

Urinary Tract Infections, Lack of Bladder and Bowel Control

People with open spina bifida often have nerve damage that prevents the bladder from completely emptying, a condition that can cause urinary tract infections and kidney damage. The child or parent can address this problem by inserting a plastic tube called a "catheter" into the bladder several times a day to allow the bladder to empty fully. Medications, injections, and surgery can also help address incontinence issues and preserve kidney and bladder function for the long-term. Children with spina bifida should see a urologist (a doctor who specializes in urinary tract problems) regularly.

Section 32.2

Living with Spina Bifida at Different Ages

This section includes text excerpted from "Spina Bifida," Centers for Disease Control and Prevention (CDC), January 30, 2019.

Living with Infants with Spina Bifida

Having a new baby is an exciting and challenging time. New parents often feel many different emotions—such as love, joy, happiness, worry, and exhaustion. The same is true for parents who have a child affected by spina bifida. However, in addition to adjusting to life with a new baby, parents of a child with spina bifida also need to learn as much as possible about the condition to prepare for the needs of their child.

Learning about Spina Bifida

When parents find out they are going to have a child with spina bifida, it can be overwhelming. It is important that they know that most children born with spina bifida reach their full potential.

It is very important for parents to take an active role in managing their child's care. Parents need to know about spina bifida and understand the health issues and treatment options to make the best possible choices for the health and happiness of their child.

- Parents should talk with a healthcare provider about any questions or concerns they have.
- Parents can start learning about spina bifida by visiting the Centers for Disease Control and Prevention's (CDC) website.
- The Spina Bifida Association provides information on spina bifida, and it can be helpful in recommending clinics or healthcare providers who are experts in the care of children and adults with spina bifida.

Physical Health—What to Expect

No two babies with spina bifida are exactly alike. Health issues will be different for each baby. Some babies have issues that are more severe than other babies. With the right care, babies born with spina bifida will grow up to reach their full potential.

Open Spina Bifida

When a baby is born with open spina bifida, in which the spinal cord is exposed (myelomeningocele), doctors will perform surgery to close it before birth or within the first few days of the baby's life.

Hydrocephalus

Many babies born with spina bifida get hydrocephalus (often called "water on the brain"). This means that there is extra fluid in and around the brain. The extra fluid can cause the spaces in the brain, called "ventricles," to become too large, and the head can swell. Hydrocephalus needs to be followed closely and treated properly to prevent brain injury.

If a baby with spina bifida has hydrocephalus, a surgeon can put in a shunt. A shunt is a small hollow tube that will help drain the fluid from the baby's brain and protect it from too much pressure. Additional surgery might be needed to change the shunt as the child grows up or if it becomes clogged or infected.

Mobility and Physical Activity

People affected by spina bifida get around in different ways. These include walking without any aids or assistance; walking with braces, crutches, or walkers; and using wheelchairs.

People with spina bifida higher on the spine (near the head) might have paralyzed legs and use wheelchairs. Those with spina bifida lower on the spine (near the hips) might have more use of their legs and use crutches, braces, or walkers, or they might be able to walk without these devices.

Doctors can start treatment for movement problems soon after a baby with spina bifida is born. A physical therapist can work with parents and caregivers to teach them how to exercise a baby's legs to increase strength, flexibility, and movement.

Regular physical activity is important for all babies, especially for those with conditions that affect movement, such as spina bifida. There are many ways for babies with spina bifida to be active. For example, they can:

- Play with toys, such as activity mats.
- Enjoy parks and recreation areas.
- Participate in community programs, such as the Early Intervention Program for Infants and Toddlers with Disabilities, which is a free program in many communities.
- Do exercises recommended by a physical therapist.

Skin

Babies with spina bifida can develop sores, calluses, blisters, and burns on their feet, ankles, and hips. Parents and caregivers can help protect the baby's skin by:

- Checking the baby's skin every day for redness, including under braces
- Trying to avoid hot bath water, hot irons, and hot or unpadded seat belt clasps that may cause burns
- Making sure the baby does not stay out in the sun too long
- Making sure the baby is not sitting or lying in one position for too long

Latex (Natural Rubber) Allergy

Many babies with spina bifida are allergic to products that contain latex, or natural rubber. This means they should not use items made of natural rubber. For babies, this would include rubber nipples and pacifiers. The baby can wear a bracelet to alert other people of the allergy. Parents and caregivers should discuss this with their baby's healthcare providers.

Health Checks

Every baby needs a primary healthcare provider (for example, a pediatrician, family doctor, or nurse practitioner). The primary healthcare provider will want to make sure that the baby is healthy; developing normally; and receiving immunization against diseases and infections, including the flu.

In addition to seeing a primary healthcare provider, shortly after birth, the baby will be checked and treated as needed by doctors who specialize in different parts of the body. These doctors might suggest treatments or surgeries to help the baby.

These specialists might include:

- An orthopedist, who will work with the baby's muscles and bones
- A urologist, who will check the baby's kidneys and bladder
- A neurosurgeon, who will check the baby's brain and spine

Finding Support

Having support and community resources can help increase confidence in managing spina bifida, enhance the quality of life (QOL), and assist in meeting the needs of all family members. It might be helpful for parents of children with spina bifida to talk with one another. One parent might have learned how to address some of the same concerns another parent has. Often, other parents of children with special needs can give advice about good resources for these children.

Remember that the choices of one family might not be best for another family, so it is important that parents understand all options and discuss them with their child's healthcare providers.

Living with Toddlers and Preschoolers with Spina Bifida

Life with a toddler or preschooler is both fun and challenging. These young children experience huge mental, social, and emotional changes. They have a lot of energy and enthusiasm for exploring and learning about their world and becoming independent. Developing independence can be especially challenging for children with spina bifida. Parents should start helping their child develop independence early in childhood.

Encouraging Independence

For toddlers and preschoolers with spina bifida, there are many ways that parents and other caregivers can help them become more active and independent, such as:

- Teaching the child about her or his body and about spina bifida
- Encouraging the child to make choices, such as between two items of clothing
- Asking the child to help with daily tasks, such as putting away toys

Children with spina bifida might need extra help at times. But it is very important that children be given the opportunity to complete a task before help is given. It is also important that parents give only the help that is needed rather than helping with the entire task. Parents must learn the difficult balance between giving the right amount of help to increase their child's independence and confidence, while at the same time being careful not to give the child tasks that cannot reasonably be completed—which might decrease their child's confidence.

Physical Health—What to Expect

No two children with spina bifida are exactly alike. Health issues will be different for each child. Some children have issues that are more severe than other children. With the right care, children born with spina bifida will grow up to reach their full potential.

Mobility and Physical Activity

Children affected by spina bifida get around in different ways. These include walking without any aids or assistance; walking with braces, crutches, or walkers; and using wheelchairs.

Children with spina bifida higher on the spine (near the head) might have paralyzed legs and use wheelchairs. Those with spina bifida lower on the spine (near the hips) might have more use of their legs and use crutches, braces, or walkers, or they might be able to walk without these devices.

A physical therapist can work with children, parents, and caregivers to teach them how to exercise the child's legs to increase strength, flexibility, and movement.

Regular physical activity is important for all children, but especially for those with conditions that affect movement, such as spina bifida. There are many ways for children with spina bifida to be active. For example, they can:

- Engage in active play with friends.
- Roll or walk in the neighborhood.
- Enjoy parks and recreation areas with playgrounds that are accessible for those with disabilities.
- Participate in community programs, such as the Early Intervention Program for Infants and Toddlers with Disabilities and Special Education Services for Preschoolers with Disabilities, which are free programs in many communities.
- Do exercises recommended by a physical therapist.

Using the Bathroom

Children with spina bifida often cannot control when they go to the bathroom (incontinence). They also can develop urinary tract infections

(UTIs). It is important to develop a plan for going to the bathroom that works and is as simple as possible. This can lead to increased health, participation, and independence at school and in the home, and avoid embarrassment for children with spina bifida. Healthcare providers can help develop a plan for the child. A tube (catheter) inserted in the child's bladder can help drain urine. In some cases, extra fiber can be added to the diet to keep bowel movements regular. Surgery also might be recommended.

Skin

Children with spina bifida can develop sores, calluses, blisters, and burns on their feet, ankles, and hips. However, they might not know when these develop because they might not be able to feel certain parts of their body. In addition, toddlers might not know how to tell their parents about issues with their skin.

Parents and caregivers can help protect the child's skin and teach the child how to do this too, by:

- Checking the child's skin every day for redness, including under braces
- Trying to avoid hot bath water, hot irons, and hot or unpadded seat belt clasps that may cause burns
- Making sure the child wears properly fitting shoes at all times
- Using sunscreen on the child and making sure the child does not stay out in the sun too long
- Making sure the child is not sitting or lying in one position for too long

Health Checks

Every child needs a primary healthcare provider (for example, a pediatrician, family doctor, or nurse practitioner). The primary healthcare provider will want to make sure that the child is healthy; developing normally; and receiving immunizations against diseases and infections, including the flu.

In addition to seeing a primary healthcare provider, a child with spina bifida will be checked and treated as needed by doctors who specialize in different parts of the body. These doctors might suggest treatments or surgeries to help the child.

These specialists might include:

- An orthopedist, who will work with the child's muscles and bones
- A urologist, who will check the child's kidneys and bladder
- A neurosurgeon, who will check the child's brain and spine

Safety

Safety is an important issue for children with spina bifida. They can be at higher risk for injuries and abuse. It is important for parents and other family members to teach them how to stay safe and what to do if they feel threatened or have been hurt in any way.

Finding Support

Having support and community resources can help increase confidence in managing spina bifida, enhance the quality of life, and assist in meeting the needs of all family members. It might be helpful for parents of children with spina bifida to talk with one another. One parent might have learned how to address some of the same concerns another parent has. Often, other parents of children with special needs can give advice about good resources for these children.

Remember that the choices of one family might not be best for another family, so it is important that parents understand all options and discuss them with their child's healthcare providers.

School-Aged Children with Spina Bifida

Starting school brings children into regular contact with the larger world. Friendships become important and physical, social, and mental skills develop rapidly during this time. Children who feel good about themselves are more able to resist negative peer pressure and make better choices.

This is an important time for children to become more responsible and independent. This is also a good time to start exploring potential lifetime interests, such as hobbies, music, or sports. Developing independence can be challenging for people affected by spina bifida. It is important to begin working on this process early in childhood.

School

Many children with spina bifida do well in school. But some can experience difficulties, especially children with shunts that are used to treat hydrocephalus. These children often have problems with learning. They might have difficulty paying attention or work slowly, be restless, or lose things. They also might have trouble making decisions. There are activities that children can do at home and at school to help with these problems. Healthcare professionals can provide information about these activities.

Individualized Education Plan

An Individualized Education Plan (IEP) is important because it will help children develop skills at school. Children who participate in special education classes will have an IEP. An IEP is a legal document that lets the school know what kinds of assistance will be needed by a child during the school day. An IEP is created by parents and school personnel, such as a psychologist, teachers, a school nurse, and a physical education teacher, as well as any other professionals that parents think might be helpful.

504 Plan

If a child does not qualify for an IEP, parents can request a 504 Plan be developed for their child at school. Usually, a 504 Plan is used by a general education student who is not eligible for special education services. By law, children may be eligible to have a 504 Plan which lists accommodations related to a child's disability. The 504 Plan accommodations may be needed to give the child an opportunity to perform at the same level as their peers. For example, a 504 Plan may include the child's assistive technology needs, such as using a tablet or laptop computer to take notes and making sure they have a wheelchair accessible environment at school.

Physical Health—What to Expect

No two children with spina bifida are exactly alike. Health issues will be different for each child. Some children have issues that are more severe than other children. With the right care, children born with spina bifida will grow up to reach their full potential.

Mobility and Physical Activity

Children with spina bifida higher on the spine (near the head) might have paralyzed legs and use wheelchairs. Those with spina bifida lower on the spine (near the hips) might have more use of their legs and use crutches, braces, or walkers, or they might be able to walk without these devices.

A physical therapist can work with children, parents, and caregivers to teach them how to exercise the child's legs to increase strength, flexibility, and movement.

Regular physical activity is important for all children, but especially for those with conditions that affect movement, such as spina bifida. The Centers for Disease Control and Prevention (CDC) recommends 60 minutes of physical activity a day. There are many ways for children with spina bifida to be active. For example, they can:

- Engage in active play with friends.
- Roll or walk in the neighborhood.
- Enjoy parks and recreation areas with playgrounds that are accessible for those with disabilities.
- Attend summer camps and recreational facilities that are accessible for those with disabilities.
- Participate in sports activities (for example, swimming) and teams for people with or those without disabilities.

Using the Bathroom

Children with spina bifida often cannot control when they go to the bathroom (incontinence). They also can develop urinary tract infections. It is important to develop a plan for going to the bathroom that works and is as simple as possible. This can lead to increased health, participation, and independence at school and in the home, and avoid embarrassment for children with spina bifida. Healthcare providers can help develop a plan. A tube (catheter) inserted in the child's bladder can help drain urine. In some cases, extra fiber can be added to the diet to keep bowel movements regular. Surgery also might be recommended.

Skin

Children with spina bifida can develop sores, calluses, blisters, and burns on their feet, ankles, and hips. However, they might not know when these develop because they might not be able to feel certain parts of their body.

Parents and caregivers can help protect the child's skin and teach the child how to do this, too, by:

- Checking the child's skin every day for redness, including under braces
- Trying to avoid hot bath water, hot irons, and hot or unpadded seat belt clasps that may cause burns
- Making sure the child wears properly fitting shoes at all times
- Using sunscreen on the child and making sure the child does not stay out in the sun too long
- Making sure the child does not sit or lie in one position for too long

Latex (Natural Rubber) Allergy

Many children with spina bifida are allergic to products that contain latex, or natural rubber. This means they should not use items made of natural rubber. A child with this type of allergy can wear a bracelet to alert other people of the allergy.

Health Checks

Every child needs a primary care provider (for example, a pediatrician, family doctor, or nurse practitioner). The primary healthcare provider will want to make sure that the child is healthy; developing normally; and receiving immunizations against diseases and infections, including the flu.

In addition to seeing a primary healthcare provider, a child with spina bifida will be checked and treated as needed by doctors who specialize in different parts of the body. These doctors might suggest treatments or surgeries to help the child.

These specialists might include:

- An orthopedist, who will work with the child's muscles and bones
- A urologist, who will check the child's kidneys and bladder
- A neurosurgeon, who will check the child's brain and spine

Safety

Safety is an important issue for children with spina bifida. They can be at higher risk for injuries and abuse. As these children become more independent, it is important for their parents and other family members to teach them how to stay safe and what to do if they feel threatened or have been hurt in any way.

Finding Support

Having support and community resources can help increase confidence in managing spina bifida, enhance the quality of life, and assist in meeting the needs of all family members. It might be helpful for parents of children with spina bifida to talk with one another. One parent might have learned how to address some of the same concerns another parent has. Often, other parents of children with special needs can give advice about good resources for these children.

Remember that the choices of one family might not be best for another family, so it is important that parents understand all options and discuss them with their child's healthcare providers.

Adolescents and Teens with Spina Bifida

Many physical, mental, emotional, and social changes are associated with the adolescent and teen years. Teens and adolescents develop their own personalities and interests and want to become more independent.

This transition period can be challenging, especially for people affected by spina bifida. It is important for the parents and caregivers of adolescents and teens with spina bifida to take active steps toward making them independent starting in childhood, so, that by the time they are older, they can develop the necessary skills to help them reach their full potential.

Physical Health

As people with spina bifida mature, they will perform more and more activities themselves. Most teens will dress and bathe themselves, manage their bathroom plans, and move about independently in their homes and communities. They might begin to make their own doctor appointments and continue to participate in updating their own Individualized Education Plan (IEP) or 504 Plan, if they have one. They also should participate in a seating or wheelchair evaluation at least once each year if they use a wheelchair. This evaluation will make sure the wheelchair fits correctly and makes moving as easy as possible.

Mobility and Physical Activity

People with spina bifida higher on the spine (near the head) might have paralyzed legs and use wheelchairs. Those with spina bifida lower on the spine (near the hips) might have more use of their legs and use crutches, braces, or walkers, or they might be able to walk without these devices.

A physical therapist can work with adolescents and teens to teach them how to exercise their legs to increase strength, flexibility, and movement.

Regular physical activity is important for all teens and adolescents, but especially for those with conditions that affect movement, such as spina bifida. The Centers for Disease Control and Prevention (CDC) recommends 60 minutes of physical activity a day. There are many ways for teens and adolescents with spina bifida to be active. For example, they can:

- Engage in physical activities with friends.
- Roll or walk in the neighborhood.
- Lift weights.
- Participate in sports activities (for example, swimming) and on teams for people with and those without disabilities.
- Attend summer camps and recreational facilities that are accessible for those with disabilities.

Sexual Health and Sexuality

Parents and caregivers of adolescents and teens with spina bifida can encourage them to talk with their healthcare professional about sexuality and sexual functioning, contraceptives, and reproductive concerns.

Spina bifida causes nerve damage that can affect sexual functioning. Most people with spina bifida are fertile and can have children.

Folic Acid

Folic acid is very important. All women who can get pregnant should be sure to take 400 micrograms (μg) of folic acid every day, even if they are not planning a pregnancy anytime soon. If a woman has enough folic acid in her body before and during pregnancy, it can help prevent major birth defects of the baby's brain and spine—including spina bifida.

A woman with spina bifida who is planning to get pregnant should talk with her doctor about getting a prescription to take 4,000 μg (4.0 milligrams) of folic acid one month before pregnancy and during early pregnancy.

Mental Health and Well-Being

Overall mental health and well-being are very important for everyone. Mental health is how people think, feel, and act as they cope with life. To be at their best, people need to feel good about their lives and value themselves.

Teens and adolescents with spina bifida might feel isolated from others or have a low self-esteem. This can cause them to become depressed. There are different ways to treat depression. Exercise can be effective. Counseling or medication also might be needed.

Everyone feels worried, anxious, sad, or stressed sometimes. If these feelings do not go away and they interfere with daily life, adolescents and teens should talk with other people, such as a family member, school counselor, or healthcare professional, about their feelings. Depression and other mental-health concerns can be treated.

If you have questions about mental health or where to get mental-health services, your doctor or a licensed mental-health professional in your community may be able to answer those questions or refer you to someone who can. A nearby health facility or your state mental-health agency also may be able to help.

Safety

Safety is important for adolescents and teens with spina bifida. They can be at higher risk for injuries and abuse. As they become more independent, it is important for them to learn how to stay safe and what to do if they feel threatened or have been hurt in any way.

Getting Around

Being safely mobile in their homes and communities will help adolescents and teens become more independent. To do this, they will need to find and use transportation safely.

Many teens with spina bifida have issues that can affect safe driving. A driver rehabilitation evaluation specialist can identify what these issues are and whether modifications to the car would make it accessible for a teen with spina bifida.

Parents and caregivers can also help teens learn to safely use buses, cabs, and ride-hailing services.

Looking to the Future

Teens with spina bifida and their families should begin planning for life after high school. This includes:

- Looking for doctors that treat adults with spina bifida
- Deciding if the person affected by spina bifida will live outside of her or his parents' home
- Choosing work
- Exploring college or vocational school opportunities
- Volunteering in the community
- Having healthy relationships

Planning early can help make the years ahead easier.

Finding Support

Having support and community resources can help increase confidence in managing spina bifida, enhance the quality of life, and assist in meeting the needs of all family members. It might be helpful for parents of children with spina bifida to talk with one another. One parent might have learned how to address some of the same concerns another parent has. Often, other parents of children with special needs can give advice about good resources for these children.

Remember that the choices of one family might not be best for another family, so it is important that parents understand all options and discuss them with their child's healthcare providers.

Young Adults

The transition from adolescence to adulthood can be a time of growth and success, as well as difficulty. For people with spina bifida, it is especially important to begin planning for transitions in childhood, so they are able to lead independent lives as adults.

Young adults affected by spina bifida can face challenges, such as:

- Learning to take care of their own health needs
- Working

- Going to school
- Volunteering
- Finding and using transportation
- Living outside their parents' home
- Developing healthy relationships

Physical Health—What to Expect

Young adults with spina bifida can provide or manage much of their own care. Some examples include:

- Finding new doctors that care for adults affected by spina bifida
- Obtaining medical insurance if they are no longer covered under their parents' health plan
- Talking to healthcare professionals about their condition
- Making doctor appointments
- Ordering or reordering medications and supplies
- Seeking immediate medical help when needed
- Managing their own bathroom plan

Mobility and Physical Activity

Regular physical activity is important for all people, but especially for those with conditions that affect movement, such as spina bifida. The Centers for Disease Control and Prevention (CDC) recommends 60 minutes of physical activity a day. There are many ways for people with spina bifida to be active. For example, they can:

- Roll or walk in the neighborhood.
- Lift weights.
- Participate in sports activities (for example, swimming) and teams for people with or those without disabilities.

Sexual Health and Sexuality

It is important that young adults with spina bifida talk with their healthcare professional about sexuality and sexual functioning, contraceptives, and reproductive concerns.

Spina bifida causes nerve damage that can affect sexual functioning. Most people with spina bifida are fertile and can have children.

Folic Acid

Folic acid is very important. All women who can get pregnant should be sure to take 400 micrograms (μg) of folic acid every day, even if they are not planning a pregnancy anytime soon. If a woman has enough folic acid in her body before and during pregnancy, it can help prevent major birth defects of the baby's brain and spine—including spina bifida.

A woman with spina bifida who is planning to get pregnant should talk with her doctor about getting a prescription to take 4,000 μg (4.0 milligrams) of folic acid one month before pregnancy and during early pregnancy.

Mental Health and Well-Being

Overall mental health and well-being are very important for everyone. Mental health is how people think, feel, and act as they cope with life. To be at their best, people need to feel good about their lives and value themselves.

Young adults with spina bifida might feel isolated from others or have a low self-esteem. This can cause them to become depressed. There are different ways to treat depression. Exercise can be effective. Counseling or medication also might be needed.

Everyone feels worried, anxious, sad or stressed sometimes. If these feelings do not go away and they interfere with daily life, adults should talk with other people, such as a family member or healthcare professional, about their feelings.

If you have questions about mental health or where to get mental-health services, your doctor or a licensed mental-health professional in your community may be able to answer those questions or refer you to someone who can. A nearby health facility or your state mental-health agency also may be able to help.

Getting Around

To be independent, young adults need to be able to find and use transportation safely. Many young adults with spina bifida have issues that can affect safe driving. A driver rehabilitation evaluation specialist can identify whether modifications to the car would make it accessible for a young adult with spina bifida.

Young adults can also learn to find and safely use buses, cabs, and ride-hailing services. As they plan for employment, college, or vocational training, young adults will need to find and use transportation safely.

Being safely mobile in their homes and communities will help young adults with spina bifida be more independent.

Looking to the Future

Many young adults are still getting used to being independent. They may have recently started working, volunteering, going to college, or living independently.

Continuing to plan for the future is very important. This includes setting goals and making a plan for how to achieve them. Unexpected problems can be challenging, and it is important for young adults to not give up and to keep working towards their goals. Sometimes, the goals need to be modified, or they take longer than planned. Either way, planning now will help young adults with spina bifida continue to succeed.

Finding Support

Finding support and resources in the community can increase a young adult's confidence in managing spina bifida, enhance their quality of life, and meet the needs of all family members.

Parents of young adults with spina bifida may want to talk to one another. One parent might have learned how to address some of the same concerns another parent has. Often, parents of other young adults with special needs can give advice and share resources about what's worked for them.

Remember that the choices of one family might not be best for another family, so it is important that parents understand all the options and discuss those with the appropriate healthcare professional.

Section 32.3

Tethered Spinal Cord Syndrome

This section includes text excerpted from "Tethered Spinal Cord Syndrome Information Page," National Institute of Neurological Disorders and Stroke (NINDS), March 27, 2019.

Tethered spinal cord syndrome is a neurological disorder caused by tissue attachments that limit the movement of the spinal cord within the spinal column. Attachments may occur congenitally at the base of the spinal cord or they may develop near the site of an injury to the spinal cord. These attachments cause an abnormal stretching of the spinal cord. The course of the disorder is progressive. In children, symptoms may include lesions, hairy patches, dimples, or fatty tumors on the lower back; foot and spinal deformities; weakness in the legs; low back pain; scoliosis; and incontinence. This type of tethered spinal cord syndrome appears to be the result of improper growth of the neural tube during fetal development and is closely linked to spina bifida. Tethered spinal cord syndrome may go undiagnosed until adulthood, when pain, sensory and motor problems, and loss of bowel and bladder control emerge. This delayed presentation of symptoms is related to the degree of strain placed on the spinal cord over time and may be exacerbated during sports or pregnancy, or may be due to narrowing of the spinal column (stenosis) with age. Tethering may also develop after spinal cord injury and scar tissue can block the flow of fluids around the spinal cord. Fluid pressure may cause cysts to form in the spinal cord, a condition called "syringomyelia." This can lead to additional loss of movement, feeling, or the onset of pain or autonomic symptoms.

Treatment of Tethered Spinal Cord Syndrome

Magnetic resonance imaging (MRI) is often used to evaluate individuals with these symptoms and can be used to diagnose the location of the tethering, lower-than-normal position of the conus medullaris, or presence of a tumor or fatty mass (lipoma). In children, early surgery is recommended to prevent further neurological deterioration. Regular followup is important; retethering may occur in some individuals during periods of rapid growth and may be seen between five to nine years of age. If surgery is not advisable, spinal cord nerve roots may be cut to relieve pain. In adults, surgery to free (detether) the spinal cord can reduce the size and further development of cysts in the cord and may restore some function or alleviate other symptoms. Other treatment is symptomatic and supportive.

Prognosis for Tethered Spinal Cord Syndrome

With treatment, individuals with tethered spinal cord syndrome have a normal life expectancy. However, some neurological and motor impairments may not be fully correctable. Surgery soon after symptoms emerge appears to improve chances for recovery and can prevent further functional decline.

Chapter 33

Spinal Tumors and Cysts

Chapter Contents

Section 33.1—Facts about Spinal Tumors 274

Section 33.2—Syringomyelia 288

Section 33.3—Tarlov Cysts 293

Section 33.1

Facts about Spinal Tumors

This section includes text excerpted from "Brain and Spinal Cord Tumors: Hope through Research," National Institute of Neurological Disorders and Stroke (NINDS), July 6, 2018.

What Are Brain and Spinal Cord Tumors?

Brain and spinal cord tumors are found in the tissue inside the skull or the bony spinal column, which makes up the central nervous system (CNS). A tumor is a mass of cells that forms a new growth or is present at birth (congenital). Tumors occur when genes that regulate cell growth become damaged or mutated, allowing cells to grow and divide out of control. Tumors can form anywhere in the body.

Depending on its type, a growing tumor can kill healthy cells or disrupt their function. It can move or press on sensitive tissue and block the flow of blood and other fluid, causing pain and inflammation. A tumor can also block the normal flow of electricity in the brain or nerve signaling to and from the brain. Some tumors cause no trouble at all.

There are more than 120 types of brain and spinal cord tumors. Some are named by the type of normal cell they most closely resemble (such as glioma) or location (such as meningioma, which form in the lining of the brain and spinal cord). The following overview explains how the CNS works and what happens when a tumor is present.

Overview of the Brain and Spinal Cord

The brain has three major parts:

- **Brain stem**. This lowest part of the brain (above the neck) connects to the spinal cord and relays information between the brain and the body using bundles of long nerves. It controls basic life-sustaining functions, including blood pressure, heartbeat, breathing, consciousness, swallowing, and body temperature.
- **Cerebrum**. This largest and outermost part of the brain processes information from our senses to tell the body how to respond. It controls functions including movement, touch, judgment, learning, speech, emotions, and thinking.
- **Cerebellum**. Located at the lower rear of the brain, above the brainstem, the cerebellum controls balance, helps maintain

equilibrium, and coordinates such complex muscle movements as walking and talking.

The brain's two halves, or hemispheres, use nerve cells (neurons) to speak with each other. Each side of the cerebrum controls movement and function on the other side of the body. In addition, each hemisphere has four sections, called "lobes," which handle different neurological functions.

The frontal lobes manage voluntary movement, such as writing, and let us set and prioritize goals. A frontal lobe tumor can cause changes in personality, intellect, reasoning, and behavior; affect coordination and walking; and cause speech loss. The temporal lobes are linked to perception, memory, and understanding sounds and words. A tumor here might cause speech and hearing problems; blackouts; seizures; or sensations, such as a feeling of fear. The parietal lobes let us simultaneously receive and understand sensations, such as pressure and pain. A parietal lobe tumor might cause difficulty understanding or speaking words, problems with coordination, seizures, and numbness or weakness on one side of the body. The occipital lobes receive and process light and visual images and detect motion. An occipital lobe tumor can affect the field of vision, usually on one side of the view, and how we understand written words.

Three layers of protective tissue (called the "meninges") cover the brain—the thick dura mater (outer layer), the arachnoid (middle), and the pia mater (innermost to the brain).

Brain tumors in infants and adults tend to be located in the cerebrum. Brain tumors in children between 1 and 12 years of age are more commonly found in the cerebellum.

The spinal cord—an extension of the brain—lies protected inside the bony spinal column. It contains bundles of nerves that carry messages between the brain and other parts of the body, such as instructions from the brain to move an arm or information from the skin that signals pain.

A tumor that forms on or near the spinal cord can disrupt communication between the brain and the nerves or restrict the cord's supply of blood. Because the spinal column is narrow, a tumor here—unlike a brain tumor—can cause symptoms on both sides of the body at the same time.

Most spinal cord tumors form below the neck. Symptoms generally strike body areas at the same level or at a level below that of the tumor. For example, a tumor midway along the spinal cord (in the thoracic spine) can cause pain that spreads over the chest and gets worse when the individual coughs, sneezes, or lies down. A tumor that grows in the cervical spine can cause pain that seems to come from the neck or arms, and a tumor that grows in the lower, lumbar spine can trigger back or leg pain.

The three major groups of spinal cord tumor describe where they are found. Extradural tumors grow between the inner surface of the spinal canal and the tough dura mater. Tumors inside the dura (intradural tumors) are further divided into those outside the spinal cord (extramedullary tumors) and those inside the spinal cord (intramedullary tumors). Other descriptors for spinal cord tumors are intrinsic, meaning the tumor forms inside the spinal cord, and extrinsic, where the tumor forms outside of and presses on the cord as it grows.

About Central Nervous System Tumor

What Are Benign and Malignant Tumors?

No matter where they are located in the body, tumors are classified as "benign" or "malignant."

Benign tumors are slow-growing, noncancerous cell masses that have a defined edge and do not spread to other parts of the body. Cells in the tumor are similar to normal cells. Often, these tumors can be removed surgically and usually do not recur.

Malignant, or cancerous, tumors have cells that look different from normal cells. They can quickly invade the surrounding tissue and often have edges that are hard to define, which makes it difficult to remove the entire tumor surgically.

What Are Primary and Metastatic Tumors?

Primary tumors of the CNS are growths that begin in the brain or spinal cord. They can be either malignant or benign and are identified by the types of cells they contain, their location, or both. Most primary CNS tumors occur in adults.

Metastatic, or secondary, tumors in the CNS are caused by cancer cells that break away from the primary tumor that developed in a non-CNS part of the body. These tumors are named after the type of cancer that causes them. Metastatic tumors (also called "metastases") to the brain occur in about one-fourth of all cancers that develop in other parts of the body, such as cancer of the lung, breast, or kidneys, or melanoma, a form of skin cancer. They are more common than primary tumors and occur more often in adults than in children.

Metastatic spine tumors usually form within the bony covering of the spinal column but may also invade the spinal canal from the chest or abdomen.

While cancers elsewhere in the body can easily cause tumors inside the brain and spinal cord, CNS tumors rarely spread outside the nervous system.

What Causes Central Nervous System Tumors

Researchers really do not know why the primary brain and spinal cord tumors develop. Possible causes under investigation include viruses, defective genes, exposure to certain chemicals and other hazardous materials, and immune system disorders. Although smoking, alcohol consumption, and certain dietary habits are associated with some types of cancers, they have not been linked to primary CNS tumors.

In a small number of individuals, CNS tumors may result from specific genetic diseases, such as neurofibromatosis and tuberous sclerosis, or exposure to radiation. It is currently unclear if nonionizing radiation (radio waves) from mobile phone use increases the risk of developing a brain tumor.

Brain and spinal cord tumors are not contagious or, at this time, preventable.

Who Is at Risk?

Anyone can develop a primary CNS tumor, although the risk is very small. Having one or more of the known risk factors does not guarantee that someone will develop a tumor. Brain tumors occur more often in males than in females and are most common in middle-aged to older persons. They also tend to occur more often in children under nine years of age than in other children, and some tumors tend to run in families. Most brain tumors in children are primary tumors.

Other risk factors for developing a primary CNS tumor include race (Caucasians are more likely to develop a CNS tumor than other races) and occupation. Workers in jobs that require repeated contact with ionizing radiation or certain chemicals, including those used to manufacture building supplies or plastics and textiles, have a greater chance of developing a brain tumor.

How Many People Have These Tumors?

More than 359,000 persons in the United States are estimated to be living with a diagnosis of primary brain or central nervous system tumor. More than 195,000 Americans are diagnosed with a brain tumor each year. Brain tumors are the most common form of solid tumor in children.

Spinal cord tumors are less common than brain tumors. Even though they affect people of all ages, spinal cord tumors are most common in young and middle-aged adults. Nearly 3,200 central nervous system tumors are diagnosed each year in children under 20 years of age.

How Are Tumors Graded?

The generally accepted scale for grading CNS tumors was approved by the World Health Organization (WHO) in 1993. Grading is based on the tumor cellular makeup and location. Tumors may also be classified as "low-grade" (slowly growing) or "high-grade" (rapidly growing). Some tumors change grades as they progress, usually to a higher grade, and can become a different type of tumor. The tumor is graded by a pathologist, following a biopsy or during surgery.

Grade I tumors grow slowly and generally do not spread to other parts of the brain. It is often possible to surgically remove an entire grade I benign tumor, but this type of tumor may be monitored periodically, without further treatment.

Grade II tumors also grow slowly, sometimes into surrounding tissue, and can become a higher-grade tumor. Treatment varies according to tumor location and may require chemotherapy, radiation, or surgery, followed by close observation.

Grade III tumors are malignant and can spread quickly into other CNS tissue. Tumor cells will look different than those in surrounding tissue. Aggressive treatment, often using a combination of chemotherapy, radiation, and/or surgery, is required.

Grade IV tumors invade nearby tissue very quickly and are difficult to treat. The cancerous tissue will look very different from surrounding tissue. Aggressive treatment is required.

What Are the Possible Symptoms?

Brain and spinal cord tumors cause many diverse symptoms, which can make detection tricky. Symptoms depend on tumor type, location, size, and rate of growth. Certain symptoms are quite specific because they result from damage to particular areas of the brain. Symptoms generally develop slowly and worsen as the tumor grows.

The most obvious sign of a brain tumor in infants is a rapidly widening head or bulging crown.

Common symptoms of a brain tumor in adults include headaches, seizures, problems with balance or coordination, loss of muscle control, hydrocephalus, and changes in personality or behavior.

Headaches are the most common symptom of a brain tumor. Headaches may progressively worsen, become more frequent or constant, and recur, often at irregular intervals. Headache pain may worsen when coughing, changing posture, or straining and may be severe upon waking.

Seizures can occur with symptoms that may include convulsions, loss of consciousness, or loss of bladder control. Seizures that first start in adulthood (in someone who has not been in an accident or who had an illness that causes seizures) are a key warning sign of brain tumors.

Nausea and vomiting may be more severe in the morning and may accompany headaches. Vision or hearing problems can include blurred or double vision, partial or total loss of vision or hearing, ringing or buzzing sounds, and abnormal eye movements. Personality, behavior, and cognitive changes can include psychotic episodes and problems with speech, language, thinking, and memory.

Motor problems can include weakness or paralysis, lack of coordination, or gradual loss of sensation or movement in an arm or leg. A sudden, marked change in handwriting may be a sign of a tumor. Balance problems can include dizziness, trouble with walking, clumsiness, or loss of the normal control of equilibrium. Hydrocephalus and increased intracranial pressure are caused when a tumor blocks the flow of the cerebrospinal fluid (CSF) that surrounds the brain and spinal cord. Symptoms may include headaches, nausea, and vomiting.

Other symptoms may include endocrine disorders or abnormal hormonal regulation, difficulty swallowing, facial paralysis and sagging eyelid, fatigue, weakened the sense of smell, or disrupted sleep and sleep pattern changes.

Common symptoms of a spinal cord tumor include pain, numbness or sensory changes, motor problems, and loss of muscle control.

Pain can feel as if it is coming from various parts of the body. Back pain may extend to the hips, legs, feet, and arms. This pain is often constant and may be severe. It is often progressive and can have a burning or aching quality. Numbness or sensory changes can include decreased skin sensitivity to temperature and progressive numbness or a loss of sensation, particularly in the legs.

Motor problems and loss of muscle control can include muscle weakness, spasticity (in which the muscles stay stiffly contracted), and impaired bladder and/or bowel control. If untreated, symptoms may worsen to include muscle wasting, decreased muscle strength, an abnormal walking rhythm known as "ataxia," and paralysis.

Symptoms may spread over various parts of the body when one or more tumors extend over several sections of the spinal cord.

How Are Central Nervous System Tumors Diagnosed?

A doctor, usually a neurologist, oncologist, or neuro-oncologist, can confirm a diagnosis of a brain or spinal cord tumor based on a patient's symptoms, personal and family medical history, and results of a physical exam and specialized tests and techniques.

A neurological exam—the first test—assesses movement and sensory skills, hearing and speech, reflexes, vision, coordination and balance, mental status, and changes in mood or behavior, among other abilities. Some tests require a specialist to perform and analyze results.

Diagnostic Imaging

The doctor will order one or more imaging techniques that show extremely detailed views of body structures, including tissues, organs, bones, and nerves. If there is a tumor, diagnostic imaging will confirm the diagnosis and help doctors determine the tumor type, detect swelling and other associated conditions, and, over time, check the results of treatment.

Computed tomography (CT) scan uses X-rays and a computer to produce fast, detailed cross-sectional images or "slices" of organs, bones, and tissues, including a tumor. It is also good for detecting the buildup of calcium, which causes tissue to harden and can develop into a tumor.

Magnetic resonance imaging (MRI) uses a computer, radio waves, and a strong magnetic field to produce two-dimensional slices or a detailed three-dimensional model of the tissue being scanned. MRI takes longer to perform than a CT scan but is more sensitive and gives better pictures of tumors located near the bone.

Both CT and MRI scans for tumors are usually performed before and after administration of a "contrast" agent (such as a dye) that is given into a vein. Many tumors become much brighter on the scan taken after the contrast is given.

Functional MRI (fMRI) creates images of areas of the brain with specific functions, such as movement and language. It can assess brain damage from head injury or degenerative disorders; identify and monitor other neurological disorders, such as stroke; and show the distance between specific brain functions and tumors in particular areas of the brain.

Magnetic resonance spectroscopy (MRS) gives doctors a chemical snapshot of tissues being studied. It uses the MRI scanner magnetic field and radio waves to measure and analyze the chemical makeup of the tissue sample.

Positron emission tomography (PET) provides computer-generated two- and three-dimensional scans of the brain's chemical activity and cellular function. PET traces and measures the brain's use of glucose (sugar, used by the brain for energy) that is attached to small amounts of radioactivity and injected into the bloodstream. Since malignant tissue uses more glucose than normal tissue, it usually shows up on the scan as brighter than surrounding tissue.

Single photon emission computed tomography (SPECT) studies blood flow to tissue. Certain tumors grow new blood vessels to increase their supply of blood and nutrients. A radioactive isotope is injected intravenously and traced as it travels into the skull. A sophisticated computer processes and stacks the data into a detailed three-dimensional image of activity within the brain.

Angiography (or arteriogram) can distinguish certain types of tumors that have a characteristic pattern of blood vessels and blood flow. A dye that deflects X-rays is injected into a major blood vessel, and a series of X-rays is taken as the dye flows to the brain. In many situations, angiography has been replaced by noninvasive tests, such as CT and MRI.

Laboratory Tests

Testing blood, urine, and other substances can provide clues about the tumor and monitor levels of therapeutic drugs.

Additional tests may include an electroencephalogram, or EEG, which monitors brain activity through the skull (tumors can disrupt the normal flow of brain wave activity and cause seizures); CSF analysis, in which a small amount of the cerebrospinal fluid is removed by a special needle and examined for abnormal cells or unusual levels of various compounds that suggest a brain or spinal cord tumor; and magnetoencephalography (MEG), which studies brain function by measuring the magnetic field generated by nerve cells in the brain.

CSF fluid analysis should be performed with extreme caution on individuals with very large brain tumors.

Diagnosing the distinct type of brain tumor is often difficult. Individuals should consider asking their primary care physician or oncologist for a second opinion, particularly from a neuro-oncologist or neurosurgeon, as there may be new information available, and some tumors can change grade or recur. Even a second opinion that confirms the original diagnosis can help people better prepare for their care and treatment.

How Are Brain and Spinal Cord Tumors Treated?

A specialized team of doctors advises and assists individuals throughout treatment and rehabilitation. These doctors may include:

- A neurologist is a specialist in nervous system disorders.
- An oncologist is a specialist in cancer.
- A neuro-oncologist is a neurologist or oncologist who specializes in nervous system tumors.
- A neuroradiologist is a doctor trained in reading diagnostic imaging results who specializes in the CNS.
- A pathologist is a clinical physician who diagnoses diseases of tissues or cells using a variety of laboratory tests.
- A neurosurgeon is a brain or spinal cord surgeon.
- A radiation oncologist is a doctor who specializes in using radiation to treat individuals with cancer.

This team will recommend a treatment plan based on the tumor's location, type, size, and aggressiveness, as well as on the individual's medical history, age, and general health.

Initial treatment for a CNS tumor may involve a variety of drugs, including anticonvulsants to treat seizures, pain medications, steroids or other anti-inflammatory drugs to reduce swelling and improve blood flow, antidepressants to treat anxiety or ease depression that might occur following a tumor diagnosis, and drugs to fight nausea caused by various treatments.

Malignant tumors require some form of treatment, while some small benign tumors may need only periodic monitoring. The three standard treatment options for malignant CNS tumors are neurosurgery, radiation therapy, and chemotherapy. Some patients may receive a combination of treatments.

Neurosurgery

Surgery is usually the first step in treating an accessible tumor—one that can be removed without unacceptable risk of neurological damage. Surgery is aimed at removing all or as much tumor as possible (called "resecting" or "excising") and can often slow the worsening of neurological function.

An inaccessible or inoperable tumor is one that cannot be removed surgically because of the risk of severe nervous system damage during the operation. These tumors are frequently located deep within the brain or near vital structures, such as the brain stem.

A biopsy is sometimes performed to help doctors determine how to treat a tumor. A brain biopsy involves surgically removing a small part of the skull to sample the tumor tissue. Biopsies can sometimes be performed by a needle inserted through a small hole. A small piece of tissue remains in the hollow needle when it is removed from the body. A pathologist will stain and examine the tissue for certain changes that signal cancer and grade it to reflect the degree of malignancy.

If the sample is cancerous, the surgeons will remove as much of the tumor as possible. For some primary brain tumors, it is not possible to surgically remove all malignant cells. Malignant brain tumors commonly recur from cells that have spread from the original tumor mass into the surrounding brain tissue. In contrast, many benign tumors and secondary metastatic tumors can be completely removed surgically.

In some cases, a surgeon may need to insert a shunt into the skull to drain any dangerous buildup of CSF caused by the tumor. A shunt is a flexible plastic tube that is used to divert the flow of CSF from the central nervous system to another part of the body, where it can be absorbed as part of the normal circulatory process.

Fortunately, research has led to advances in neurosurgery that make it possible for doctors to completely remove many tumors that were previously thought to be inoperable. These new techniques and tools let neurosurgeons operate within the tight, vulnerable confines of the CNS. Some tools used in the operating room include a surgical microscope, the endoscope (a small viewing tube attached to a video camera), and miniature precision instruments that allow surgery to be performed through a small incision in the brain or spine.

Intraoperative MRI uses a special type of MRI to provide a real-time evaluation of the surgery. Constantly updated images that are provided during surgery let doctors see how much tumor material has been removed. Intraoperative MRI can also help doctors choose the best surgical approaches and monitor any complications during surgery.

Navigation equipment used in computer-guided, or stereotactic, neurosurgery gives doctors a precise, three-dimensional map of an individual's spine or brain as the operation progresses. A computer uses preoperative diagnostic images of the individual to reduce the risk of damage to surrounding tissue.

Intraoperative nerve monitoring tests, such as evoked potentials, use real-time recordings of nerve cell activity to determine the role of specific nerves and monitor brain activity as the surgery progresses. Small electrodes are used to stimulate a nerve and measure its electrical response (or evoked potential). Some surgeries may be done while the individual is awake under monitored anesthesia care, rather than under general anesthesia. This allows doctors to monitor the individual's speech and motor functions as a tumor is being removed.

A possible side effect of surgery is swelling around the site of the tumor, and this can be treated with steroids. Bleeding into the tumor site or infection are other serious risks of brain surgery.

In the case of metastatic tumors, doctors usually treat the original cancer. However, if there are only one or two metastases to the brain or if a metastatic tumor causes serious disability or pain, doctors may recommend surgery—even if the original cancer has not been controlled.

Surgery may be the beginning and end of your treatment if the biopsy shows a benign tumor. If the tumor is malignant, doctors often recommend additional treatment, including radiation and chemotherapy, or one of several experimental treatments.

Radiation Therapy

Radiation therapy usually involves repeated doses of X-rays or other forms of radiation to kill cancer cells or keep them from multiplying. When successful, this therapy shrinks the tumor mass but does not actually remove it. Radiation therapy can be used to treat surgically inaccessible tumors or tumor cells that may remain following surgery.

Depending on tumor type and stage, radiation treatment might be delivered externally, using focused beams of energy or charged particles that are directed at the tumor, or internally, using a surgically implanted device. The stronger the radiation, the deeper it can penetrate to the target site. Healthy cells may also be damaged by radiation therapy, but most are able to repair themselves, while the damaged tumor cells cannot.

A radiation oncologist will explain the therapy and how much radiation is needed. Treatment often begins a week after surgery and may continue for several weeks. Depending on tumor type and location, individuals may be able to receive a modified form of therapy to lessen damage to healthy cells and improve the overall treatment.

Externally-delivered radiation therapy poses no risk of radioactivity to the patient or family and friends. Types of external radiation therapy include:

- Whole brain radiation is generally used to shrink multiple cancerous tumors, rather than to target individual tumors. It may be given as the sole form of treatment or in advance of other forms of radiation therapy and microsurgery. Whole brain radiation is generally used for metastatic tumors and rarely for primary tumors.
- Conventional external beam radiation aims a uniform dose of high-energy radiation at the tumor and surrounding tissue from outside the body. It is used to treat large tumors or those that may have spread into surrounding tissue.
- Three-dimensional conformal radiotherapy (3D-CRT) uses diagnostic imaging to prepare an accurate, computer-generated three-dimensional image of the tumor and surrounding tissue. The computer then coordinates and sends multiple beams of radiation to the tumor's exact shape, sparing nearby organs and surrounding tissue.
- Intensity-modulated radiation therapy (IMRT) is similar to 3D-CRT but varies the intensity of the hundreds of individual radiation beams to deliver more precise doses to the tumor or to specific areas within it. IRMT can provide a highly effective dose of radiation to the tumor, with less exposure to surrounding tissue.
- Hyperfractionation involves giving two or more smaller amounts of radiation a day instead of a larger, single dose. It can deliver more radiation to certain tumors and reduce damage to normal cells.
- Radiosurgery is usually a one-time treatment involving a large amount of sharply focused radiation that is aimed at the brain tumor. Stereotactic radiosurgery uses computer imaging to direct precisely focused radiation into the tumor from multiple angles. It does not actually cut into the person but, similar to other forms of radiation therapy, harms a tumor cell's ability to grow and divide. Stereotactic radiosurgery is commonly used to treat surgically inaccessible tumors. It also may be used

at the end of conventional radiation treatment. Two common stereotactic radiosurgery procedures are:

- Linear-accelerated radiosurgery (LINAC) uses radar-like technology to prepare and fire a single beam of high-energy X-rays into the tumor. Also called "high linear-energy-transfer radiation," LINAC forms the beam to match the tumor's shape, avoiding surrounding tissue. A special machine that rotates around the head then fires a uniform dose of radiation into the tumor.
- Gamma knife® radiosurgery focuses more than 200 beams of gamma radiation into one intersecting beam that is fired into the tumor. It also uses computer imaging to prepare a model of the tumor. This single treatment takes between 1 and 4 hours and is often recommended for inaccessible or hard to treat tumors.

Both procedures may be given on an outpatient basis, but an overnight stay in the hospital is often recommended.

- Proton beam therapy directs a beam of high-energy protons directly at the tumor site, leaving surrounding healthy tissue and organs intact. It is best used to treat tumors that are solid and have not spread to other parts of the body. Proton beam therapy can be used as a stand-alone treatment or in combination with chemotherapy or as followup to surgery.
- Internal tumor radiation therapy, also called "brachytherapy" or "interstitial radiation therapy," involves placing a small amount of radioactive material into or near the tumor (or its cavity, if the tumor has been surgically removed). In most cases, the radiation is inserted at the time of surgery or using imaging and a catheter. The radiation may be left in place for several days and, if more than one treatment is needed, the doctor may leave the catheter in place for a longer period.

Individuals may need to be hospitalized for a few days following this procedure, as the radiation may extend outside their body and could possibly harm others. The radiation becomes less active each day until it is safe for individuals who have been treated to be around others.

Side effects of radiation therapy vary from person to person and are usually temporary. They typically begin about two weeks after treatment starts and may include fatigue, nausea, vomiting, reddened or sore skin in the area receiving treatment, headache, hearing loss, problems with sleep, and hair loss (although the hair usually grows back once the treatment has stopped). Radiation therapy in young children, particularly those children three years of age or younger, can cause problems with learning, processing information, thinking, and growing.

Chemotherapy

Chemotherapy uses powerful drugs to kill cancer cells or stop them from growing or dividing. These drugs are usually given by pill or injection and travel through the body to the brain, or they can be inserted surgically using dissolvable wafers that have been soaked in a chemotherapeutic drug. These wafers slowly release a high concentrate of the drug to kill any remaining malignant cells. Chemotherapy may also be given to kill cancer cells in the spinal column.

Chemotherapy is given in cycles to more effectively harm cancer cells and give normal cells time to recover from any damage. The oncologist will base the treatment on the type of cancer, drug(s) to be used, the frequency of administration, and the number of cycles needed.

Individuals might receive chemotherapy to shrink the tumor before surgery (called "neo-adjuvant therapy"), in combination with radiation therapy, or after radiation treatment (called "adjuvant therapy") to destroy any remaining cancer cells. Metronomic therapy involves giving continuous low-dose chemotherapy to block mechanisms that stimulate the growth of new blood vessels needed to feed the tumor. Chemotherapy is also used to treat CNS lymphoma and inaccessible tumors or tumors that do not respond to radiation therapy.

Not all tumors are vulnerable to the same anticancer drugs, so a person's treatment may include a combination of drugs. Common CNS chemotherapeutics include temozolomide, carmustine (also called "BCNU"), lomustine, tamoxifen, carboplatin, methotrexate, procarbazine, and vincristine. Individuals should be sure to discuss all options with their medical team.

Side effects of chemotherapy may include hair loss, nausea, digestive problems, reduced bone marrow production, and fatigue. The treatment can also harm normal cells that are growing or dividing at the same time, but these cells usually recover and problems stop once the treatment has ended.

Alternative and complementary approaches may help tumor patients better cope with their diagnosis and treatment. Some of these therapies, however, may be harmful if used during or after cancer treatment and should be discussed with a doctor beforehand. Common approaches include nutritional and herbal supplements, vitamins, special diet, and mental or physical techniques to reduce stress.

What Is the Prognosis?

Each person is different. Prognosis depends greatly on prompt diagnosis and treatment, the individual's age and general health, whether the tumor is malignant or benign, tumor size and location, tumor grade, and response to therapy. An individual whose entire tumor has been removed successfully may recover completely. Generally, prognosis is poorer in very young children and in older individuals. Rehabilitation and counseling can help patients and family members better cope with the disorder and improve quality of life (QOL).

Continued monitoring and long-term follow-up is advised, as many tumors resist treatment and tend to recur.

Normal tissue and nerves that may have been damaged or traumatized by the tumor or its treatment will need time to heal. Some posttreatment symptoms will disappear over time. Physical therapy can help people regain motor skills, muscle strength, and balance. Some individuals may need to relearn how to swallow or speak if the brain's cognitive areas have been affected. Occupational therapy can teach people new ways to perform tasks. Supportive care can help people manage any pain and other symptoms.

Section 33.2

Syringomyelia

This section includes text excerpted from "Syringomyelia Fact Sheet," National Institute of Neurological Disorders and Stroke (NINDS), July 6, 2018.

What Is Syringomyelia?

Syringomyelia is a disorder in which a fluid-filled cyst (called a "syrinx") forms within the spinal cord. This syrinx can get bigger and elongate over time, damaging the spinal cord and compressing and injuring the nerve fibers that carry information to the brain and from the brain to the rest of the body.

A watery liquid known as "cerebrospinal fluid" (CSF) normally surrounds and protects the brain and spinal cord. CSF also fills connected cavities within the center of the brain called the "ventricles," which continue to a small central canal that runs the length of the spinal cord. When a person has syringomyelia, this fluid collects within the tissue of the spinal cord, expands the central canal, and forms a syrinx. Generally, a syrinx develops when the normal flow of CSF fluid around the spinal cord or lower brain stem is disturbed. When syrinxes affect the brain stem, the condition is called "syringobulbia."

What Causes Syringomyelia

Syringomyelia may have several possible causes, but most cases are associated with Chiari malformation—an abnormal condition in which brain tissue extends through the hole at the bottom of the skull (foramen magnum) and into the spinal canal, obstructing the flow of CSF. Syringomyelia may also be caused by spinal cord injuries, spinal cord tumors, and damage caused by inflammation around the spinal cord. In some cases, the cause is unknown (idiopathic).

What Are the Forms of Syringomyelia?

There are two major forms of syringomyelia.

- **Congenital syringomyelia (also known as "communicating syringomyelia").** In most cases, syringomyelia is caused by a Chiari malformation which may allow a syrinx to develop, most often in the cervical spine (neck) region. Symptoms usually begin between the ages of 25 and 40. People with congenital syringomyelia may also have hydrocephalus, a buildup of excess CSF in the brain with an enlargement of the cerebral ventricles. Straining or coughing can force CSF into the ventricles, causing the person to develop a headache or even lose consciousness (so called "cough syncope"). In addition, they may have a disorder called "arachnoiditis"—an inflammation of the arachnoid, one of the three membranes that surrounds the spinal cord.
- **Acquired syringomyelia (also known as "primary spinal syringomyelia" or "noncommunicating syringomyelia").** Causes of acquired syringomyelia include spinal cord injury (SCI), meningitis (an inflammation of brain and spinal cord

membranes usually caused by an infection), arachnoiditis, tethered cord syndrome (a condition that is present at birth that causes the spinal cord to abnormally attach to the tissues in the lower spine, limiting its movement), a spinal cord tumor, and bleeding into the cord (hemorrhage).

What Are Symptoms of Syringomyelia?

Symptoms of damage to the spinal cord vary among individuals according to where the syrinx forms, how large it is, and how long it extends. Symptoms develop slowly over time and may occur on one or both sides of the body. Sometimes coughing and straining can trigger symptoms, but they do not cause syringomyelia. Symptoms may include:

- Pain
- Progressive weakness in the arms and legs
- Stiffness in the back, shoulders, neck, arms, or legs
- Headaches
- Loss of sensitivity to pain or hot and cold, especially in the hands
- Numbness or tingling
- Imbalance
- Loss of bowel and bladder control
- Problems with sexual function
- Curvature of the spine (scoliosis). This may be the only symptom in children.

How Is Syringomyelia Diagnosed?

To diagnose syringomyelia, a physician will review the person's medical history and perform a physical exam, focusing on neurological function. The physician will also likely order imaging of the spine or brain. Sometimes, syringomyelia may be found during diagnostic imaging for another disorder.

Magnetic resonance imaging (MRI) is the most reliable way to diagnose syringomyelia. Computer-generated radio waves and a powerful magnetic field produce clear images of the brain and spinal cord. Using this test, a physician will be able to determine if there is a syrinx in the spine or another abnormality, such as a tumor.

In some cases, a dynamic MRI may be performed to show the flow of fluid around the spinal cord and within the syrinx. Many images are taken in rapid succession to provide such dynamic views. A dye or contrast agent may be injected to enhance the MRI images.

How Is Syringomyelia Treated?

The type of treatment for syringomyelia depends on the severity and progression of an individual's symptoms.

Monitoring

In the absence of symptoms, syringomyelia is usually not treated. In addition, a physician may recommend not treating the condition in individuals of advanced age or in cases where there is no progression of symptoms. However, people should be carefully monitored by a neurologist or neurosurgeon, as symptoms can worsen over time. Individuals may also want to avoid activities that involve straining (e.g., lifting heavy objects, jumping) since these actions can trigger symptoms. People with an associated Chiari malformation are especially apt to experience headache with straining.

Surgery

Surgery is usually recommended for individuals with symptomatic or progressive syringomyelia. There are two general forms of treatment: restoration of normal CSF flow around the spinal cord and direct drainage of the syrinx. The type of treatment depends on what is causing the symptoms.

- **Treating the Chiari malformation**. The main goal of Chiari surgery is to provide more space at the base of the skull and upper neck. This reduces pressure on the brain and spinal cord and restores the normal flow of CSF. Surgery can allow the syrinx to drain, sometimes becoming smaller or even disappearing entirely. Symptoms may improve even if the syrinx remains the same size or is reduced only slightly. Individuals should get treated sooner rather than later, since delaying treatment can cause irreversible spinal cord damage. Syringomyelia can recur after surgery, making additional operations necessary.

- **Preventing a syrinx from forming or expanding after an injury**. In the case of trauma-related syringomyelia, the primary strategy is to prevent a syrinx from developing or growing in the first place. This somewhat controversial procedure (called "expansive duraplasty") is done in a surgical operation on the spine that involves removing scar tissue around the spinal cord and sometimes adding a patch to expand the "dura," the membrane that surrounds the spinal cord. By clearing and expanding the space around the spinal cord, the normal flow of CSF may be restored.
- **Removing the obstruction**. Surgical removal of obstructions, such as scar tissue, bone from the spinal canal, or tumors, can help restore the normal flow of CSF. If a tumor is causing syringomyelia, removing the tumor almost always eliminates the syrinx. Occasionally, radiation may also be used to shrink the tumor.
- **Draining the syrinx**. Especially if there is no associated Chiari malformation or tumor, it may be necessary to drain the syrinx. This is usually done in cases where the syrinx is growing, or the cause of the CSF obstruction cannot be identified. To perform this procedure, a surgeon inserts a drain called a "stent" or "shunt." A stent consists of a small tube that is inserted into the syrinx fluid and allows fluid from within the cord to drain into the space just outside the spinal cord. Similarly, a shunt consists of a flexible tube and a valve that drains the syrinx fluid into another part of the body, usually the abdomen. By draining the syrinx, both of these procedures can halt the progression of symptoms and relieve headache. However, these procedures carry the risk of spinal cord injury, infection, or bleeding, and may not help all individuals.

Section 33.3

Tarlov Cysts

This section includes text excerpted from "Tarlov Cysts," Genetic and Rare Diseases Information Center (GARD), National Center for Advancing Translational Sciences (NCATS), August 9, 2018.

What Are Tarlov Cysts?

Tarlov cysts are fluid-filled sacs that most commonly are found at the base of the spine (the sacrum). They affect the nerve roots in the sacrum, whereas the spinal nerve roots are embedded within the cyst wall or within the cyst cavity.

What Are the Symptoms of Tarlov Cysts?

A person can have one Tarlov cyst or multiple cysts, and symptoms may or may not be present, depending on the size and location of the cyst(s). In general, the larger the cyst is, the more likely it is to cause symptoms. In some cases, a cyst begins to cause symptoms following trauma or in response to a buildup of cerebrospinal fluid (CSF). Examples of symptoms caused by a Tarlov cyst include pain when moving or changing position (especially in the buttocks or lower back), muscle weakness, headaches, impaired reflexes, numbness or other sensation abnormalities, loss of bladder or bowel control, sexual dysfunction (impotence), or other neurologic problems. Symptoms generally occur in the area of the body served by the involved nerves.

How Is a Tarlov Cyst Diagnosed?

Diagnosing a Tarlov cyst can take a long time because there is limited awareness among primary care physicians, and symptoms are similar to those of many other disorders or health problems. In some cases, a person may be misdiagnosed as having herniated discs, arachnoiditis, or gynecological conditions (in females). The diagnosis may ultimately be made following an magnetic resonance imaging (MRI) and/or computerized tomography (CT) myelogram due to pain, or sometimes following tests performed by a urologist due to bladder problems. The exact cause of Tarlov cysts is not currently known.

What Is the Treatment for Tarlov Cysts?

While there is no standard accepted treatment for individuals with symptomatic Tarlov cysts, many different therapies have been tried. Tarlov cysts may be drained and shunted to relieve pressure and pain, but relief is often only temporary and fluid buildup in the cysts will recur. Corticosteroid injections may also temporarily relieve pain. Non-steroidal anti-inflammatory drugs (NSAIDs) may be prescribed to treat chronic pain and inflammation. Injecting the cysts with fibrin glue (a combination of naturally occurring substances based on the clotting factor in blood) may provide temporary relief of pain. Microsurgical removal of the cyst wall may be an option in select individuals who do not respond to conservative treatments and who continue to experience pain or progressive neurological damage.

Transcutaneous electrical nerve stimulation (TENS) has been proven useful for some in pain management. TENS devices deliver electrical impulses through the skin to the nerves to control pain. Unlike medications and topical ointments, TENS does not have any known side effects, other than skin irritation from the electrodes in some patients.

A recent review analyzed the different surgical options, including the following:

- Sacral laminectomy with microsurgical cyst fenestration and cyst imbrication
- Sacral laminectomy with resection of the sacral cyst
- Microsurgical excision of the cyst, along with duraplasty or plication of the cyst
- Release of the valve and imbrication of the sacral cysts with laminectomies
- Total or partial cyst wall removal, arranging the remaining nerve sheath, and repairing the local defect with muscle, gelfoam, and fibrin glue
- Removal of the cyst and closure of defect by fibrin glue
- Microscopic cyst resection and closure of defect by fibrin glue
- Microsurgical fenestration from the cyst to the thecal sac
- Fenestration of the cyst and closure of the opening by stitches and glue

- Cyst remodeling around the root using titanium clips
- Cyst excision and occlusion of its neck

The authors of this review concluded that the best results are obtained with the complete removal of the cyst and closure of the defect by fibrin glue, microscopic cyst resection, and closure of the defect by fibrin glue, or cyst removal with closure of its neck.

What Is the Prognosis for a Tarlov Cyst?

The long-term outlook (prognosis) varies from person to person, depending on the severity of symptoms and effectiveness of treatment. Following surgery, some people have considerable relief of pain, while others have no change in symptoms. In some cases, surgery causes different symptoms or worsens existing symptoms. Residual symptoms following treatment may require continued pain management and changes in lifestyle. If left untreated, a Tarlov cyst can cause permanent neurological damage.

Chapter 34

Cervical Disc Disease

Cervical disc disease is a condition in which the nerves and spinal cord are compressed. In the cervical spine, there are six gel-like discs in between the cervical vertebrae; each disc acts as a shock absorber and prevents cervical vertebrae rubbing against each other while you move. Aging and other factors cause these discs to lose water content, collapse, and, sometimes, break. The structure of the vertebrae is affected when the disc deteriorates. These structural changes put unwanted pressure on the cervical spine, causing pain and a loss of function.

Causes and Symptoms

The aging process, severe trauma, and other activities, such as gymnastics, weight lifting, and smoking, seem to lead to cervical disc disease. Doctors suspect that genetic inheritance and autoimmune and environmental conditions may also be a cause of this disease.

- Symptoms of cervical disc disease are:
- Stiffness in the neck
- Neck pain
- Numbness
- Tingling in the hands and arms

- Weakness
- Pain in the back of the shoulder
- Decreased flexibility

Diagnosis

The presence of cervical disc disease is determined by your doctor after they assess your flexibility, range of motion, and strength of your neck, legs, and arms. The doctor provides a treatment plan based upon the physical examination.

Your doctor orders diagnostic tests after the physical examination to confirm the diagnosis of cervical disc disease. The diagnostic tests may include:

- **X-rays** help identify any misalignment of the bones in the neck region. It also detects bone spurs and degenerative bones.
- **Magnetic resonance imaging (MRI)** scans are helpful to see in-depth and higher quality images of soft tissues, bones, nerves, discs, and the spinal cord.
- **Computed tomography (CT)** scans show a more detailed image of the neck's anatomy and from different angles. The CT scans are taken in conjunction with a myelogram in order to obtain better results.
- A **myelogram** is a type of detailed CT scan that utilizes a contrast dye to help differentiate bones and nerves more clearly than other scans.
- **Electromyography (EMG)** is used to determine the muscles' impulses during contraction and rest. The EMG tests are used for nerve conduction studies (NCS) to check if the nerves in the spinal cord are working properly.

Treatment

Nonsurgical Treatment

Most often, nonsurgical treatment is chosen for cervical disc disease in hope to relieve pain and modify muscle activities. Nonsurgical treatments include the following:

- **Physical therapy** has a set of specific exercises that focus on strengthening strained or weakened muscles. Sometimes, physical therapy includes posture therapy, in which the patient has to stretch their neck muscles by using traction. The time period for physical therapy varies upon the condition of the patient's disc disease. On average, the duration of physical therapy lasts from six to eight weeks, with two to three sessions per week.

- **Medications** include over-the-counter (OTC) and prescription drugs that ease and reduce the patient's neck pain.
- A **soft cervical collar** is suggested by a doctor to decrease the pain and relax the muscles around the neck. These collars are worn for a short time, since long-term usage may weaken the muscles around the neck.
- **Heat and cold therapy** around the neck is conducted by a doctor or therapist in order to relieve the symptoms.
- **Manual manipulation** is when the cervical spine is adjusted in hope of improving a patient's range of motion and/or reducing their pain. This treatment is completed by a chiropractor or qualified health professional.

Surgical Treatment

If physical therapy and medications do not help, a surgical treatment is considered. Surgery is done to lessen pain and weakness and prevent further damage. The two common types of surgical treatment for cervical disc disease are:

- **Anterior cervical discectomy and fusion (ACDF).** This procedure is done in the front of the neck. It includes the removal of the damaged disc, the decompression of the nerve root, and the insertion of a cage or bone graft to maintain height and stability.
- **Cervical artificial disc replacement.** This procedure involves the removal of the damaged disc and replacing it with an artificial disc. The goal of this surgical treatment is to preserve motion at the spine level.

After the surgery, the doctor will restrict you from doing certain physical activities, such as lifting heavy objects, general housework, etc. Once the neck is healed, the physiotherapists will teach strengthening and flexibility exercises, along with proper postures while standing, sitting, and lifting objects.

Physical exercises and postures can help in reducing pain during daily activities. Consult your doctor before taking any medicines to reduce pain as it may cause side effects.

References

1. Shim, John H. "Cervical Degenerative Disc Disease," SPINE-health, October 6, 2016.
2. "Cervical Degenerative Disc Disease—Spinal Cord and Nerve Compression," The Spine Diagnostic & Pain Treatment Center, n.d.
3. "Cervical Disc Degeneration Conditions," Medtronic, November 6, 2016.
4. "Cervical Disc Disease," Baylor Scott & White Neurosurgery Associates, June 21, 2017.

Chapter 35

Other Musculoskeletal Conditions of Back and Neck

Chapter Contents

Section 35.1—Sacroiliac Joint Syndrome 302
Section 35.2—Spondylolisthesis... 305
Section 35.3—Torticollis 309
Section 35.4—Chronic Myofascial Pain 312
Section 35.5—Klippel-Feil Syndrome 315

Section 35.1

Sacroiliac Joint Syndrome

Sacroiliac joints (SI joints) are a critical linkage system that is situated between the two iliac bones (large pelvic bones) and the sacrum (tailbone). The sacrum is the triangular shaped bone located in the lower spine. Unlike other vertebrae in spine, these five vertebrae are fused together and do not move. There are two sacroiliac joints that connect the spine to the pelvis, and these joints are responsible for support and stability. Ligaments and muscles in the SI joints provide enough flexibility to allow for four degrees of rotation and 2mm for translation.

When your SI joints are not moving normally because of stiffness or overexertion, it can result in sacroiliac (SI) joint pain. SI joint pain is felt in the lower back and the buttocks. This pain can mimic other conditions, such as a herniated disc or hip problem.

Types of Sacroiliac Joint Syndrome

There are two main types of sacroiliac joint syndrome, and they depend upon the severity of pain.

- **Acute pain,** lasts from several days to weeks
- **Chronic pain,** persists more than three months

Causes of Sacroiliac Joint Syndrome

The most common causes of SI joint pain are:

- Aging
- Pregnancy
- Childbirth
- High-energy trauma, such as falling on the buttocks, an accident, a work injury, etc.

Previous lower back surgery can also lead to this condition. People who have arthritis are more likely to have this condition. If someone has one leg that is longer or weaker than their other leg, this uneven movement may also cause SI pain.

SI joint syndrome occurs when the ligaments are damaged or torn; this condition causes inflammation in the joints, which disrupts them.

Symptoms of Sacroiliac Joint Syndrome

The symptoms of SI joint pain are as follows:

- Lower back pain
- Pain in the hips, buttocks, and/or groin
- Numbness and tingling in the buttocks and/or back
- Stiffness in the lower back
- Swelling in the SI joint
- Difficulties with sitting, sleeping, standing, walking, or climbing stairs

Diagnosis of Sacroiliac Joint Syndrome

Diagnosis of SI joint syndrome begins with a review of your medical history and is followed by a physical examination. The medical history includes information about your diet, sleeping habits, any previous injuries and/or surgeries, and other activities in your daily life. The physical examination is done using orthopedic provocation tests, such as:

- **Distraction test,** which includes applying pressure on the front part of the hip while lying face up.
- **Sacral thrust test,** which involves applying pressure on the back of the hip while lying face down
- **Patrick test,** which involves pressing the heel of the foot, while crossing one leg over the other. The doctor also presses the top knee to check for the development of pain in the SI joints.
- **Palpation test,** which involves pressing the thumb into each side of the SI joints in order to find any tenderness over the problematic SI joint.

Imaging tests are conducted after the physical examination. Tests, such as X-rays, magnetic resonance imaging (MRI), and computerized tomography (CT), are taken to confirm the syndrome. Sacroiliac joint injection, also known as "sacroiliac joint block," consists of injecting a numbing solution (bupivacaine or lidocaine) into the SI joint. If the pain is relieved after this procedure, the patient will be diagnosed with SI joint syndrome.

Treatments of Sacroiliac Joint Syndrome

Nonsurgical Procedure

The main goal of the treatment is to relieve pain and to restore motion in the joint. Most often, SI joint syndrome is treated by nonsurgical procedures. These procedures may include:

- **Physical therapy:** This includes physical exercises that are recommended by your physiotherapist, and they mostly focus on your joint movement. These exercises reduce pain and help with the motion of the tight sacroiliac joint.
- **Manual manipulation:** An osteopathic doctor, chiropractor, or other qualified health professional adjusts the SI joint by using controlled and sudden forces. The goal of this treatment is to reduce joint fixation and increase mobility of the joint.
- **Usage of braces:** Pelvic braces are used around the hip when the SI joint is too loose. The braces stabilize the area and provide support to the SI joint.
- **Medications:** Over-the-counter (OTC) medicines and anti-inflammatory drugs (naproxen or ibuprofen) can help with mild or moderate pain relief.
- **Sacroiliac joint injections:** A local anesthetic, in conjunction with anti-inflammatory drugs, is injected into the SI joint to reduce pain for a short period of time.
- **Massages:** Treatments such as dry needling, trigger point therapy, and massages can ease the SI joint pain.

Surgical Procedure

Surgical treatment is chosen if nonsurgical treatment fails to provide pain relief for a long period of time. SI joint fusion is the standard surgical procedure for SI joint syndrome. This surgery eliminates movement at the SI joint by fusing together the two sides of the joint (sacrum and ilium). This fusion is usually achieved with the use of screws or rods, as well as a bone graft across the SI joint.

The risk involved in SI joint fusion is the possibility that the procedure will not completely alleviate pain in the SI joint and/or will result in unsuccessful fusion. The surgery may even put pressure on the lower back, causing more pain and discomfort.

Prognosis of Sacroiliac Joint Syndrome

Physical exercises and therapies may be followed in order to alleviate the pain caused in the sacroiliac joint. Wearing hip braces can also help support and stabilize the joint. Maintain a proper posture as recommended by your doctor or physiotherapist while sitting, standing, walking, sleeping, and lifting weights. Weight reduction can prevent excessive stress of the SI joint.

References

1. “Sacroiliac Joint Pain,” Mayfield Brain & Spine, December 4, 2004.
2. Yeomans, Steven G. “Surgical Treatment for Sacroiliac Joint Pain,” SPINE-health, February 7, 2018.
3. “Sacroiliac Joint Syndrome,” Physiopedia, January 1, 2014.
4. Miller, John. “Sacroiliac Joint Pain,” Physio Works, April 18, 2019.
5. Burt Driver, Catherine. “Sacroiliac Joint Dysfunction (SI Joint Pain),” MedicineNet, November 2, 2007.

Section 35.2

Spondylolisthesis

Spondylolisthesis is a spinal condition, in which one vertebra slips forward onto the vertebra directly below it. It most often occurs in the lower back, but it can also happen in the mid- or upper back, or at the back of your neck.

Types of Spondylolisthesis

The most common types of spondylolisthesis are as follows:

- **Congenital or dysplastic spondylolisthesis** is described as a physical abnormality or disease that is present from birth. It is caused by a birth defect in the processes of the spine that are meant to control movements, such as in the facet joints. The facet joints act as hinges and run in pairs—one on each side throughout the spine. These joints are responsible for movement and stability of the spine, and they keep the bone aligned. However, in the case of type I spondylolisthesis, the facet joints do not work properly and allow vertebrae to slip over the other.
- **Isthmic spondylolisthesis** mostly occurs in adults and is due to extreme wear and tear of the vertebrae from repetitive stress. In some cases, the microfracture causes the bone to slip out of place. It causes problems in the pars interarticularis, which is a section of bone that is located behind the vertebrae. It is more common in athletes, gymnasts, and football linemen.
- **Degenerative spondylolisthesis** is the most common form of the disorder. With aging, the discs in between the vertebrae loose water content and slip out of place.

The following are the less common types of spondylolisthesis:

- **Pathological spondylolisthesis** is a condition in which the spine's strength is weakened by a disease, such as osteoporosis, tumor, etc.
- **Postsurgical spondylolisthesis** is a type of spondylolisthesis that results from spinal surgery and causes vertebrae slippage.
- **Traumatic spondylolisthesis** is a full fracture of the pars interarticularis due to high-energy trauma.

Causes of Spondylolisthesis

Causes of spondylolisthesis vary based on one's age, genes, and lifestyle. If it is determined that a patient's condition is heredity, family members of all ages are susceptible to spondylolisthesis.

People who engage in high-intensity sports, such as wrestling, weightlifting, football, diving, gymnastics, etc., are more likely to have spondylolisthesis because their spine is subjected to constant stress. Sudden injuries also lead to the slippage of vertebrae.

Symptoms of Spondylolisthesis

People with spondylolisthesis have either minimal or no symptoms at all during the initial stages. Low back pain is the most common symptom, in which pain spreads across the lower back and feels similar to a muscle strain. Other symptoms of spondylolisthesis include:

- Weakness in one or both legs
- Tight hamstrings
- Increased inward curve, known as "lordosis"
- Pain spreading across the lower back
- Difficulty in walking and/or running

Diagnosis of Spondylolisthesis

Physical Examination

Your doctor will conduct a physical examination in order to diagnose spondylolisthesis. The physical examination includes looking for:

- Areas of pain
- A limited range of motion
- Spasms in muscles
- Muscle weakness

The doctor will observe your posture while standing, sitting, and walking in order to locate muscle tightness. The patient's previous medical history is also taken into consideration for the physical examination.

Imaging Tests

Imaging tests help to identify the exact location and extent of the damaged vertebrae in the spine. These include:

- **X-rays:** Provide accurate images of bones. To find the stress fracture, X-rays are taken at various angles.
- **Computed tomography (CT) scan:** Provides more accuracy than X-ray images, which helps the doctor to learn more about the fracture.
- **Magnetic resonance imaging (MRI) scan:** The MRI-scan images display a clear picture of the body's soft tissues, which

helps in finding any damages to the intervertebral discs between the vertebrae.

Treatment of Spondylolisthesis

The treatment for spondylolisthesis depends upon the severity of the pain and vertebra slippage.

Nonsurgical Treatment

The doctor plans for nonsurgical treatment initially. The primary goal of nonsurgical treatment is to relieve the pain and to restore the position of the vertebrae. Common nonsurgical treatment methods include the following:

- Usage of back braces
- Physical therapy exercises
- Over-the-counter (OTC) prescription drugs and/or other medications
- Usage of epidural steroid injections

Surgical Treatment

Surgical procedures are contemplated for people who have:

- Severe back pain that has not improved after nonsurgical treatment
- More slippage of the vertebrae that worsens over time
- A compressed nerve in the spine

There are several surgical treatments available for spondylolisthesis, and your surgical procedure is selected based upon your condition of spondylolisthesis. Spinal fusion is the most common surgical procedure used for treating spondylolisthesis. The spinal fusion involves fusing the damaged vertebrae with the adjacent one with rods, screws, and a piece of bone extracted from a nearby area. If nerve compression is found in the spine, the doctor opens up the spinal canal and relieves pressure before the spinal fusion procedure.

Whether the treatment is nonsurgical or surgical, it is important to follow the physical exercises and postures mentioned by your physiotherapist. People who had their spondylolisthesis cured are free from pain, however, and they can resume sports and other activities gradually with few recurrences or complications.

References

1. "Spondylolisthesis," Cleveland Clinic, October 4, 2005.
2. Moore, Kristeen. "Spondylolisthesis," Healthline, November 30, 2017.
3. "Spondylolysis and Spondylolisthesis," OrthoInfo, September 30, 2016.
4. "Spondylolisthesis," Atlantic Brain and Spine, February 17, 2017.
5. Fletcher, Jenna. "Spondylolisthesis: Causes, Symptoms, and Treatments," Medical News Today, August 14, 2017.

Section 35.3

Torticollis

Congenital torticollis, also known as "wryneck" or "twisted neck," is a condition in which an infant's neck is twisted as the neck muscle is shortened, making it difficult for the child to turn his or her head. It usually occurs at birth or shortly after birth and normally takes six to eight weeks to discover the condition as the baby begins to gain control over the head and neck; however, it can take up to three months to develop. Infants with torticollis do not feel any pain, and it happens in both boys and girls. Some babies with congenital torticollis also have hip dysplasia.

Causes of Torticollis

The exact cause of congenital torticollis is unknown; however, a common belief is that the condition can be caused because of the abnormal positioning of the fetus inside the uterus (a breech position, where the buttocks of the baby would face the birth canal). Congenital torticollis can also happen after a difficult birth. If forceps or vacuum devices were used during childbirth, it is more likely that the baby would develop this condition. These devices put pressure on the sternocleidomastoid muscle (SCM), the neck muscle. This muscle extends from the jawbone to the collarbone and breastbone; when the muscle is pulled or stretched, it might tear, which causes bleeding or bruising within the muscle. The bruised muscle develops scar tissue (fibrosis) that shortens and tightens the neck muscle, which pulls the child's head to a side. The scar tissue forms a lump that can be felt on the side of the neck. In few cases, congenital malformation of the cervical spine is another cause of congenital torticollis.

Symptoms of Torticollis

Each child may experience symptoms differently. The torticollis may be seen at birth or several weeks after birth.

Here are the most common symptoms for congenital torticollis:

- The head is tilted to one side and the chin faces the opposite shoulder. A majority of infants are affected on the right side of the neck.
- The baby finds it difficult to turn her or his head to the sides and up and down because of a limited range of motion. The baby looks over one shoulder instead of using his or her eyes to follow movements near them.
- If the baby is breastfed, then she or he may prefer breastfeeding only on one breast.
- In the first few weeks after birth, the baby may have a lump in the affected neck muscle; it is not painful, but it can be felt.
- Some babies develop a flat head on one or both sides due to sleeping on the same side always.

Diagnosis of Torticollis

If an infant has difficulty in turning the head or the head is tilted, a pediatrician needs to be consulted. The healthcare provider would discuss the infant's general health, ask specifically about torticollis symptoms, and do a complete physical examination. Diagnostic procedures for congenital torticollis are as follows:

- **X-ray.** A test using electromagnetic energy beams that captures and produces images of internal tissues, bones, and organs. It helps check abnormality in the neck muscles.
- **Ultrasound examination.** An imaging technique that examines the function of internal organs and assesses blood flow through various vessels. It uses high-frequency sound waves and a computer to produce images of tissues and blood vessels to check the muscle around the mass.

Treatment of Torticollis

If congenital torticollis is not treated, it may result in the child not being able to move the head properly, or it could cause permanent tightening of the muscle with uneven development of the neck and face. The healthcare provider will determine the treatment based on the child's overall health, age, and medical history; the extent of the condition; the child's tolerance toward different treatment methods; and the parent's opinion or preference.

The basic treatment for congenital torticollis is a gentle exercise program to stretch the sternocleidomastoid muscle (neck muscle). The healthcare provider will teach exercises that can be performed on the baby. The exercises are as follows:

- **Stretching exercises**. The baby's neck is turned from side to side gently so that the chin touches each shoulder. The head is tilted downward on the unaffected side to help relieve tension and lengthen the neck muscle.
- **Infant stimulation.** This enables the baby to learn to stretch the muscle. The baby is encouraged to turn both ways by placing toys or offering the milk bottle, so that her or his head is turned to see them.

Surgical treatments are also available if the condition cannot be corrected with these exercises. Almost 10 percent of kids with congenital torticollis need surgery. It is a minor procedure and is usually done once the child reaches preschool years.

There is no prevention possible for this condition.

References

1. "Congenital Muscular Torticollis," American Academy of Orthopaedic Surgeons (AAOS), n.d.

2. "Congenital Muscular Torticollis," Children's Hospital of Philadelphia, n.d.
3. "Congenital Torticollis," WebMD, n.d.
4. Solo-Josephson, Patricia. "Infant Torticollis," The Nemours Foundation/KidsHealth®, July 2017.

Section 35.4

Chronic Myofascial Pain

Chronic myofascial pain (CMP), also known as "myofascial pain syndrome" (MPS), is a chronic, painful condition that affects the muscles, particularly the covering layer of the muscle, known as the "fascia." When repetitive or excessive stress is placed on a muscle, it can create sensitive areas called "myofascial trigger points" (MTrPs) that can cause pain throughout the muscle. These trigger points can also cause pain in unrelated parts of the body, a phenomena called "referred pain."

Myofascial pain is dull, aching, and deep. Along with pain, individuals may experience sleep problems, as well as decreased muscle flexibility and strength. The trigger point may be active (consistently painful) or latent (pain and tenderness only when touched).

Possible Causes of Trigger Points

Although what causes trigger points is not completely understood, potential contributing factors include:

- Poorly conditioned muscles
- Chronic overload of muscles associated with repetitive movements
- Poor ergonomics and postural stress, such as sitting for prolonged duration of time

- A difference in length between the patient's legs
- Lifting or moving objects without using proper techniques
- Increased muscle tension due to anxiety or depression
- Fatigue, trauma, and cold weather

Diagnosing Chronic Myofascial Pain

Healthcare providers diagnose CMP by completing a physical examination of the painful areas and collecting a detailed history from the patient. During the examination, the doctors may apply gentle pressure in a certain way to the trigger points to check for a referred pattern of pain or a muscle twitch. They will also feel for the texture of the muscle fibers and do tests to determine the strength and flexibility of the muscles.

Chronic myofascial pain is common in people between the ages of 30 and 60, affecting both men and women equally. Recent research has identified myofascial trigger points as a contributing factor in chronic headaches, tension-type headaches, neck pain, and shoulder disorders.

Managing Myofascial Pain Syndrome

Treatment consists of three main components:

1. Reduce the chronic overload of the muscles. Identify the factors and correct it.
2. Eliminate the trigger point. There are several methods used to do this.
3. Strengthen the affected group of muscles.

Treatment Options for Chronic Myofascial Pain

Medications

- Pain relievers. Over-the-counter pain relievers, including ibuprofen (Advil, Motrin IB, others) and naproxen sodium (Aleve), may relieve pain.
- Antidepressants can reduce pain and improve sleep.
- Sedatives can help to relax muscles; however, they should be used under a doctor's supervision since they can be addictive.

Physical Therapy

A physical therapist may treat chronic myofascial pain using one or more of the following methods:

- Stretching exercises loosen tight muscles and release the trigger point.
- Strengthening exercises build up muscle strength and prevents early muscle fatigue.
- Massage therapy helps muscles relax and prevents spasms or cramps.
- Hot packs or hot shower
- Ultrasound uses high-frequency sound waves to promote healing in the muscle tissue and helps release triggers.

Needle procedures

There are two types of needle procedures:

- Wet needling is a therapeutic practice in which a numbing agent or steroid is injected by needle into the trigger point to relieve the pain.
- Dry needling involves inserting an acupuncture needle into the trigger point. This results in a reduction of substances that interact with nearby nociceptors (the parts of nerves that sense pain) and ultimately provides pain relief.

Self-Care Measures

Along with the treatment, patients can employ a variety of measures that can prevent recurrence and aid in better treatment outcomes.

- **Exercise.** Regular exercise and an active lifestyle can help patients cope with pain.
- **Relaxation.** Various relaxation methods can help reduce tension and stress. Deep breathing exercises, listening to soothing music, meditation, and talking with friends can help.
- **Taking time for yourself.** Taking care of yourself by eating healthy and getting enough sleep will help relieve pain and the associated stress.

- **Support group.** Talking to a counselor or joining a support group can help patients cope with pain.

References

1. "Chronic Myofascial Pain (CMP)," Cleveland Clinic, March 1, 2013.
2. "Dry Needling," Physiopedia, n.d.
3. "Myofascial Pain Syndrome," MayoClinic, December 9, 2014.

Section 35.5

Klippel-Feil Syndrome

This section includes text excerpted from "Klippel Feil Syndrome," Genetic and Rare Diseases Information Center (GARD), National Center for Advancing Translational Sciences (NCATS), May 20, 2015. Reviewed April 2019.

What Is Klippel-Feil Syndrome?

Klippel-Feil syndrome (KFS) is a congenital, musculoskeletal condition characterized by the fusion of at least two vertebrae of the neck. Common symptoms include a short neck, low hairline at the back of the head, and restricted mobility of the upper spine. This syndrome can cause chronic headaches, as well as pain in both the neck and the back. Other features may involve various other body parts or systems. Sometimes, KFS occurs as a feature of another disorder or syndrome, such as Wildervanck syndrome or hemifacial microsomia. In these cases, people have the features of both KFS and the additional disorder. KFS may be caused by mutations in the *GDF6* or *GDF3* gene and inherited in an autosomal dominant manner; or, it may be caused by mutations in the *MEOX1* gene and inherited in an autosomal recessive manner. Treatment is symptomatic and may include medications, surgery, and/or physical therapy (PT).

What Are the Symptoms of Klippel-Feil Syndrome?

Klippel-Feil syndrome is characterized by the fusion of two or more spinal bones in the neck (cervical vertebrae). The condition is present from birth (congenital). The three most common features include a low posterior hairline (at the back of the head), a short neck, and limited range of motion in the neck. However, not all people with KFS have these features.

Klippel-Feil syndrome has been reported in people with a very wide variety of other conditions and abnormalities, including:

- Scoliosis (curvature of the spine)
- Cervical dystonia (painful, involuntary tensing of the neck muscles)
- Genitourinary abnormalities (those of the reproductive organs and/or urinary system, including the kidneys)
- Sprengel deformity
- Cardiac (heart) defects, such as ventricular septal defect
- Pulmonary abnormalities (relating to the lungs) and respiratory problems
- Hearing deficits
- Facial asymmetry, or other abnormalities of the head and face (such as cleft palate or hemifacial microsomia)
- Torticollis
- Central nervous system (CNS) abnormalities (including Chiari malformation (CM), spina bifida, or syringomyelia), and/or neurological symptoms
- Other skeletal abnormalities (including those of the ribs, limbs, and/or fingers)
- Situs inversus
- Short stature
- Synkinesia (where movement in one hand involuntarily mimics the deliberate movement of the other hand)
- Wildervanck syndrome
- Duane syndrome or other eye (ocular) abnormalities

What Are the Causes of Klippel-Feil Syndrome?

The exact underlying causes and mechanisms of KFS are not well understood. In general, medical researchers believe KFS happens when the tissue of the embryo that normally develops into separate vertebrae does not divide correctly.

Isolated KFS (meaning that it is associated with another syndrome) can be sporadic or inherited. Although KFS may, in some cases, be caused by a combination of genetic and environmental factors, mutations in at least three genes have been linked to KFS: *GDF6*, *GDF3*, and *MEOX1*.

When KFS is a feature of another disorder, such as fetal alcohol syndrome (FAS), Goldenhar syndrome (GS), Wildervanck syndrome, or hemifacial microsomia, among others, it is caused by mutations in genes involved in the other disorder.

Is Klippel-Feil Syndrome Inherited?

In some cases, KFS appears to occur randomly for unknown reasons (sporadically). In other cases, the condition appears to be genetic and may occur in more than one person in a family. Both autosomal dominant and autosomal recessive inheritance patterns have been reported, with different responsible genes.

When KFS is caused by mutations in the *GDF6* or *GDF3* genes, it is inherited in an autosomal dominant manner. This means that having a mutation in only one copy of the responsible gene is enough to cause features of the condition. When a person with an autosomal dominant condition has children, each child has a 50 percent (1 in 2) chance of inheriting the mutated copy of the gene.

When KFS is caused by mutations in the *MEOX1* gene, it is inherited in an autosomal recessive manner. This means that a person must have mutations in both copies of the responsible gene to be affected. The parents of a person with an autosomal recessive condition usually each carry one mutated copy of the gene and are referred to as "carriers." Carriers are usually unaffected. When two carriers of the same autosomal recessive condition have children, each child has a 25 percent (1 in 4) risk of being affected; a 50 percent (1 in 2) chance of being an unaffected carrier, similar to each parent; and a 25 percent risk of being unaffected and not being a carrier.

When KFS occurs as a feature of another condition, the inheritance pattern follows that of the other condition.

How Is Klippel-Feil Syndrome Diagnosed?

Klippel-Feil syndrome is typically diagnosed when X-rays or other imaging techniques show the fusion of cervical vertebrae. X-rays of the entire spine should be performed to detect other spinal abnormalities, and additional imaging studies may be needed to assess the extent of the abnormality.

Klippel-Feil syndrome can be associated with a wide range of other abnormalities involving many parts of the body. Therefore, other initial exams are needed to detect additional physical abnormalities or underlying conditions. These include:

- Examination of the chest to rule out involvement of the heart and lungs
- Examination of the chest wall to detect possible rib anomalies
- Magnetic resonance imaging (MRI) for spinal stenosis or neurological deficits
- Ultrasound of the kidneys for renal abnormalities
- Hearing evaluation due to high incidence of hearing loss
- Various lab tests to assess organ function
- Additional tests or consultations with specialists may be recommended depending on the features present in each person with KFS.

What Treatment Options Are Available for Klippel-Feil Syndrome?

There is no cure for KFS. Treatment is generally symptomatic and supportive. Management depends on the features and severity in each person and can be lifelong. Careful evaluation, consistent follow-up, and coordination with various specialists are needed to improve outcome and make sure that no related diagnosis is missed.

There are various conservative therapies available, including the use of cervical collars, braces, traction, physical therapy, nonsteroidal anti-inflammatory drugs (NSAIDs), and various pain medications. However, for many people with KFS, symptoms are progressive due to degenerative changes that occur in the spine.

Surgery may be indicated for a variety of reasons, including persistent pain, neurologic deficits, cervical or craniocervical instability, constriction of the spinal cord, or to correct severe scoliosis. Some people with KFS may need surgery to repair other skeletal abnormalities or those related to the heart, kidneys, ears, eyes, or other parts of the body.

Those at an increased risk for neurological complications should be regularly monitored by their healthcare providers and may be advised to avoid activities that could lead to trauma or injury to cervical vertebrae.

What Is the Prognosis for Klippel-Feil Syndrome?

The long-term outlook (prognosis) for people with KFS varies depending on the specific features and severity in each affected person. While all affected people have fusion of at least two vertebrae of the neck, additional signs and symptoms (if present) can vary greatly. In general, people with minimal involvement can lead normal, active lives and may have no significant restrictions or symptoms. People with additional abnormalities and/or severe forms of the condition may require careful and routine follow-up, but they can have a good prognosis if symptoms and complications are treated early.

Part Five

Medications and Rehabilitative Therapies for Spinal Problems

Chapter 36

Managing Chronic Pain

Most people experience some kind of pain during their lives. Pain serves an important purpose: it warns the body when it is in danger, such as when your hand touches a hot stove. But, ongoing pain causes distress and affects the quality of life (QOL). Pain is the number one reason people see a doctor.

A class of drugs called "opioids" is often used to treat pain. One reason, explains National Institutes of Health's (NIH) pain expert Dr. Michael Oshinsky, is that opioids work well for many people. Opioids can stop the body from processing pain on many levels, from the skin to the brain. Because they work throughout the body, he says, "Opioids can be very effective for multiple types of pain."

But, opioids also produce feelings of happiness and well-being. They are also reinforcing; the more people take them, the more they crave them. This can lead to addiction, or continuing to take opioids despite negative consequences. Scientists have not yet been able to develop opioids that reduce pain without producing these addicting effects, Oshinsky explains.

The longer someone takes opioids, the more they may need to take to get the same effect. This is called "tolerance." Having a high tolerance does not always mean you will become addicted. However, taking higher doses of opioids increases the risk for both addiction and overdose.

This chapter includes text excerpted from "Managing Pain," *NIH News in Health*, National Institutes of Health (NIH), October 2018.

The United States is now in the grip of an opioid crisis. Every day, more than 100 Americans die from an opioid overdose. This number includes deaths from prescription opioids.

"We do not need 'better' opioids. We need to move away from the reliance on opioids for developing pain treatments," Oshinsky says.

The NIH is funding research focused on new and more precise ways to treat pain. It is also working to develop new treatments to combat opioid misuse and addiction.

Opioids Are Not Always Needed

Opioids are often prescribed for acute pain. Acute pain is short-term pain, the kind experienced after an accident or an operation. But other drugs may be just as effective for acute pain, even after surgery, explains Dr. Dena Fischer, a dental health expert at the NIH. Some of these drugs, such as acetaminophen or ibuprofen, do not require a prescription.

People may think that prescription drugs work better for acute pain. Although, that is often not the case, Fischer says. Using something other than an opioid first can be especially important to manage acute pain in fields such as dentistry, she adds.

Many people receiving opioid prescriptions from dentists are teens or young adults who have never been prescribed an opioid before.

"Research is starting to tell us that people who receive an opioid prescription as a teenager have a tendency to continue to take opioids for nonmedical purposes in the long term," Fischer says.

Healthcare providers who decide their patient needs an opioid are now being encouraged to give only a few pills at a time. People who receive shorter prescriptions are less likely to misuse their pills by taking more than prescribed or taking them after the pain is gone. This also cuts down the chance that the pills could be taken by others.

When Pain Is Chronic

Managing chronic pain is more complicated than treating acute pain. More than 25 million people in the United States alone live with chronic pain, which is pain that lasts for more than three months.

Many things can cause chronic pain. For example, Oshinsky says, a muscle that was damaged in an accident may heal relatively quickly. But if a nerve was also hurt, it can continue to send pain signals long after the body has repaired the muscle.

Other types of chronic pain are driven by brain changes, explains Dr. David Williams, an NIH-funded pain researcher at the University of Michigan. When these changes happen, the brain continues to perceive pain even though the injury has healed.

For people with this type of chronic pain, sometimes called "central pain," opioids and some other kinds of pain medications can actually make the pain worse.

Research has shown that talk therapies, such as cognitive behavioral therapy (CBT), can help many people with chronic central pain. These types of therapies "emphasize behaving in different ways or thinking in different ways that alter the perception of pain," Williams explains. "Pain is a combination of a sensory and an emotional experience."

Cognitive behavioral therapy can also help people with chronic pain management related health problems, such as problems sleeping, feeling tired, or trouble concentrating. This can increase the QOL for people with chronic pain. It can also have overlapping effects.

"Pain processing and sleep and thinking and mood all share the same neurotransmitters in the brain," Williams says. "So, by improving something like sleep, you are also improving pain."

Nonopioid drugs can help some people with chronic pain too, Oshinsky says. Many of these drugs were first developed to treat different health conditions, such as seizures, depression, or anxiety, but they can also change the way the brain processes pain.

Some people benefit from devices that stimulate the nerves directly to block pain signals from reaching the brain, Oshinsky adds. Different devices can work on different parts of the nervous system, from the nerves in the skin to the spinal cord.

People with certain types of pain have also been shown to benefit from exercise, acupuncture, massage therapy, or yoga.

Expanding the Options

The alternatives to opioids we have now do not work for everyone's pain. More nonopioid, nonaddictive treatment options could help reduce the number of opioids prescribed each year.

The NIH launched the Helping to End Addiction Long-Term (HEAL) Initiative to address the shortage of effective medications for chronic pain and other issues contributing to the opioid crisis.

Some of the research funded by the HEAL Initiative will focus on understanding how chronic pain develops. A better understanding of how acute pain becomes chronic could reveal new treatment targets.

Researchers funded by the HEAL Initiative also hope to learn how to predict who will develop chronic pain from acute pain. This information could be used to guide early pain management, Oshinsky explains. The HEAL Initiative will fund research on new treatments for opioid misuse and addiction as well.

More options for pain management could help doctors better personalize pain treatment. "It could be a little more like precision medicine, where you try to identify what flavor of pain the patient has and then match the treatments we have available to the needs of that patient," Williams explains.

Chapter 37

All about Medications for Spinal Pain

If you have ever been treated for severe pain from surgery, an injury, or an illness, you know just how vital pain relief medications can be.

Pain relief treatments come in many forms and potencies, are available by prescription or over-the-counter (OTC), and treat all sorts of physical pain—including pain brought on by chronic conditions, sudden trauma, and cancer.

Pain relief medicines (also known as "analgesics" and "painkillers") are regulated by the U.S. Food and Drug Administration (FDA). Some analgesics, including opioid analgesics, act on the body's peripheral and central nervous systems (CNS) to block or decrease sensitivity to pain. Others act by inhibiting the formation of certain chemicals in the body.

Among the factors, healthcare professionals consider in recommending or prescribing pain relief medications are the cause and severity of the pain.

Types of Pain Relievers

Over-the-Counter Medications

OTC medications relieve the minor aches and pains associated with conditions such as headaches, fever, colds, flu, arthritis, toothaches, and menstrual cramps.

This chapter includes text excerpted from "A Guide to Safe Use of Pain Medicine," U.S. Food and Drug Administration (FDA), February 9, 2009. Reviewed April 2019.

There are basically two types of OTC pain relievers: acetaminophen and nonsteroidal anti-inflammatory drugs (NSAIDs).

Acetaminophen is an active ingredient found in more than 600 OTC and prescription medicines, including pain relievers, cough suppressants, and cold medications.

NSAIDs are common medications used to relieve fever and minor aches and pains. They include aspirin, naproxen, and ibuprofen, as well as many medicines are taken for colds, sinus pressure, and allergies. They act by inhibiting an enzyme that helps make a specific chemical.

Prescription Medications

Typical prescription pain relief medicines include opioids and non-opioid medications.

Derived from opium, opioid drugs are very powerful products. They act by attaching to a specific "receptor" in the brain, spinal cord, and gastrointestinal tract. Opioids can change the way a person experiences pain.

Types of prescription opioid medications include:

- **Morphine**, which is often used before and after surgical procedures to alleviate severe pain
- **Oxycodone**, which is also often prescribed for moderate to severe pain
- **Codeine**, which comes in combination with acetaminophen or other nonopioid pain relief medications and is often prescribed for mild to moderate pain
- **Hydrocodone**, which comes in combination with acetaminophen or other nonopioid pain relief medications and is prescribed for moderate to moderately severe pain

The FDA has recently notified makers of certain opioid drugs that these products will need to have a risk evaluation and mitigation strategy (REMS) to ensure that the benefits continue to outweigh the risks.

Affected opioid drugs, which include brand name and generic products, are formulated with the active ingredients; fentanyl, hydromorphone, methadone, morphine, oxycodone, and oxymorphone.

The FDA has the authority to require a REMS under the FDA Amendments Act of 2007.

Types of nonopioid prescription medications include ibuprofen and diclofenac, which treat mild to moderate pain.

Use Pain Medications as Directed

Pain medications are safe and effective when used as directed. However, misuse of these products can be extremely harmful and even deadly.

Consumers who take pain relief medications must follow their healthcare professional's instructions carefully. If a measuring tool is provided with your medicine, use it as directed.

Do not change the dose of your pain relief medication without talking to your doctor first. Also, pain medications should never be shared with anyone else. Only your healthcare professional can decide if a prescription pain medication is safe for someone.

The following are other key points to remember.

With acetaminophen:

- Taking a higher dose than recommended will not provide more relief and can be dangerous.
- Too much can lead to liver damage and death. The Risk for liver damage may be increased in people who drink three or more alcoholic beverages a day while using acetaminophen-containing medicines.
- Be cautious when giving acetaminophen to children. Infant drop medications can be significantly stronger than regular children's medications. Read and follow the directions on the label every time you use a medicine. Be sure that your infant is getting the infants' pain formula and your older child is getting the children's pain formula.

With nonsteroidal anti-inflammatory drugs:

- Too much can cause stomach bleeding. This risk increases in people who are over 60 years of age, are taking prescription blood thinners, are taking steroids, have a history of stomach bleeding or ulcers, and/or have other bleeding problems.
- Use of NSAIDs can also cause kidney damage. This risk may increase in people who are over 60 years of age, are taking a diuretic (a drug that increases the excretion of urine), have high blood pressure, heart disease, or pre-existing kidney disease.

With opioids:

- Use of opioids can lead to drowsiness. Do not drive or use any machinery that may injure you, especially when you first start the medication. The dose of an opioid pain medication that is safe for you could be high enough to cause an overdose and death in someone else, especially children.

Know the Active Ingredients

A specific area of concern with OTC pain medicines is when products sold for different uses have the same active ingredient. A cold and cough remedy may have the same active ingredient as a headache remedy or a prescription pain reliever.

To minimize the risks of an accidental overdose, consumers should avoid taking multiple medications with the same active ingredient at the same time.

All OTC medicines must have all of their active ingredients listed on the package. For prescription drugs, the active ingredients are listed on the container label.

Talk with your pharmacist or another healthcare professional if you have questions about using OTC medicines, especially before using them in combination with dietary supplements or other OTC or prescription medicines.

Misuse and Abuse of Pain Medications

Misuse and abuse of pain medications can be extremely dangerous. This is especially so in regard to opioids. These medications should be stored in a place where they cannot be stolen.

According to National Institutes of Health (NIH), studies have shown that properly managed medical use of opioid analgesic compounds (taken exactly as prescribed) is safe, can manage pain effectively, and rarely causes addiction.

But the abuse of opioids is a significant public safety concern. Abusers ingest these drugs orally, and they also crush the pills in order to snort or inject them.

Commonly abused opioid pain medicines include prescription drugs, such as codeine, and the brand-name products Oxycontin (oxycodone), Vicodin (hydrocodone with acetaminophen), and Demerol (meperidine).

Addiction is just one serious danger of opioid abuse. A number of overdose deaths have resulted from snorting and injecting opioids, particularly the drug OxyContin, which was designed to be a slow-release formulation.

Use Opioids Safely: Three Key Steps

Step 1: Keep your doctor informed. Inform your healthcare professional about any past history of substance abuse. All patients treated with opioids for pain require careful monitoring by their healthcare professional for signs of abuse and addiction, and to determine when these analgesics are no longer needed.

Step 2: Follow directions carefully. Opioids are associated with significant side effects, including drowsiness, constipation, and depressed breathing, depending on the amount taken. Taking too much could cause severe respiratory depression or death. Do not crush or break pills. This can alter the rate at which the medication is absorbed and lead to overdose and death.

Step 3: Reduce the risk of drug interactions. Do not mix opioids with alcohol, antihistamines, barbiturates, or benzodiazepines. All of these substances slow breathing, and their combined effects could lead to life-threatening respiratory depression.

Chapter 38

What You Need to Know about Nonsteroidal Anti-Inflammatory Medications

What Are Nonselective Nonsteroidal Anti-Inflammatory Drugs and COX-2 Selective Nonsteroidal Anti-Inflammatory Drugs?

Nonsteroidal anti-inflammatory drugs (NSAIDs) are a group of drugs used to temporarily relieve pain and inflammation. They work by blocking the production of prostaglandins, or chemicals believed to be associated with pain and inflammation.

What Are Nonsteroidal Anti-Inflammatory Drugs?

Prescription NSAIDs are important to help manage many debilitating conditions, such as osteoarthritis and rheumatoid arthritis. Some prescription NSAIDs also are used to treat pain. Over-the-counter (OTC) versions of some NSAIDs are used to treat pain associated with dental problems, tendonitis, strains, sprains, and other injuries.

This chapter includes text excerpted from "The Benefits and Risks of Pain Relievers: Q and A on NSAIDs with Sharon Hertz, M.D." U.S. Food and Drug Administration (FDA), September 24, 2015. Reviewed April 2019.

NSAIDs are also commonly used to treat fever and to reduce pain associated with menstrual cramps.

What Conditions Do Nonsteroidal Anti-Inflammatory Drugs Treat?

Nonselective NSAIDs work by inhibiting two enzymes that are involved with inflammation—cyclooxygenase-1 and cyclooxygenase-2 (COX-1 and COX-2).

There are several nonselective NSAIDs on the market, including diclofenac, ibuprofen, ketoprofen, meloxicam, naproxen, and oxaprozin. Ibuprofen and naproxen are available in both prescription and OTC versions. The doses in OTC NSAIDs are lower than the doses of prescription versions and should only be used for up to 10 days without seeing a doctor. So, if you take OTC ibuprofen (Advil and Motrin) or naproxen (Aleve), the doses are about half the doses of prescription versions.

COX-2 selective inhibitors are a newer type of medicine that blocks the COX-2 enzyme more than the COX-1 enzyme. The only COX-2 selective inhibitor currently on the market in the United States is the prescription drug Celebrex (celecoxib), which is marketed by Pfizer. It was believed that COX-2 inhibitors may be less likely to cause the stomach problems associated with the older NSAIDs, but all NSAIDs carry the risk of stomach problems.

What Are the Risks of Taking Nonsteroidal Anti-Inflammatory Drugs?

As with all drugs, there is the potential for an allergic reaction to NSAIDs. Symptoms might include hives, facial swelling, wheezing, and skin rash.

There is the potential for gastrointestinal bleeding (bleeding in the stomach or elsewhere in the digestive tract) associated with all NSAIDs. The risk of bleeding is low for people who use NSAIDs intermittently. The risk of stomach problems increases for people who take them every day or regularly, especially for people who are older than 65 years of age, people with a history of stomach ulcers, and people who take blood thinners or corticosteroids (prednisone). Alcohol use can also increase the risk of stomach problems.

In addition, using all NSAIDs, except for aspirin, increases the risk of heart attack or stroke. These serious side effects can occur as early as the first few weeks of using an NSAID, and the risk might rise the longer people take nonaspirin NSAIDs.

All NSAIDs also carry the risk of potential skin reactions. Patients should be alert for symptoms, such as skin reddening, rash or blisters.

Aspirin is a nonselective NSAID and has been shown in clinical trials to reduce the risks of certain cardiovascular events in patients who have cardiovascular disease (CVD) or who have already had a heart attack or ischemic stroke. Aspirin is sold in generic forms and under brand names, such as Bayer and St. Joseph's.

Which People Are at Highest Risk for Cardiovascular Adverse Events Associated with Nonsteroidal Anti-Inflammatory Drugs?

People who have cardiovascular disease—particularly those who recently had a heart attack, cardiac bypass surgery, or stroke—are at the highest risk for adverse events. According to studies, people who have already had a heart attack are at an increased risk of having another heart attack or dying of heart attack-related causes if they are treated with NSAIDs, other than aspirin.

Which COX-2 Selective Inhibitors Have Been Taken off the Market?

Merck voluntarily withdrew Vioxx (rofecoxib) in 2004 after finding out the results of a study that showed patients who took Vioxx had a higher risk for heart attacks than patients who took a placebo. The U.S. Food and Drug Administration (FDA) asked Pfizer to withdraw Bextra (valdecoxib) from the market in 2005 because the overall risk/benefit profile was unfavorable. The request was based on many factors. Along with the other risks associated with NSAIDs, there was a higher than expected number of reports of serious and potentially life-threatening skin reactions, including death.

An increased risk of cardiovascular adverse events has been shown for all COX-2 inhibitors, including Celebrex, which is still on the market in the United States. Based on available data, the FDA determined that the benefits of Celebrex outweigh the potential risks in properly selected and informed patients. The FDA asked Pfizer to include a boxed warning on the Celebrex label, and asked manufacturers of all prescription NSAIDs to revise their labeling with a boxed warning too. The boxed warning highlights the potential for increased risk of cardiovascular events as well as serious, potentially life-threatening gastrointestinal bleeding. It is important to know that the FDA also determined that the risk for cardiovascular events was most likely present for the nonselective NSAIDs as well, and all of the manufacturers of these drugs were asked to add important warnings to their labels.

What Can Consumers Do to Lower Their Risks with Nonsteroidal Anti-Inflammatory Drugs?

Tell your doctor about your complete medical history, including any history of cardiovascular disease or stomach ulcers. This will help you and your doctor weigh the risks and benefits. You can also ask your doctor what you can do to lessen the chance for stomach irritation such as taking the medication with a meal. Also, ask what steps you can take to lower the risk of cardiovascular disease and report medication side effects to your doctor. Whether you are taking a prescription NSAID or an OTC NSAID, following directions is important. Available scientific data do not suggest an increased risk of serious cardiovascular events for short-term, low-dose use of OTC NSAIDs, but it is not known if that is because there is no risk or because there are many challenges when trying to study the use of OTC NSAIDs. Be aware that the OTC labeling states that if you take an NSAID for longer than 10 days, you should see your doctor. The lowest effective dose should be used for the shortest time.

Chapter 39

Spinal Injections

The spine is made up of several small rectangular bones, called "vertebrae," which stack on each other. These bones are connected and supported by intervertebral cushion-like structures called "discs," and they are surrounded by nerves. This entire structure of the spine can wear down due to various reasons, such as aging, injury, spinal disorders, etc., causing mild to severe pain. In such cases, spinal injections are used to deliver medicines into or around the spine in order to relieve the pain. In general, two kinds of medications are used in therapeutic spinal injections.

1. **Local anesthetics:** They are used to create numbness and block the pain in the infected area temporarily. Lidocaine and bupivacaine are some of the most commonly used local anesthetics.
2. **Steroids:** They are used to reduce the inflammation in the affected area. Cortisone is a well-known anti-inflammatory steroid medication. The steroids are usually injected in conjunction with the use of local anesthetics.

Apart from the therapeutic purposes, spinal injections are also used as diagnostic tools to determine the exact source of the pain. During the diagnostic process, if pain is relieved after injecting in a particular area, then that area is considered to be the source of pain.

Fluoroscopy

The spinal injections are usually performed under the guidance of X-rays. Initially, a liquid contrast dye is injected into the spine, and its flow is monitored with X-rays. This method is called "fluoroscopy" and helps to locate the source of the pain. The procedure may be repeated until the exact location is identified, and no medication will be injected until then.

Types of Spinal Injections

There are different types of spinal injection techniques, and each are discussed below.

Epidural Injections

The epidural space is the area around the sheath (dura) that protects the spinal nerves. It runs throughout the length of the spine; thus, when a medicine is injected into the epidural space, it can flow freely and cover all of the nerve roots. Epidural injections are used to treat radiating kind of pains, such as pain that begins in the spine and spreads to the arms and legs. This kind of pain usually occurs in the conditions, such as a slipped disc, sciatica, and spinal stenosis, in which the spinal nerves are compressed or irritated. In the epidural injection technique, an anesthetic is injected into the epidural space with or without an anti-inflammatory medication. The medication helps to reduce the inflammation and relieve the pain.

For diagnostic purposes, the epidural injection is targeted at a specific nerve with a local anesthetic, such as lidocaine. If the pain is relieved completely, then the doctor may conclude that the particular nerve is the source of the problem.

Facet Joint Injections

Facet joints are the links that connect each vertebra on the back of the spine. These joints are responsible for the flexibility of the spine. The injections that are targeted at these joints are called "facet joint injections." They are commonly used to treat pains caused by joint degeneration and arthritis in the neck, middle back, and lower back regions. For diagnostic purposes, the facet joint injections can be injected in two different ways.

- The anesthetic is directly injected into the joint. If the pain is relieved, then the particular joint will be considered problematic. So, as a therapeutic process, the doctor may inject steroids into the same joint to provide lasting pain relief.
- The anesthetic is injected into the nerve carrying signals from the joint. If the result shows that the nerve is the problem source, then the doctor may use radiofrequency ablation or a burning technique to block the pain signals from the nerve.

Sacroiliac Joint Injections

Sacroiliac (SI) joints lie between the sacrum and pelvic bones. Problems in SI joints can cause pain in the lower body parts, including the low back, buttocks, and legs. The SI joint injection technique helps to diagnose, as well as treat, such pains. The procedure of this technique is more similar to that of facet joint injections.

Discography

Discography is targeted on the intervertebral discs. This is a less common method when compared to other spinal injection techniques. It is extensively used for diagnosis rather than treatment. In discography, a fluid is injected into the jelly-like central portion (nucleus) of the spine to assess the pressure exerted by the disc. The results are used to identify the problematic disc before spinal surgery so that the surgery can be planned accordingly.

Who Cannot Have Spinal Injections?

Not everyone is a good candidate for spinal injections. People with the following medical conditions are prohibited from having spinal injections.

- Active systemic infections—dental infections, skin infections, blood poisoning, etc.
- Allergy to anesthetics and steroids
- Anticoagulation or bleeding disorders
- Diabetes
- Hypertension
- Cardiovascular diseases

Risks and Complications

Any medical intervention comes with its own risks, and spinal injections are no exceptions. The various risks and complications associated with spinal injections include:

- Infections
- Bleeding
- Muscle weakness
- Paralytic attack
- Spinal headache
- Spinal nerve injury

In addition to the risks listed above, the anesthetics and steroids used in these injections may also cause some side effects, such as:

- Excessive appetite
- Diarrhea
- Nausea and vomiting
- Facial flushing
- Irregular menstrual cycle in women

Therefore, before having any spinal injections, discuss your condition with your doctor to ensure that you are a good fit.

References

1. Park, Daniel K. "Spinal Injections," OrthoInfo, August 2018.
2. "Spinal Injections," Guy's and St Thomas' NHS Foundation Trust, October 2016.
3. "Spinal Injections," Allaboutbackandneckpain.com, DePuy Synthes Spine, n.d.

Chapter 40

Physical Therapy for Back and Neck Disorders

Physical therapy is one of the most effective approaches for the treatment of back and neck pain. Most doctors and patients consider physical therapy as the first line of treatment before resorting to expensive medications and invasive procedures. With physical therapy, the main focus is on strengthening the support structures of the spine and its joints, namely the muscles, tendons, and ligaments.

What Does Physical Therapy Do?

There are five main goals of physical therapy, and they are as follows:

1. Educating the patients about the benefits of regular stretching and strengthening exercises, which will aid in pain relief and the tissue healing process
2. Educating the patients on the importance of maintaining proper postures in various positions, and reinforcing the ergonomic principles
3. Using appropriate modalities to reduce pain and to control the inflammatory cycle, thereby accelerating the healing

---

process. The physical therapist may choose to use ice, heat, traction, ultrasound, or electrical stimulation based on their examination and findings.

4. Teaching the patients about how to prevent future occurrences of back and neck pain
5. Educating the patients on how to handle an acute exacerbation of back and neck pain symptoms

Components of Physical Therapy

There are two main components that physical therapists use when treating back and neck pain. They are:

1. Passive physical therapy using electrotherapy modalities
2. Active physical therapy in the form of exercises

Passive Physical Therapy

This is called "passive" because the patient remains passive, and the therapy is carried out on the patient externally. This is done by using various electrotherapy modalities, such as:

Heat / Ice Packs

Heat/ice packs are inexpensive and easily available modalities of treatment. They reduce muscle spasms and control the inflammation, which modulates pain effectively. Some patients prefer heat and some prefer cold, but they can be applied alternatively. A 20-minute application every 2 hours will be effective, especially in the acute phase of pain.

Ultrasound

Ultrasound uses high-frequency sound waves, which can result in localized deep heating of the injured tissues. This therapy is effective for acute pains, as it promotes healing.

Transcutaneous Electrical Nerve Stimulation (TENS)

Transcutaneous electrical nerve stimulation uses electrical stimulation, which modulates the pain sensation at the spinal cord and masks it from the brain. Most of the patients with back and neck pain respond with substantial pain relief. TENS unit can be also prescribed for home use.

Spinal Traction

Spinal traction is used when the spine needs a decompression that will relieve pressure on the nerves. This can be applied both manually and mechanically. When the traction is on, it stretches the spine and takes the pressure off of the compressed intervertebral discs. This allows the disc to heal itself. Traction is used mainly with disc disorders and other back problems.

Active Physical Therapy

Physical therapists will prescribe various stretching and strengthening exercises based on their patient evaluation. While the passive modalities take care of acute pain and inflammation, active exercises are needed to stretch tight muscles and to strengthen weak muscles.

Stretching Exercises

The hamstring muscle, which is at the back of the thigh, needs to be stretched in almost every back pain. Corner stretches, which stretch the neck and shoulder muscles, is very effective with neck pain. These stretches will not take much time and can be performed every day for better results. There are also other stretches for tight back and neck muscles, which physical therapists will be able to teach.

Strengthening Exercises

Back and neck muscles have to be strengthened so that they are able to keep the spine in a stable position to function. Spending 15 to 20 minutes every day on regular strengthening exercises is important in the prevention of future occurrences of back and neck pain. Exercises can be learned from a qualified physical therapist so that they are performed at the right intensity, frequency, and duration.

Low-Intensity Aerobic Exercises

Aerobic exercises can be carried out through various activities, such as walking, cycling, or swimming. These can be done for 30 to 40 minutes three times a week or on alternate days.

If patients with back pain can carry out this exercise regime even with a busy schedule, the exercises will help with pain relief and prevent reccurrence.

References

1. Ullrich Jr, Peter F. "Physical Therapy: Passive PT (Modalities) for Back Pain," SPINE-health, March 21, 2014.
2. Dickerman, Rob D. "Physical Therapy for Neck Pain Relief," SPINE-health, May 3, 2018.
3. "Back and Neck Pain: Physical Therapy: Procedure Details," Cleveland Clinic, November 8, 2013.
4. "Can Physical Therapy Treat Back Pain?" University of Utah Health, n.d.
5. "Spinal Traction," Healthline Media, n.d.

Chapter 41

Back and Neck Braces

Your physician may recommend braces as a part of treatment if you are diagnosed with a spinal disorder or deformity, or you are recovering from a surgery. The braces, also known as "orthotics," offer a noninvasive way of healing your current condition/problem; they prevent further problems from occurring in the spine. The braces help your spine heal faster by immobilizing it. The braces are made up of materials, such as molded plastic, elastic cotton/nylon, and foam rubber.

There are more than 30 types of back braces available for spine disorders, and the most commonly used braces are as follows.

Cervical (Neck) Braces

Cervical braces are used for stabilization of the neck (cervical spine). Doctors recommend cervical braces as an alternative treatment for spinal disorders or for postsurgical recovery. There are several types of cervical braces available, and a few of the more common types are mentioned below:

- **A soft cervical collar** is a flexible brace that is made from thick foam rubber and covered in cotton. It is placed around the cervical spine and reduces pain by supporting the neck.
- **A rigid cervical collar** also is known as a "Philadelphia collar." This collar is more rigid, or stiff, than the soft collar. The rigid

---

cervical collar consists of front and back pieces that are attached with velcro on each side. It is usually worn 24 hours a day to treat a cervical fracture, provide support after surgery, or ease strain.

- **A halo ring** consists of a titanium ring that is secured to the skull by four metal pins. Four bars are attached to a vest that is worn on the chest, which holds the ring and neck in place. The halo ring restricts neck and head movements after a cervical fusion surgery or a fracture.
- **Sterno-occipital mandibular immobilization device (SOMI)** is a cervical-thoracic brace that supports a damaged neck and keeps the head from moving by holding the neck in alignment with the spine. It is used for stable fractures, postsurgical stabilization, degenerative pathologies, and arthritis.

Back Braces

Sacroiliac and Lumbosacral Braces

The sacroiliac braces are used for preventing motion in the sacroiliac (SI) joint by exerting a compressed force on the region between the sacrum (base of the spine) and the hipbone. The lumbosacral brace stabilizes the lower back (lumbar) and consists of splints that provide comfortable support, alleviating lower back pain. The sacroiliac and lumbosacral braces are made up of heavy cotton that is reinforced by lightweight stays.

Trochanteric Belts

Trochanteric belts are used to treat pelvic fractures or SI joint pain. It limits movement and alleviates pain in the SI joint. It is made of an elastic, stretchable material that is worn around the pelvis, between the trochanter (bony part towards the end of the thigh bone) and the iliac (pelvis) ridges/crests.

Corset Braces

Corset braces provide rigidity and support for the spine. These corsets extend over the buttocks and are held up by shoulder straps. The length of the corset brace varies, depending upon your condition. A shorter corset is used for low back pain, whereas the longer corset is used for problems in the mid- and/or thoracic spine.

Hyperextension Braces

The hyperextension braces are commonly used to treat compression fractures and for recovery after a spinal surgery. These braces prevent excessive bending of the spine during any activity. The hyperextension brace puts pressure on the pelvic bone and chest in order to keep the spine extended.

Rigid Braces

Rigid braces are generally prescribed for low back pain. It is also used for stabilizing the spine after surgery. These braces have plastic or metal uprights (vertical posts) that mimic the shape of the lower back and pelvis. The brace transfers the weight of the spine by exerting pressure on your abdomen. There are many types of rigid braces available, and the most common types are:

- **A chair-back brace** immobilizes the lumbar spine by restricting the ability to bend (front, back, and sideways) and rotate.
- **A raney flexion jacket** reduces the pressure that is applied on the lower back by securing the lumbar spine in a neutral tilt. The fixed tilt prevents lordosis (an inward curve of the lumbar spine).
- **A Williams brace** is used to treat the condition of spondylolisthesis by limiting movement of the spine. This type of brace allows front bending, but side-to-side bending is limited by side uprights.

Molded Jackets

These jackets provide rigid stabilization to treat conditions, such as spinal fractures and scoliosis. The molded jackets support a large area—it covers the thoracic spine (upper back), the lumbar spine (low back), and the sacrum (bony part below lumbar spine). The jacket distributes pressure evenly, preventing excess pressure on unstable areas of the spine. It is made of molded plastic.

Lifting Belts

Lifting belts reduce muscle fatigue and low back strain during heavy lifting. This belt is worn around the waist, covering the lumbar region, and it closes in front. Generally, lifting belts are made up of cloth or canvas and do not have stays.

Complications

Even though the effects of back and neck braces are positive, wearing them over a period of time causes loss of muscle function. Sometimes, back braces shift the stress to other areas of the body, which can cause injury to other muscles or ligaments. Also, using braces for a long period of time has a psychological effect to it—removing braces makes you feel uncomfortable even after the condition is healed. Consult your doctor or physiotherapist before wearing a brace.

References

1. "Braces for Your Neck and Back," Mayfield Brain & Spine, November 8, 2003.
2. "Brace Treatments for Neck and Back Conditions," Virginia Spine Institute, February 1, 2001.
3. Eidelson, Stewart G. "Spinal Bracing Center," SpineUniverse, May 30, 2018.
4. "Hyperextension Braces: Healing Compression Fractures of the Spine," Trulife, August 31, 2018.
5. Sinicropi, Stefano. "The Benefits and Drawbacks of Back Braces," Dr. Stefano Sinicropi, January 6, 2016.

Chapter 42

Spinal Manipulation for Low Back Pain

Low back pain (LBP) (often referred to as "lower back pain") is a common condition that usually improves with self-care (practices that people can do by themselves, such as remaining active, applying heat, and taking pain-relieving medications). However, it is occasionally difficult to treat. Some healthcare professionals are trained to use a technique called "spinal manipulation" to relieve low back pain and improve physical function (the ability to walk and move).

About Low Back Pain

Back pain is one of the most common health complaints, affecting 8 out of 10 people at some point during their lives. The lower back is the area most often affected. For many people, back pain goes away on its own after a few days or weeks. But for others, the pain becomes chronic and lasts for months or years. Low back pain can be debilitating, and it is a challenging condition to diagnose, treat, and study. The total annual costs of low back pain in the United States—including lost wages and reduced productivity—are more than $100 billion.

This chapter includes text excerpted from "Spinal Manipulation for Low Back Pain," National Center for Complementary and Integrative Health (NCCIH), April 2013. Reviewed April 2019.

About Spinal Manipulation

Spinal manipulation—sometimes called "spinal manipulative therapy"—is practiced by healthcare professionals, such as chiropractors, osteopathic physicians, naturopathic physicians, physical therapists, and some medical doctors. Practitioners perform spinal manipulation by using their hands or a device to apply a controlled force to a joint of the spine. The amount of force applied depends on the form of manipulation used. The goal of the treatment is to relieve pain and improve physical functioning.

Side Effects and Risks Associated with Spinal Manipulation

Reviews have concluded that spinal manipulation for low back pain is relatively safe when performed by a trained and licensed practitioner. The most common side effects are generally minor and include feeling tired or temporary soreness.

Reports indicate that cauda equina syndrome (CES), a significant narrowing of the lower part of the spinal canal in which nerves become pinched and may cause pain, weakness, loss of feeling in one or both legs, and bowel or bladder problems, may be an extremely rare complication of spinal manipulation. However, it is unclear if there is actually an association between spinal manipulation and CES, since CES usually occurs without spinal manipulation. In people whose pain is caused by a herniated disc, manipulation of the low back appears to have a very low chance of worsening the herniation.

What the Science Says about Spinal Manipulation for Low Back Pain

Overall, studies have shown that spinal manipulation is one of several options—including exercise, massage, and physical therapy—that can provide mild-to-moderate relief from low back pain. Spinal manipulation also appears to work, as well as more conventional treatments, such as applying heat, using a firm mattress, and taking pain-relieving medications.

In their 2007 guidelines, the American College of Physicians (ACP) and the American Pain Society (APS) included spinal manipulation as one of several treatment options for practitioners to consider when low back pain does not improve with self-care. A 2010 Agency for Healthcare Research and Quality (AHRQ) report noted that complementary health therapies, including spinal manipulation, offer additional options to conventional treatments, which often have limited benefit in managing back and neck pain. The AHRQ analysis also found that spinal manipulation was more effective than placebo and as effective as medication in reducing low back pain intensity. However, the researchers noted inconsistent results when they compared spinal manipulation with a massage or physical therapy to reduce low back pain intensity or disability.

Researchers continue to study spinal manipulation for low back pain.

- A review of 26 clinical trials looked at the effectiveness of different treatments, including spinal manipulation, for chronic low back pain. The authors concluded that spinal manipulation is as effective as other interventions for reducing pain and improving function.
- A review that looked at various manual therapies, such as spinal manipulation and massage, for a range of conditions found strong evidence that spinal manipulation is effective for chronic low back pain and moderate evidence of its effectiveness for acute low back pain.
- An analysis looked at the evidence from 76 trials that studied the effects of several conventional and complementary health practices for low back pain. The researchers found that the pain-relieving effects of many treatments, including spinal manipulation, were small and were similar in people with acute or chronic pain.
- A review that focused on spinal manipulation for chronic low back pain found strong evidence that spinal manipulation works as well as a combination of medical care and exercise instruction, moderate evidence that spinal manipulation combined with strengthening exercises works as well as prescription nonsteroidal anti-inflammatory drugs (NSAIDs) combined with exercises, and limited-to-moderate evidence that spinal manipulation works better than physical therapy and home exercise.

Researchers are investigating whether the effects of spinal manipulation depend on the length and frequency of treatment. In one study funded by the National Center for Complementary and Integrative Health (NCCIH), that examined long-term effects in more than 600 people with low back pain, results suggested that chiropractic care involving spinal manipulation was at least as effective as conventional medical care for up to 18 months. However, less than 20 percent of participants in this study were pain free at 18 months, regardless of the type of treatment used.

Researchers are also exploring how spinal manipulation affects the body. In an NCCIH-funded study of a small group of people with low back pain, spinal manipulation affected pain perception in specific ways that other therapies (stationary bicycle and low back extension exercises) did not.

Chapter 43

Spinal Manipulation or Home Exercise Is More Effective than Medication for Acute Neck Pain

Spinal manipulation or home exercise was more effective than medication for treatment of acute to subacute neck pain, according to a recent National Center for Complementary and Integrative Health (NCCIH)-funded study published in the *Annals of Internal Medicine*. Researchers from Northwestern Health Sciences University (NWHSU) and the Minneapolis Medical Research Foundation (MMFR) randomly assigned 272 participants with neck pain, between the ages of 18 and 65, to receive either spinal manipulation therapy, medication, or home exercise instruction.

In the study, spinal manipulation therapy consisted of various techniques, including spinal adjustments (low amplitude, high velocity) and mobilization (low velocity) of areas of the spine. Participants in the medication group received nonsteroidal anti-inflammatory drugs (NSAIDs), acetaminophen, or both; those who did not respond to these medications or could not tolerate them received narcotic medications.

This chapter includes text excerpted from "Spinal Manipulation or Home Exercise More Effective Than Medication for Acute Neck Pain, Study Finds," National Center for Complementary and Integrative Health (NCCIH), September 24, 2017.

Home exercise with instruction focused on gentle, self-controlled movement of the neck and shoulder joints, and participants were instructed to do the exercises six to eight times each day. In addition, participants in this group received two individualized hour-long sessions of one-on-one exercise instruction, as well as written directions for exercise at home.

The researchers observed significant short- and long-term improvements in participant-rated pain in the spinal manipulation group compared with those receiving medication. At 12 weeks, 82 percent of participants in the spinal manipulation group (compared to 69% in the medication group) experienced reductions of pain of at least 50 percent. Similar findings occurred at 26 and 52 weeks. Additionally, the spinal manipulation group reported greater global improvement, participant satisfaction, and function than the medication group. Home exercise with instruction was just as effective as spinal manipulation at each time point.

Few studies exist to date regarding the management of neck pain with noninvasive methods, such as spinal manipulation, home exercise, or medications. According to the researchers, the findings from this study suggest that both spinal manipulation and home exercise may be viable treatment options for managing neck pain.

Chapter 44

Chiropractic Care for Back Pain

Chapter Contents

Section 44.1—Overview of Chiropractic Care 356

Section 44.2—What to Expect at Your First Chiropractic Visit 360

Section 44.1

Overview of Chiropractic Care

This section includes text excerpted from "Chiropractic: In Depth," National Center for Complementary and Integrative Health (NCCIH), November 8, 2018.

The term "chiropractic" combines the Greek words "cheir" (hand) and "praxis" (practice) to describe a treatment done by hand. Hands-on therapy—especially adjustment of the spine—is central to chiropractic care. Chiropractic is based on the notion that the relationship between the body's structure (primarily that of the spine) and its function (as coordinated by the nervous system) affects one's health.

Spinal adjustment/manipulation is a core treatment in chiropractic care, but it is not synonymous with chiropractic. Chiropractors commonly use other treatments in addition to spinal manipulation, and other healthcare providers (e.g., physical therapists or some osteopathic physicians) may use spinal manipulation.

Chiropractic Care in the United States

In the United States, chiropractic is often considered a complementary health approach. According to the 2017 National Health Interview Survey (NHIS), which included a comprehensive survey of the use of complementary health approaches by Americans, the use of chiropractic care by adults increased from 9.1 percent in 2012 to 10.3 percent in 2017. Among children, however, there was no significant difference in the use of chiropractic care during this same time period (3.5 percent in 2012 and 3.4 percent in 2017). Additionally, an analysis of 2012 NHIS cost data found that adults in the United States spent approximately $11.9 billion out-of-pocket on visits to complementary health practitioners—$3.9 billion of which was spent on visits to practitioners for chiropractic or osteopathic manipulation.

Many people who seek chiropractic care have low back pain. People also commonly seek chiropractic care for other kinds of musculoskeletal pain (e.g., neck, shoulder), headaches, and extremity (e.g., hand or foot) problems.

An analysis of the use of complementary health approaches for back pain, based on data from the 2002 NHIS, found that chiropractic was by far the most commonly used therapy. Among survey respondents who had used any of these therapies for their back pain, 74 percent (approximately 4 million Americans) had used chiropractic. Among those who had used chiropractic for back pain, 66 percent perceived "great benefit" from their treatments.

Treatment Method

During the initial visit, chiropractors typically take a health history and perform a physical examination, with a special emphasis on the spine. Other examinations or tests, such as X-rays, may also be performed. If chiropractic treatment is considered appropriate, a treatment plan will be developed.

During follow-up visits, practitioners may perform one or more of the many different types of adjustments and other manual therapies used in chiropractic care. Given mainly to the spine, a chiropractic adjustment involves using the hands or a device to apply a controlled, rapid force to a joint. The goal is to increase the range and quality of motion in the area being treated and to aid in restoring health. Joint mobilization is another type of manual therapy that may be used.

Chiropractors may combine the use of spinal adjustments and other manual therapies with several other treatments and approaches such as:

- Heat and ice
- Electrical stimulation
- Relaxation techniques
- Rehabilitative and general exercise
- Counseling about diet, weight loss, and other lifestyle factors
- Dietary supplements

What the Science Says about Chiropractic Treatment

Researchers have studied spinal manipulation for a number of conditions ranging from back, neck, and shoulder pain to asthma, carpal tunnel syndrome (CTS), fibromyalgia (FM), and headaches. Much of the research has focused on low back pain and has shown that spinal manipulation appears to benefit some people with this condition.

A 2010 review of scientific evidence on manual therapies for a range of conditions concluded that spinal manipulation/mobilization may be helpful for several conditions in addition to back pain, including migraine and cervicogenic (neck-related) headaches, neck pain, upper- and lower-extremity joint conditions, and whiplash-associated disorders. The review also identified a number of conditions for which spinal manipulation/mobilization appears not to be helpful (including asthma, hypertension, and menstrual pain) or the evidence is inconclusive (e.g., fibromyalgia, mid-back pain, premenstrual syndrome, sciatica, and temporomandibular joint disorders).

Safety

- Side effects from spinal manipulation can include temporary headaches, tiredness, or discomfort in the parts of the body that were treated.
- There have been rare reports of serious complications, such as stroke, cauda equina syndrome (a condition involving pinched nerves in the lower part of the spinal canal), and worsening of herniated discs, although cause and effect are unclear.
- Safety remains an important focus of ongoing research:
  - A 2007 study of treatment outcomes for 19,722 chiropractic patients in the United Kingdom concluded that minor side effects (such as temporary soreness) after cervical spine manipulation were relatively common, but that the risk of a serious adverse event was "low to very low" immediately or up to seven days after treatment.
  - A 2009 study that drew on nine years of hospitalization records for the population of Ontario, Canada analyzed 818 cases of vertebrobasilar artery (VBA) stroke (involving the arteries that supply blood to the back of the brain). The study found an association between visits to a healthcare practitioner and subsequent VBA stroke, but there was no evidence that visiting a chiropractor put people at greater risk than visiting a primary care physician. The researchers attributed the association between healthcare visits and VBA stroke to the likelihood that people with VBA dissection (torn arteries) seek care for related headache and neck pain before their stroke.

Practitioners: Education and Licensure

Chiropractic colleges accredited by the Council on Chiropractic Education (CCE) offer Doctor of Chiropractic (D.C.) degree programs. (The CCE is the agency certified by the U.S. Department of Education (ED) to accredit chiropractic colleges in the United States.) Admission to a chiropractic college requires a minimum of 90-semester hour credits of undergraduate study, mostly in the sciences.

Chiropractic training is a four-year academic program that includes both classroom work and direct experience caring for patients. Coursework typically includes instruction in the biomedical sciences, as well as in public health and research methods. Some chiropractors pursue a two- to three-year residency for training in specialized fields.

Chiropractic is regulated individually by each state and the District of Columbia (DC). All states require completion of a Doctor of Chiropractic degree program from a CCE-accredited college. Examinations administered by the National Board of Chiropractic Examiners (NBCE) are required for licensing and include a mock patient encounter. Most states require chiropractors to earn annual continuing education credits to maintain their licenses. Chiropractors' scope of practice varies by state in areas such as the dispensing or selling of dietary supplements and the use of other complementary health approaches, such as acupuncture or homeopathy.

Seeking Chiropractic Care

If you are thinking about seeking chiropractic care:

- Ask about the chiropractor's education and licensure.
- Mention any medical conditions you have, and ask whether the chiropractor has specialized training or experience in the condition for which you are seeking care.
- Ask about typical out-of-pocket costs and insurance coverage. (Chiropractic is covered by many health maintenance organizations and private health plans, Medicare, and state workers' compensation systems.)
- Tell the chiropractor about any medications (prescription or over-the-counter (OTC)) and dietary supplements you take. If the chiropractor suggests a dietary supplement, ask about potential interactions with your medications or other supplements.
- Tell all of your healthcare providers about any complementary health approaches you use. Give them a full picture of what you do to manage your health. This will help ensure coordinated and safe care.

Section 44.2

What to Expect at Your First Chiropractic Visit

Patients usually visit a chiropractor through a referral of any specialist or through personal reference. A thorough chiropractic consultation will typically take an hour's time or more. The chiropractic visit includes the following:

- A discussion of the patient's history and symptoms
- A chiropractic examination
- A diagnostic study
- Diagnosis
- Treatment plan

Patient's History and Symptoms

During your first visit, the chiropractor will make a comprehensive assessment, regarding your problem, and provide the right treatment plan. In order to assess the problem you have, the chiropractor will ask certain questions in relation to your medical history and symptoms of the problem, such as:

- Reason for the pain
- Location of the pain
- Severity of the pain
- Whether the pain is a result of a previous injury
- Major illnesses you have experienced
- Medications you take
- Surgeries you have had
- Sleeping habits

Background information, including your family's medical history, is also essential for the chiropractor to determine the type of problem you have.

Chiropractic Examination

After the chiropractor gathers your medical history, a complete chiropractic examination is completed. It includes general tests, such as heart rate, respiration, reflex, and blood pressure tests. The examination also consists of other tests, such as neurological and orthopedic tests, which assess motion of the affected area(s), reflexes, muscle tone, and muscle strength.

Diagnostic Study

Diagnostic studies reveal structural ruptures (bone) and abnormalities. Based on the patient's medical history and physical examination, diagnostic studies may or may not be necessary. Diagnostic studies provide more information about the affected part than a normal chiropractic examination does. The commonly conducted diagnostic tests are:

- Magnetic resonance imaging (MRI)
- X-rays
- Other laboratory tests

Diagnosis

The diagnosis of a patient is determined by consolidating the data gathered from the patient's medical history, chiropractic examination, and diagnostic studies (if any). Once the diagnosis is determined, the chiropractor will decide if the condition will respond to chiropractic care or not. The chiropractor will explain the results of the diagnoses, including:

- The diagnosed condition
- The treatment plan
- The time period of the chiropractic treatment

Treatment Plan

The treatment plan of a diagnosed condition depends upon the following:

- General health
- Age
- Severity of the injury

Generally, chiropractors will provide treatment plans during the patient's first visit, but some patients may have to wait until their next appointment. The chiropractic treatment plan will include some, or all, of the following:

- Exercises to improve strength, coordination, and balance of muscles
- Ways to improve healing of the soft tissue and pain control
- Adjustments to dysfunctions of joints
- Massages, hot/cold application, and nutrition education

The chiropractor will organize a treatment plan based upon the goal. There are two types of goals in chiropractic treatment, and they are:

- **Short-term goal**—to restore muscle balance by reducing the pain and restoring the function of the joint.
- **Long-term goal**—to improve the patient's general health and restore the joint's functional independence.

In order to attain these goals, your chiropractor will schedule one or two visits per week for two to four weeks. In your later visits, the chiropractor will determine whether to continue the treatment or not.

During your visit, typical adjustments of the joints will be carried out by your chiropractor. Typical adjustments are the therapeutic manipulations of joints through a controlled force and with the appropriate velocity in the right direction for a number of times. These are done to restore structural alignment of the damaged joint.

After your first visit, you might feel slight discomfort or fatigue. However, this will resolve later. If you are feeling any pain, contact your chiropractor.

References

1. Levine, Michael. "What to Expect during Your First Chiropractic Visit," ChiroCare of Florida, July 27, 2017
2. Schubbe, Peter J. "Chiropractic Treatment Plan," SPINE-health, January 2017.

3. "What Happens at the Chiropractor?" University of Minnesota, February 8, 2007.

4. "What to Expect from Your First Chiropractic Visit," Canadian Chiropractic Association (CCA), February 13, 2019.

Chapter 45

Meditation and Cognitive-Behavioral Therapy to Ease Low Back Pain

Most people experience low back pain at some point in their lives. Treatment choices include over-the-counter (OTC) and prescription drugs, cold and hot compresses, exercise, and, in some cases, surgery. Some complementary health practices—such as spinal manipulation, acupuncture, massage, and yoga—may also be helpful in relieving chronic low back pain.

A team led by Dr. Daniel Cherkin at the Group Health Research Institute (GHRI) in Seattle compared different approaches to treating chronic low back pain. They enrolled 342 people, between the ages of 20 and 70, who had back pain for more than 3 months that could not be attributed to a specific cause. Participants were randomly assigned to 1 of 3 treatment groups: cognitive behavioral therapy (CBT), mindfulness-based stress reduction (MBSR), or usual care.

CBT is a form of psychotherapy that trains people to modify specific thoughts and behaviors. It is previously been shown to be effective for alleviating back pain in a variety of age groups. CBT group participants focused on changing dysfunctional thoughts, setting and

---

This chapter includes text excerpted from "Meditation and Cognitive-Behavioral Therapy Ease Low Back Pain," National Institutes of Health (NIH), March 29, 2016.

working toward behavioral goals, relaxation skills, and pain coping strategies.

MBSR focuses on increasing awareness and acceptance of moment-to-moment experiences—including physical discomfort and difficult emotions—without trying to change them. MBSR group members engaged in mindfulness practices that included yoga and both sitting and walking meditation.

The CBT and MBSR groups attended weekly two-hour sessions for eight weeks. They received workbooks and audio compact discs (CDs) for home practice. The usual care group could seek whatever treatment, if any, they wanted.

At 6 months, functional improvement—measured with an established questionnaire—was higher for 61 percent of those in the MBSR group and 58 percent of those in the CBT group, compared to 44 percent of those in the usual care group. The percentage of those with improvement in self-reported back pain was also greater with MBSR (44%) and CBT (45%) than usual care (27%). Both treatments continued to show moderate benefits after 1 year.

"The research suggests that training the brain to respond differently to pain signals may be more effective—and last longer—than traditional physical therapy and medication," Cherkin says. "The results from this research affirm that nondrug/nonopioid therapies, such as meditation, can help manage chronic low back pain. Physicians and their patients can use this information to inform treatment decisions," says National Center for Complementary and Integrative Health (NCCIH) Director Dr. Josephine Briggs.

The research was supported by the National Institutes of Health's (NIH) National Center for Complementary and Integrative Health. Results appeared online on March 22, 2016, in the *Journal of the American Medical Association (JAMA)*.

Further research will be needed to determine whether the treatment benefits extend beyond a year, to identify mechanisms that underlie their effectiveness, and to assess their cost-effectiveness.

Chapter 46

Yoga May Help Treat Back Pain

Many people experience low back pain over their lifetime. For those who do not recover quickly, the discomfort can become chronic, lasting for months or even years.

Researchers funded by the National Institutes of Health (NIH) have been looking for new ways to treat long-lasting low back pain. A new study shows that yoga (a mind and body practice) may help relieve moderate to severe low back pain. The research team recruited 320 people with chronic low back pain from diverse backgrounds and underserved communities. More than half of the study's participants were non-Hispanic Black individuals and earned less than $30,000 per year.

The participants were randomly assigned to 3 groups. The first group took 12 weekly yoga classes designed for people with low back pain. The second group had 15 physical therapy (PT) sessions over 12 weeks. These included exercises to strengthen back and core muscles. The third group received a self-help book and newsletters to learn how to deal with back pain.

The results suggested that a structured yoga class may be an option for treating chronic low back pain. All three groups reported improvement in physical function and pain reduction. However, people in the yoga and physical therapy treatment groups were more likely than

---

This chapter includes text excerpted from "Yoga May Help Treat Back Pain," *NIH News in Health*, National Institutes of Health (NIH), August 2017.

those in the education-only group to stop taking pain relievers after a year.

"Chronic low back pain disproportionately impacts those who are economically disadvantaged," says research team leader Dr. Robert Saper of the Boston University School of Medicine (BUSM) and Boston Medical Center (BMC). "Therefore, we feel that it was important to test whether the yoga would be received well by an underserved population as well as being effective."

Chapter 47

Acupuncture for Back Pain

Chapter Contents

Section 47.1—The Use of Acupuncture to Treat Pain 370
Section 47.2—Acupuncture and Low Back Pain 373

Section 47.1

The Use of Acupuncture to Treat Pain

This section includes text excerpted from "Understanding Acupuncture," *NIH News in Health*, National Institutes of Health (NIH), February 2011. Reviewed April 2019.

Acupuncture is a traditional medicine that has been practiced in China and other Asian countries for thousands of years. Its proponents say it can do everything from relieving pain to bringing a general sense of wellness. Others think the only benefits you get from acupuncture are in your head. Studies have found that both sides may have a point. Acupuncture can be effective for certain health problems, such as some types of chronic pain. But, how it works is something of a mystery.

Acupuncture is the stimulation of specific points on the body. The methods can vary, but the most well-known type in the United States is the insertion of thin metal needles through the skin. At least three million adults nationwide use acupuncture every year, according to the latest estimates.

Acupuncture is part of a family of procedures that originated in China. According to traditional Chinese medicine, the body contains a delicate balance of two opposing and inseparable forces: yin and yang. Yin represents the cold, slow, or passive principle. Yang represents the hot, excited, or active principle. Health is achieved by balancing the two. Disease comes from an imbalance that leads to a blockage in the flow of qi—the vital energy or life force thought to regulate your spiritual, emotional, mental, and physical health. Acupuncture is intended to remove blockages in the flow of qi and restore and maintain health.

Researchers do not know how these ideas translate to our Western understanding of medicine, explains Dr. Richard L. Nahin of the National Institutes of Health's (NIH) National Center for Complementary and Alternative Medicine (NCCAM), now renamed as National Center for Complementary and Integrative Health (NCCIH). However, the fact is that many well-designed studies have found that acupuncture can help with certain conditions, such as back pain, knee pain, headaches, and osteoarthritis.

"In many research studies, it is clear that if you are comparing acupuncture to usual care, the acupuncture group almost always does better," Nahin says. The problem, he explains, is that when researchers have compared acupuncture to carefully designed "control" treatments, the picture becomes more complicated.

Well-designed clinical trials need control groups—people who get a sham or simulated treatment called a "placebo." Placebos might come in the form of a sugar pill or a saline injection. They give researchers something to compare the real treatment with. Although, designing a placebo for acupuncture is a challenge.

"I don't really think you can come up with a great placebo needling," says Dr. Karen J. Sherman, an NIH-funded acupuncture researcher at the Group Health Research Institute in Seattle.

For example, when researchers have compared inserting needles with just pressing a toothpick onto acupuncture points, they have often found both treatments to be successful. But Sherman questions whether these are really controlled. Many traditional acupuncturists would consider them true treatments too. The important thing, in their view, is to hit the right spot, not necessarily how deep you go.

Another option for a placebo would be to test a different location. However, Sherman says that would be inappropriate for treating pain because acupuncturists traditionally needle tender points. "To me, there's no place on the back, if you have back pain, where you can say you have a great control," Sherman says, "so I don't think that's a really solid idea."

Further complicating things is that acupuncture treatments are about more than just needles. "There'll be needles," Sherman says, "but there'll probably be other things they do in the course of the treatment. Acupuncturists will talk to you in a particular way. They might give you dietary advice or exercise advice that stems from a non-Western theoretical construct. They'll try to engage you in your own healing. They might give you a different model for thinking about your health."

"It's hard to design placebo-controlled studies of acupuncture when we don't understand what the active component of the intervention is," explains Dr. Richard E. Harris, an NIH-funded researcher at the Chronic Pain and Fatigue Research Center in Ann Arbor, Michigan.

Treatment for pain is the best-studied aspect of acupuncture. Many parts of the brain are connected in the processing of pain, and how much pain you feel partly depends on context. "If a person has an injury in battle, they might not feel it," Sherman explains, "but if they have a similar injury just walking down the street, they might just think it was dreadful."

"If you look at some of the data, what you find is that sham acupuncture and true acupuncture both produce some pain relief in whatever condition they're looking at," Nahin says. "But while both treatments turn on areas of the brain, they turn on different areas of the brain."

Harris and his colleagues, in studies of fibromyalgia (FM) patients, have found differences at the molecular level as well. "We were able to show that sham acupuncture and real acupuncture both reduced pain in fibromyalgia patients equally," he says, "but they do it by different mechanisms."

If acupuncture truly works by a different mechanism than sham acupuncture, Harris says, then they are not the same thing, even if they both help relieve pain. Harris and others are now trying to get to the bottom of what acupuncture is actually doing. Their ultimate goal is to see if other treatments might pair well with acupuncture to reduce pain better than either alone.

Should you try acupuncture? Studies have found it to be very safe, with few side effects. If you are thinking about it, talk to your doctor. "We tell people they really need to talk to their primary care provider (PCP) and discuss whether acupuncture is a viable option for them," Nahin says. "While you could go to an acupuncturist independent of a medical practitioner, we feel that an integrated approach to care is always the best approach."

"Find somebody who's dealt with your problem before," Sherman advises. "Talk to the practitioner about your specific situation and then see if it's something you can live with because it might not be the right treatment for you."

If you do decide to try acupuncture, she adds, "You need to know that you should give it some time. You can't expect one session will tell you whether it works or not. Be open minded and willing to at least entertain some of the notions that the acupuncturist brings up. Give it a try if you're open to it."

Section 47.2

Acupuncture and Low Back Pain

This section includes text excerpted from "Acupuncture: In Depth," National Center for Complementary and Integrative Health (NCCIH), January 2016.

What the Science Says about the Effectiveness of Acupuncture

Results from a number of studies suggest that acupuncture may help ease types of pain that are often chronic, such as low back pain, neck pain, and osteoarthritis/knee pain. It also may help reduce the frequency of tension headaches and prevent migraine headaches. Therefore, acupuncture appears to be a reasonable option for people with chronic pain to consider. However, clinical practice guidelines are inconsistent in recommendations about acupuncture.

The effects of acupuncture on the brain and body and how best to measure them are only beginning to be understood. The available evidence suggests that many factors—such as expectation and belief—that are unrelated to acupuncture needling may play important roles in the beneficial effects of acupuncture on pain.

For Low Back Pain

A 2012 analysis of data on participants in acupuncture studies looked at back and neck pain together and found that actual acupuncture was more helpful than either no acupuncture or simulated acupuncture.

A 2010 review by the Agency for Healthcare Research and Quality (AHRQ) found that acupuncture relieved low back pain immediately after treatment but not over longer periods of time.

A 2008 systematic review of studies on acupuncture for low back pain found strong evidence that combining acupuncture with usual care helps more than usual care alone. The same review also found strong evidence that there is no difference between the effects of actual and simulated acupuncture in people with low back pain.

Clinical practice guidelines issued by the American Pain Society (APS) and the American College of Physicians (ACP) in 2007 recommend acupuncture as one of several nondrug approaches physicians should consider when patients with chronic low back pain do not respond to self-care (practices that people can do by themselves, such as remaining active, applying heat, and taking pain-relieving medications).

Chapter 48

M6-C™ Artificial Cervical Disc

What Is M6-C™ Artificial Cervical Disc?

The M6-C™ Artificial Cervical Disc is an implant (device) that replaces the function of a damaged or diseased disc of the neck in the spine (C3 to C7). The M6-C™ contains a series of polymer (ultra-high molecular weight polyethylene) fibers wound in a specific pattern. The fiber is wound around a polymer (polycarbonate urethane) core and through the slots in two titanium alloy inner endplates. The two titanium alloy inner endplates are welded to two titanium alloy outer endplates. The endplates attach to the patient's spinal bone, and the implant is designed to maintain the natural movement of the spine.

How Does It Work?

The implanted device replaces a damaged or diseased disc of the neck in the spine. It is intended to relieve pain and allow motion in all directions (like a pivoting joint) at the operated spinal level.

This chapter includes text excerpted from "M6-C™ Artificial Cervical Disc—P170036," U.S. Food and Drug Administration (FDA), February 20, 2019.

When Is It Used?

The M6-C™ Artificial Cervical Disc is used for people who have fully formed and fully grown bones (are skeletally mature) to replace a disc in the neck, following the removal of the disc for conditions that result from a diseased or bulging disc for one disc.

What Will It Accomplish?

The device is designed to help stabilize the spine. Unlike a fusion procedure, the M6-C™ Artificial Cervical Disc is designed to allow motion at the operated spinal level, although not all patients will achieve motion after treatment. The device may lessen neck and/or arm pain, and it may help patients return to their normal activities. In the clinical study of 152 patients, there was an 86.8 percent overall success rate at 24 months.

Some of the most common problems experienced by study patients were difficulty swallowing; neck and/or arm pain; or neurological adverse events, such as numbness or tingling in the upper extremities.

When Should It Not Be Used?

The M6-C™ Artificial Cervical Disc should not be used in patients with:

- An unnatural shape (deformity) of the neck
- Advanced abnormal changes at the proposed surgery level
- Advanced degeneration to the joints on the back of the spine
- An active systemic (whole body) infection or infection at the surgery site
- History of osteoporosis
- A known allergy to titanium, stainless steel, polyurethane, polyethylene, or ethylene oxide residuals

Part Six

Information about Spinal Surgeries

Chapter 49

What You Should Know before Your Surgery

Having any type of surgery can be stressful. You might be asking yourself: What is the recovery process? How long will I be out of work? What do I do after leaving the hospital or surgery center?

An important question you might not have thought of is: How do I avoid getting a surgical site infection (SSI)?

An SSI is an infection patient can get during or after surgery. Surgical site infections can happen on any part of the body where the surgery takes place and can sometimes involve only the skin. Other SSIs are more serious and can involve tissues under the skin, organs, or implanted material.

These infections can make recovery from surgery more difficult because they can cause additional complications, stress, and increased medical costs. It is important that healthcare providers, patients, and loved ones work together to prevent these infections.

What Can Healthcare Providers Do to Ensure That the Surgical Site Is Clean?

The healthcare providers can do the following to ensure that the surgical site is clean:

This chapter includes text excerpted from "What You Should Know before Your Surgery," Centers for Disease Control and Prevention (CDC), March 14, 2016.

- Clean their hands and arms up to the elbows with an antiseptic agent just before the surgery.
- Wear hair covers, masks, gowns, and gloves during surgery to keep the surgery area clean.
- Give the patient antibiotics before surgery starts and when indicated.
- Clean the skin at the surgery site with a special soap that kills germs.

How Can You and Your Loved Ones Prevent Surgical Site Infections?

In order to prevent yourself and your loved ones from SSIs you can:

- **Inform your doctor about your health problems.** Before the surgery, discuss other health problems, such as diabetes, with your doctor. These issues can affect your surgery and treatment.
- **Quit smoking.** Patients who smoke get more infections.
- **Follow instructions.** Follow your doctor's instructions for cleaning your skin before your surgery. For example, if your doctor recommends using a special soap before surgery, make sure you do so.
- **Avoid shaving near where you will have surgery.** Shaving with a razor can irritate your skin and make it easier to develop an infection. If someone tries to shave you before surgery, ask why this is necessary.

After surgery, be sure to follow the recommendations below to protect against surgical site infection.

- Ask your provider to clean their hands before they examine you or check your wound.
- Do not allow visitors to touch the surgical wound or dressings.
- Ask family and friends to clean their hands before and after visiting you.
- Make sure you understand how to care for your wound before you leave the medical facility.
- Always clean your hands before and after caring for your wound.

- Make sure you know who to contact if you have questions or problems after you get home.
- If you have any symptoms of an infection, such as redness and pain at the surgery site, drainage, or fever, call your doctor immediately.

Chapter 50

Questions to Ask Your Doctor before You Have Surgery

Asking questions and providing information to your doctor and other healthcare providers can improve your care. Talking with your doctor builds trust and leads to better results, quality, safety, and satisfaction.

Quality healthcare is a team effort. You play an important role. One of the best ways to communicate with your doctor and healthcare team is by asking questions. Because time is limited during medical appointments, you will feel less rushed if you prepare your questions before your appointment.

Doctors know a lot about a lot of things, but they do not always know everything about you or what is best for you.

Your questions give your doctor and healthcare team important information about you, such as your most important healthcare concerns.

That is why they need you to speak up.

This chapter includes text excerpted from "Questions to Ask Your Doctor," Agency for Healthcare Research and Quality (AHRQ), U.S. Department of Health and Human Services (HHS), September 2018.

Before Your Appointment

Asking questions about your diagnoses, treatments, and medicines can improve the quality, safety, and effectiveness of your healthcare. Taking steps before your medical appointments will help you to make the most of your time with your doctor and healthcare team.

Prepare Your Questions

Time is limited during doctor visits. Prepare for your appointment by thinking about what you want to do during your next visit.

Do you want to:

- Talk about a health problem?
- Get or change a medicine?
- Get medical tests?
- Talk about surgery or treatment options?

Write down your questions to bring to your appointment. The answers can help you make better decisions, get good care, and feel better about your healthcare.

Other Helpful Tips

These steps will also help prepare for your appointment:

- Ask someone to go to your appointment with you to help you understand and remember answers to your questions.
- Create a health history that includes your current conditions and past surgeries or illnesses. Bring it to your appointment.
- Know your family's health history, such as your parents' health conditions.
- Bring all your medicines with you.

During Your Appointment

During your appointment, make sure to ask the questions you prepared before your appointment. Start by asking the ones that are most important to you.

To get the most from your visit, tell the nurse or person at the front desk that you have questions for your doctor. If your doctor does not ask you if you have questions, ask your doctor when the best time would be to ask them.

Understand the Answers and Next Steps

Asking questions is important but so is making sure you hear—and understand—the answers you get. Take notes, or bring someone to your appointment to help you understand and remember what you heard. If you do not understand or are confused, ask your doctor to explain the answer again.

It is very important to understand the plan or next steps that your doctor recommends. Ask questions to make sure you understand what your doctor wants you to do.

The questions you may want to ask will depend on whether your doctor gives you a diagnosis; recommends a treatment, medical test, or surgery; or gives you a prescription for medicine.

Questions could include:

- What is my diagnosis?
- What are my treatment options? What are the benefits of each option? What are the side effects?
- Will I need a test? What is the test for? What will the results tell me?
- What will the medicine you are prescribing do? How do I take it? Are there any side effects?
- Why do I need surgery? Are there other ways to treat my condition? How often do you perform this surgery?
- Do I need to change my daily routine?

Find out what you are to do next. Ask for written instructions, brochures, videos, or websites that may help you learn more.

After Your Appointment

After you meet with your doctor, you will need to follow her or his instructions to keep your health on track.

Your doctor may have you fill a prescription or make another appointment for tests, lab work, or a follow-up visit. It is important for you to follow your doctor's instructions.

It also is important to call your doctor if you are unclear about any instructions or have more questions.

Prioritize Your Questions

Create a list of follow-up questions to ask if you:

- Have a health problem
- Need to get or change a medicine
- Need a medical test
- Need to have surgery

Other Times to Call Your Doctor

There are other times when you should follow up on your care and call your doctor. Call your doctor:

- If you experience any side effects or other problems with your medicines
- If your symptoms get worse after seeing the doctor
- If you receive any new prescriptions or start taking any over-the-counter (OTC) medicines
- To get results of any tests you have had. Do not assume that no news is good news.
- To ask about test results you do not understand

Your questions help your doctor and healthcare team learn more about you. Your doctor's answers to your questions can help you make better decisions, receive a higher level of care, avoid medical harm, and feel better about your healthcare. Your questions can also lead to better results for your health.

Chapter 51

Minimally Invasive Spinal Surgery

What Is Minimally Invasive Spine Surgery?

Minimally invasive spine surgery (MISS) is a type of surgery that uses smaller incisions on the bones of the spine. In a traditional open spine surgery, an incision is typically five or six inches in length. The muscles around the spine retract, and this often causes harm to nearby muscles and other tissues. As a result, patients may have postsurgical pain, which extends the time of recovery.

With MISS, a smaller incision is made, and a tubular retractor is inserted. The necessary tools are then passed through the tunnel for the procedure, which ensures less injury to the neighboring muscles and tissues. This helps the surgeon access the exact location of the problem in the spine and allows her or him to view real-time X-ray images.

The other advantages of MISS are:

- A lower risk of infection
- Less bleeding
- Less postsurgical pain

"Minimally Invasive Spinal Surgery," © 2019 Omnigraphics. Reviewed April 2019.

- Smaller incisions and better cosmetic results
- A faster recovery time

MISS can be used for specific types of spine surgery, such as lumbar discectomy, laminectomy, and spinal fusion.

When Do I Need Minimally Invasive Spine Surgery?

Most of the time, patients do not need surgery for back pain, as it can be corrected with pain medications, corrective exercises, and other physical therapy modalities. When the pain is not controlled with these modalities, your doctor may recommend surgery. Spine surgery may be suggested if you have any of the following diagnoses:

- Protruded disc
- Narrowing of the spinal canal (spinal stenosis)
- Spinal deformities
- Spinal instability
- Spondylolysis (stress fracture in a lower vertebra)
- Vertebral fractures
- Tumour or infection in the spine

Not all of the above-listed conditions can be treated with MISS. You should discuss your options with your healthcare provider as it requires expertise and hospital facilities.

Commonly Performed Minimally Invasive Spine Surgeries

Spinal Decompression

When there is a narrowing of the spinal column, the nerve roots are compressed. This can result in symptoms such as pain, numbness, and muscle weakness. With MISS, using a tubular retractor, microscope, and endoscope, the bone and the tissue causing the nerve compression are removed. The most commonly done decompressive surgeries are laminectomy and foraminotomy.

Discectomy

Spinal discs are essentially jelly-like elastic rings with a soft gel on the inside. This acts as shock absorbers and cushions between the vertebral bones. If this structure becomes weakened due to overuse or injuries, the soft gel-like tissue can come outside of the elastic ring. A herniated disc can compress the nerves that are causing the pain. With MISS, the surgeon can trim or remove the herniated disc, using tubular dilators and a microscope or endoscope.

Transforaminal Lumbar Interbody Fusion

Transforaminal lumbar interbody fusion (TLIF) is performed in patients with mechanical low back pain and in patients with low back pain that is caused by postlaminectomy instability and/or spinal trauma. TLF is performed from the posterior (back) approach, and the patient is lying on her or his stomach.

Complications of Minimally Invasive Spine Surgery

Before MISS, discuss the potential complications of MISS with your healthcare provider, which may include:

- **Infection.** Antibiotics will be prescribed before, during, and after surgery to reduce the risk of infections.
- **Bleeding.** However, it may not be significant.
- **Pain.** Some patients may experience pain at the operated site.
- **Blood clots.** This is, again, a rare complication after surgery, but they are dangerous if they break and travel to the lungs.
    - In some patients, there may be a recurrence of their earlier symptoms.
    - In rare conditions, nerve damage can occur during the procedure.

What Happens after a Minimally Invasive Spine Surgery

- Some types of MISS can be done as an outpatient procedure, and some may need one or more night's stay in the hospital.
- The postoperative pain will be treated with effective pain medications.

- As soon as the patient is able to, they may resume their normal diet.
- Call your healthcare provider if you have severe symptoms, pain, difficulty breathing, or headache.
- The physical therapist will give instructions about how to use the back cautiously after surgery. Lifting or bending may be limited, and you may need to wear a back brace for some time after the surgery. Strengthening exercises will be prescribed by the therapist for muscles around the spine.
- Normal activities of daily living can be resumed in a few weeks' time.
- Make sure to carry out the healthcare provider's instructions about treatment and follow-up appointments so that the recovery is smooth, effective, and fast.

References

1. "Minimally Invasive Spine Surgery," American Association of Neurological Surgeons (AANS), n.d.
2. "Minimally Invasive Spine Surgery," The Johns Hopkins Medicine, n.d.
3. "Minimally Invasive Spine Surgery," American Academy of Orthopaedic Surgeons (AAOS), n.d.

Chapter 52

Neck Surgery

The spinal column consists of 33 vertebrae that extend from the base of the skull to the pelvis. The cervical spine (neck) comprises 8 pairs of spinal nerves and 7 vertebrae, which are separated by intervertebral discs. These discs act as a shock absorber and allow the spine to move freely during any activity.

The spinal cord runs through the hollow space known as "spinal canal," which is located between the vertebrae and the arch (situated behind each vertebra). A pair of nerves exit from the spinal cord through small openings called "foramina" (one to the left and one to the right) at each vertebral level.

The purpose of neck surgery is to treat spinal instability and nerve or spinal compression. Most often, neck surgeries are suggested for the following conditions and/or problems:

- **Cervical disc disease** is a condition in which one or more discs located between the vertebrae degenerates and ruptures. This break down of the outer covering of the disc causes the inner gel-like substance (nucleus pulposus) to herniate and compress the spinal nerve roots. This compression causes pain in the neck, which sometimes spreads to the arm.
- **Cervical stenosis** is caused by age-related degenerative changes in which the spinal canal narrows. This will lead to a compression of the spinal cord and/or nerves.

When Do We Need Surgery?

Conventional treatment will be the initial treatment method recommended by doctors. This treatment usually includes over-the-counter (OTC) medicines, prescription drugs, and physical therapy. Neck surgery is only recommended when the conventional treatment is ineffective, if symptoms persist, and if the pain starts to affect the activities of daily living.

Surgical Treatments

The primary goals of surgery are to relieve pain and restore the functional stability of the cervical spine. There are many types of surgical treatments; however, the choice regarding which surgical treatment is used is influenced by the diagnosis and severity of the problem. Most cervical spine surgeries can be performed with noninvasive techniques, such as with the use of an endoscope or laser. The most common surgical procedures are listed below.

Anterior Cervical Discectomy and Fusion

Anterior cervical discectomy and fusion (ACDF) is a surgery used to remove a degenerated or herniated disc in the neck. The surgeon reaches the damaged disc from the anterior (front) of the spine. The trachea, esophagus, and the muscles are moved aside to expose the cervical vertebrae. Depending on the symptoms, one or more discs may be removed.

After the removal of the damaged disc, a bone graft is placed in between the vertebrae to fill the empty space. This prevents the vertebrae from collapsing or rubbing against other vertebra. There are three types of bone grafts used in spinal fusion surgery. They are as follows:

- **Autograft bone** is a type of bone graft that is extracted from your own bones. The surgeon takes bone cells from the iliac crest (hip) for spinal fusion surgery. The autograft bone has the highest fusion rate because it has bone-growing cells and proteins.
- **Allograft bone** is a type of bone graft in which the bone cells are extracted from a donor (cadaver). This bone graft does not contain bone-growing cells, but it eliminates the need of extracting the bone from the same person.
- **Bone graft substitutes** are human-made materials, such as ceramics and plastics. This bone graft is also known as "cages," and involves shaving of the bone tissue taken from your spine during surgery.

The range of motion of the cervical spine decreases with the number of fusions performed on your cervical spine.

Anterior Cervical Corpectomy

Anterior cervical corpectomy is performed in conjunction with ACDF. A corpectomy is a surgical procedure in which a surgeon removes one or more vertebral bodies to relieve compression and pressure on the spinal cord due to bone spurs. This procedure is done by making an incision at the anterior (front) side of the spine. The incision is typically large and requires a longer time to heal than the anterior cervical discectomy. The gap between the vertebrae is filled using bone grafts.

Posterior Cervical Laminectomy

This procedure involves a small incision at the posterior (back) of the neck to remove the lamina (bony part behind vertebra). Posterior cervical laminectomy is done to relieve excess pressure on the spinal cord and/or nerves.

Posterior Microdiscectomy

Posterior microdiscectomy is performed through an incision in the back of the neck, typically in the middle of your neck. This surgical treatment may be considered for a disc herniation that is located on the side of the spinal cord. A high-speed burr is used for removing some of the facet joint, and this is done to identify the nerve root under the facet joint. The nerve root is moved aside to free up the space and remove the disc herniation.

Arthroplasty

Arthroplasty (artificial disc), also known as "cervical artificial disc surgery," is a procedure in which the surgeon inserts an artificial disc in the intervertebral space between two vertebrae. This is performed after the removal of the cervical disc.

Postsurgical Complications

The risks and complications associated with neck surgery are as follows:

- Chronic pain in the neck or arm

- Inadequate symptom relief
- Infection
- Excessive bleeding
- Cerebral fluid leakage
- Damage to the trachea, esophagus, or vocal cords
- Spinal instability

After the surgery, the doctor will give specific postsurgical instructions, such as therapy and medications, in order to relieve pain and restore the flexibility of the cervical spine. Discomfort is expected while you return to day-to-day activities; however, it is advised to stop what you are doing when you feel pain in the surgical area.

References

1. "Anterior Cervical Discectomy and Fusion (ACDF)," Mayfield Brain & Spine, November 2018.
2. "Cervical Spine Surgeries," The American Center for Spine and Neurosurgery (ACSN), November 28, 2011.
3. Ullrich, Peter F. "Controversies about Spinal Fusion Surgery: Allografts, Autografts, and Fusion Levels," SPINE-health, January 2010.
4. "Cervical Disc Surgery: Disc Replacement or Fusion?" WebMD, July 7, 2018.
5. "Cervical Spine," American Association of Neurological Surgeons (AANS), July 1, 2010.

Chapter 53

Low Back Surgery

Chapter Contents

Section 53.1—What Is Lumbar Spinal Surgery? 396
Section 53.2—Surgical versus Nonsurgical Therapy for Chronic Low Back Pain 399

Section 53.1

What Is Lumbar Spinal Surgery?

This section contains text excerpted from the following sources: Text in this section begins with excerpts from "Back Pain Information Page," National Institute of Neurological Disorders and Stroke (NINDS), March 27, 2019; Text under the heading "Indications for Lumbar Surgery" is excerpted from "Back Pain," National Institute of Arthritis and Musculoskeletal and Skin Diseases (NIAMS), August 30, 2016; Text under the heading "Types of Surgical Procedures" is excerpted from "Low Back Pain Fact Sheet," National Institute of Neurological Disorders and Stroke (NINDS), August 7, 2018.

Most low back pain can be treated without surgery. Treatment involves using over-the-counter (OTC) pain relievers to reduce discomfort and anti-inflammatory drugs to reduce inflammation. The goal of treatment is to restore proper function and strength to the back and prevent recurrence of the injury. Medications are often used to treat acute and chronic low back pain. Effective pain relief may involve a combination of prescription drugs and over-the-counter remedies. Although the use of cold and hot compresses has never been scientifically proven to quickly resolve low back injury, compresses may help reduce pain and inflammation and allow greater mobility for some individuals. Bed rest is recommended for only one to two days at most. Individuals can resume activities as soon as possible. Exercise may be the most effective way to speed recovery from low back pain and help strengthen back and abdominal muscles. In the most serious cases, when the condition does not respond to other therapies, surgery may relieve pain caused by back problems or serious musculoskeletal injuries.

Indications for Lumbar Surgery

Back pain is a symptom of a medical condition. Many times, the cause of back pain is never known. Back pain can get better even if you do not know the cause. Surgical treatments may be necessary in some cases, including:

- **Herniated (ruptured) discs**, where one or more of the discs that cushion the bones of the spine are damaged. The jelly-like center of the disc leaks, causing pain.
- **Spinal stenosis**, a narrowing of the spinal column that puts pressure on the spinal cord and nerves

- **Spondylolisthesis**, where one or more bones in the spine slip out of place
- **Vertebral fractures** caused by injury to the bones in the spine or by osteoporosis
- **Degenerative disc disease (DDD),** or damage to the spine's discs as a person gets older
- In rare cases, back pain is caused by a tumor, an infection, or a nerve root problem called "cauda equina syndrome." In these cases, surgery is needed right away to ease the pain and prevent more problems.

Types of Surgical Procedures

Surgical procedures are not always successful, and there is little evidence to show which procedures work best for their particular indications. Patients considering surgical approaches should be fully informed of all related risks. Surgical options include:

- **Vertebroplasty and kyphoplasty** are minimally invasive treatments to repair compression fractures of the vertebrae caused by osteoporosis. Vertebroplasty uses three-dimensional (3-D) imaging to assist in guiding a fine needle through the skin and into the vertebral body, the largest part of the vertebrae. A glue-like bone cement is then injected into the vertebral body space, which quickly hardens to stabilize and strengthen the bone and provide pain relief. In kyphoplasty, prior to injecting the bone cement, a special balloon is inserted and gently inflated to restore height to the vertebral structure and reduce spinal deformity.
- **Spinal laminectomy** (also known as "spinal decompression") is performed when spinal stenosis causes a narrowing of the spinal canal that causes pain, numbness, or weakness. During the procedure, the lamina—or bony walls of the vertebrae—along with any bone spurs, are removed. The aim of the procedure is to open up the spinal column to remove pressure on the nerves.
- **Discectomy or microdiscectomy** may be recommended to remove a disc in cases where it has herniated and presses on a nerve root or the spinal cord, which may cause intense and enduring pain. A microdiscectomy is similar to a conventional discectomy; however, this procedure involves removing the

herniated disc through a much smaller incision in the back and a more rapid recovery. Laminectomy and discectomy are frequently performed together, and the combination is one of the more common ways to remove pressure on a nerve root from a herniated disc or bone spur.

- **Foraminotomy** is an operation that "cleans out" or enlarges the bony hole (foramen) where a nerve root exits the spinal canal. Bulging discs or joints thickened with age can cause narrowing of the space through which the spinal nerve exits and can press on the nerve, resulting in pain, numbness, and weakness in an arm or leg. Small pieces of bone over the nerve are removed through a small slit, allowing the surgeon to cut away the blockage and relieve pressure on the nerve.
- **Intradiscal electrothermal therapy (IDET)** is a treatment for discs that are cracked or bulging as a result of degenerative disc disease. The procedure involves inserting a catheter through a small incision at the site of the disc in the back. A special wire is passed through the catheter, and an electrical current is applied to heat the disc, which helps strengthen the collagen fibers of the disc wall, reducing the bulging and the related irritation of the spinal nerve. IDET is of questionable benefit.
- **Nucleoplasty**, also called "plasma disc decompression" (PDD), is a type of laser surgery that uses radiofrequency energy to treat people with low back pain associated with mildly herniated discs. Under X-ray guidance, a needle is inserted into the disc. A plasma laser device is then inserted into the needle and the tip is heated to 40 to 70 degrees Celsius, creating a field that vaporizes the tissue in the disc, reducing its size and relieving pressure on the nerves. Several channels may be made depending on how tissue needs to be removed to decompress the disc and nerve root.
- **Radiofrequency denervation** is a procedure using electrical impulses to interrupt nerve conduction (including the conduction of pain signals). Using X-ray guidance, a needle is inserted into a target area of nerves and a local anesthetic is introduced as a way of confirming the involvement of the nerves in the person's back pain. Next, the region is heated, resulting in localized destruction of the target nerves. Pain relief associated with the technique is temporary, and the evidence supporting this technique is limited.

- **Spinal fusion** is used to strengthen the spine and prevent painful movements in people with degenerative disc disease or spondylolisthesis (following laminectomy). The spinal disc between two or more vertebrae is removed, and the adjacent vertebrae are "fused" by bone grafts and/or metal devices secured by screws. The fusion can be performed through the abdomen, a procedure known as an "anterior lumbar interbody fusion," or through the back, called "posterior fusion." Spinal fusion may result in some loss of flexibility in the spine and requires a long recovery period to allow the bone grafts to grow and fuse the vertebrae together. Spinal fusion has been associated with an acceleration of disc degeneration at adjacent levels of the spine.
- **Artificial disc replacement** is considered an alternative to spinal fusion for the treatment of people with severely damaged discs. The procedure involves removal of the disc and its replacement by a synthetic disc that helps restore height and movement between the vertebrae.

Section 53.2

Surgical versus Nonsurgical Therapy for Chronic Low Back Pain

This section includes text excerpted from "Low Back Pain Fact Sheet," National Institute of Neurological Disorders and Stroke (NINDS), August 7, 2018.

Studies funded by the National Institute of Neurological Disorders and Stroke (NINDS) are contributing to a better understanding of why some people with acute low back pain recover fully, while others go on to develop chronic low back pain. Brain imaging studies suggest that people with chronic low back pain have changes in brain structure and function. In one study, people with subacute back pain were followed for one year. Researchers found that certain patterns of functional connectivity across brain networks correlated with the likelihood of pain becoming chronic. The findings suggest that such patterns may help predict who is most likely to transition from subacute to chronic back pain. Other research seeks to determine the role of brain circuits important for emotional and motivational learning and memory in this transition, in order to identify new preventive interventions.

Disc degeneration remains a key cause of chronic low back pain, and the pain often persists despite surgery. National Institutes of Health (NIH)-funded basic science and preclinical studies are investigating molecular-level mechanisms that cause discs in the spine to degenerate, as well as protective mechanisms involved in disc remodeling that may diminish with advancing age. Such studies may help identify future therapeutic strategies to block degenerative mechanisms or promote remodeling processes. The NIH also is funding early research on stem cell approaches to promote disc regeneration and rejuvenate cells of the nucleus pulposus, the jelly-like substance in the center of intervertebral discs that loses water content as people age.

Several NIH-funded clinical trials and other studies in patients aim to improve treatment options and prevention strategies for chronic low back pain, as well as add to the evidence base about existing treatments. A multi-year multicenter study called the "Spine Patient Outcomes Research Trial" (SPORT) compared the most commonly used surgical and nonsurgical treatments for patients with the three most common diagnoses for which spine surgery is performed: intervertebral disc herniation, spinal stenosis, and degenerative spondylolisthesis (DS). SPORT represented the largest clinical investigation to date looking at treatment results for these disabling and costly causes of chronic low back pain.

Results after four years of follow-up showed that in general, otherwise healthy people who have surgery for one of these three conditions are likely to fare better than those who receive nonoperative care. However, the results also indicated that people who are reluctant to have surgery may also recover with nonoperative treatments if their conditions are not progressing and their pain is tolerable, and importantly, delaying or avoiding surgery did not cause additional damage in most cases. Researchers are continuing to track SPORT patient cohorts over a nine-year follow-up period to assess longer-term treatment results and cost-effectiveness across treatment options. In the interest of improving surgical techniques, NIH also is funding research on factors that contribute to the success or failure of artificial disc replacement surgery, including studies to compare discs on the market for significant differences in their durability rates over time.

Epidural injections of steroid drugs are frequently used to treat sciatica, despite limited evidence for their effectiveness. Moreover, these treatments are based on the assumption that reducing local inflammation in the vertebral column will relieve pain, but an association between structural abnormalities, inflammation, and sciatica symptoms has not been clearly demonstrated. NINDS-funded researchers are using a new imaging technique that can detect inflammation to better understand what causes chronic sciatica pain and to provide evidence to inform treatment selection.

Other NIH-funded studies are investigating physical therapy (PT) and chiropractic approaches. For example, researchers are studying whether therapy programs that emphasize certain types of exercises, such as core stabilization exercises, provide benefit to people who experience recurrent low back pain.

The increasing use of spinal manipulation and mobilization, despite lacking evidence for more than small or moderate benefit, has prompted NIH-funded researchers to study the mechanisms of these two techniques and to conduct a randomized controlled trial to assess and compare their effectiveness for the treatment of chronic low back pain.

Finally, NIH-funded researchers are studying various complementary and alternative therapies for low back pain, including those aimed at reducing stress and negative emotions believed to aggravate the experience of pain. For example, virtual reality programs are being studied for their ability to help people cope with persistent pain.

Chapter 54

Spinal Fusion Surgery

Spinal fusion surgery, also called spondylodesis or spondylosyndesis, is a procedure in which two or more vertebrae of the spine are fused together to eliminate movement between them. It is generally performed in the cervical (neck) or lumbar (lower back) region. This surgery is somewhat similar to a welding process; however, the spinal fusion surgery does not weld the vertebrae immediately. Rather, bone grafts are placed in between the vertebrae and fused together with the help of metal plates, screws, and rods.

When Is the Surgery Recommended?

Spinal fusion surgery is usually considered as a last option when other treatment methods, such as physical therapy, medications, etc., fail. The doctors recommend this surgery only if they know the exact cause of the problem.

The spinal fusion surgery can relieve pain caused by:

- Motion of the vertebrae
- Vertebral fracture
- Degenerative disc diseases
- Herniated or slipped discs
- Instability or weakness of the spine

- Scoliosis
- Spinal stenosis
- Spondylolisthesis
- Spinal infection
- Spinal tumor

How to Prepare for the Surgery

Before the surgery, the doctor may recommend several imaging tests, such as X-rays, computed tomography (CT) scan, and magnetic resonance imaging (MRI) scan, etc. These images help the doctor plan the surgery. It is important to talk about the medications that you can and cannot take before surgery with your doctor. Certain drugs, such as aspirin and anti-inflammatory drugs, can be unsafe; therefore, your doctor may recommend to stop such medications a few days prior to the surgery. Other preparations include trimming hair around the surgical site and cleaning the area with special antiseptics.

How Is the Surgery Performed?

The spinal fusion surgery is usually performed under general anesthesia. There are a number of techniques for performing this surgery. The general procedures involved are:

Incision

The doctor makes an incision in the patient's body to gain access to the spine. There are different approaches that can be utilized in order to reach the spine.

- **Anterior approach:** The spine is accessed from the front. The incision is made in the abdomen, in order to reach the spine in the lumbar region, and in the throat, to reach the spine in the cervical region.
- **Posterior approach:** The spine is accessed directly by making incisions on the back.
- **Lateral approach:** The spine is approached from the side. This approach is less common when compared to the other two approaches.

The best approach is decided based on various factors, such as the location of the vertebrae to be fused, the nature of the pain, the patient's general health condition, and the body shape of the patient.

Bone Grafts

All spinal fusions involve some kind of bone materials, called "bone grafts," that are placed in between the vertebrae. These bone grafts increase bone production, help the vertebrae heal, and promote fusion. The bone required for bone grafting can be harvested from the patient's own body. This procedure is called an "autograft." Usually, in an autograft, a healthy bone is extracted from the pelvis. An alternative to this method is called an "allograft," where the bone is obtained from another person. This is usually done through bone banks. However, today, several artificial bone graft materials have been developed to act as a substitute for both autografts and allografts. Some examples of such artificial bone grafts are:

- Demineralized bone matrices (DBMs)
- Bone morphogenetic proteins (BMPs)
- Synthetic bone

Fusion

After the process of bone grafting, the vertebrae needs to be held together to promote the fusion. The doctor uses metallic plates, screws, and rods to keep the vertebrae intact. This is called "internal fixation." In addition, the doctor may recommend the use of neck and back braces for an external support. These supports can help patients recover faster and move earlier after the surgery.

Recovery after the Surgery

The spinal fusion surgery generally causes greater pain when compared to other spinal surgeries. Medications, such as opioids, nonsteroidal anti-inflammatory drugs (NSAIDs), and local anesthetics, can offer short-term pain relief. Doctors may also prescribe the use of postoperative pain control pumps. When the patient presses a button, these pumps deliver a predetermined amount of narcotic pain medication into the intravenous line.

After the surgery, the bones may take months to solidify and heal. The recovery may take anywhere between six weeks to six months.

The time period varies depending on several factors, such as the patient's age, health condition, and type of employment. During the recovery period, the movement and general activities of the patient are restricted. The patient will be taught how to sit, stand, and move properly to keep the spine aligned. The doctor may also recommend rehabilitation programs and physical therapy for faster recovery. As the patient regains strength, she or he can gradually increase the activity level.

Complications of the Surgery

As with any medical procedure, spinal fusion surgery also has its own risks and complications. The major complications associated with spinal fusion surgery are:

- Pain
- Bleeding
- Drainage from the wound
- Blood clots
- Infections
- Pseudarthrosis
- Nerve injury
- Shaking chills
- Fever over 100°F

It is important to strictly follow the postsurgical instructions given by the doctor to avoid serious complications. Contact your doctor immediately if you find any warning signs related to blood clots or infections.

References

1. Park, Daniel K. "Spinal Fusion," OrthoInfo, June 2018.
2. "Spinal Fusion," Mayo Clinic, February 28, 2019.
3. "What Is Spinal Fusion?" WebMD, January 8, 2018.
4. "Spinal Fusion," North American Spine Society (NASS), February 1, 2002.

Chapter 55

Bone Graft and Bone Allografts

What Is a Bone Graft?

A bone graft transplants bone tissue. Surgeons use bone grafts to repair and rebuild diseased bones in your hips, knees, spine, and sometimes other bones and joints. Grafts can also repair bone loss caused by some types of fractures or cancers. Once your body accepts the bone graft, it provides a framework for the growth of new, living bone.

What Is a Bone Allograft?

If the transplanted bone comes from another person, it is called an "allograft." Most allograft bone comes from donors who have died. Tissue banks screen these donors and disinfect and test the donated bone to make sure it is safe to use. If the transplanted bone comes from another part of your own body, it is called an "autograft." Autograft bone often comes from your ribs, hips, or a leg.

This chapter contains text excerpted from the following sources: Text beginning with the heading "What Is a Bone Graft?" is excerpted from "Bone Graft," Medline Plus, National Institutes of Health (NIH), December 31, 2016; Text beginning with the heading "How Many Types of Bone Allograft Are There?" is excerpted from "Frequently Asked Questions—Bone Allografts," Centers for Disease Control and Prevention (CDC), October 25, 2013. Reviewed April 2019.

How Many Types of Bone Allografts Are There?

An allograft is a graft between genetically dissimilar members of the same species. An allograft may be obtained from living donors who are having bone removed during surgery or cadaveric donors. Allograft material has been used for more than 30 years in periodontal therapy. There are several types of allografts:

- Fresh; fresh-frozen allograft
- Freeze-dried bone allograft (FDBA)
- Demineralized freeze-dried bone allograft (DFDBA)

What Is the Risk of Disease Transmission with Bone Allografts?

Both FDBA and DFDBA materials are widely used in periodontal therapy, and there are no reports of disease transmission during the 30-year history of using freeze-dried bone allografts. However, there have been 4 cases of human immunodeficiency virus (HIV) infection following procedures using fresh-frozen bone allografts. These cases involved surgeries of the spine, hip, and knee. It is important to note, however, that fresh-frozen and fresh allografts are not typically used in periodontal therapy. Also, when using FDBA and DFDBA, the delay in processing ensures adequate time for testing for potential pathogens.

Most bone banks adhere to the guidelines of the American Association of Tissue Banks (AATB), with respect to procurement, processing, and sterilization of bone grafts. The AATB advocates excluding the collection of bone under the following circumstances:

- Donors from high-risk groups, as determined by medical testing and behavioral risk assessments
- Donors test positive for HIV antibody by enzyme-linked immunosorbent assay (ELISA).
- Autopsy of donor reveals occult disease.
- Donor bone tests positive for bacterial contamination.
- Donor and bone test positive for hepatitis B surface antigen (HBsAg) or hepatitis C virus (HCV).
- Donor tests positive for syphilis.

Using donor screening recommendations, it has been calculated that the chance of obtaining a bone graft from an HIV-infected donor (e.g., one who failed to be excluded by one of the exclusionary techniques) is 1 in 1.67 million. Furthermore, the probability that DFDBA might contain HIV has been calculated to be one in 2.8 billion. Therefore, the established exclusionary criteria combined with recommended processing procedures (harvesting in a sterile manner, repeated washings, immersion in ethanol, freezing in liquid nitrogen, freeze-drying, demineralization, and vacuum sealing) render DFDBA and FDBA grafts safe for human implantation.

Part Seven

Cancers of the Back and Neck

Chapter 56

Childhood Brain and Spinal Cord Tumors

The Brain, the Spinal Cord, and Their Functions[1]

Together, the brain and spinal cord make up the central nervous system (CNS). The brain controls many important body functions.

The brain has three major parts:

- The **cerebrum** is the largest part of the brain. It is at the top of the head. The cerebrum controls thinking, learning, problem-solving, emotions, speech, reading, writing, and voluntary movement.
- The **cerebellum** is in the lower back of the brain (near the middle of the back of the head). It controls movement, balance, and posture.
- The **brain stem** connects the brain to the spinal cord. It is in the lowest part of the brain (just above the back of the neck). The brain stem controls breathing, heart rate, and the nerves

---

This chapter includes text excerpted from documents published by two public domain sources. Text under the headings marked 1 are excerpted from "Childhood Brain and Spinal Cord Tumors Treatment Overview (PDQ®)—Patient Version," National Cancer Institute (NCI), January 15, 2019; Text under the heading marked 2 is excerpted from "Brain and Spinal Tumors Information Page," National Institute of Neurological Disorders and Stroke (NINDS), March 27, 2019.

and muscles used in seeing, hearing, walking, talking, and eating.

The spinal cord connects the brain with nerves in most parts of the body. The spinal cord is a column of nerve tissue that runs from the brain stem and down the center of the back. It is covered by three thin layers of tissue called "membranes." These membranes are surrounded by the vertebrae (back bones). Spinal cord nerves carry messages between the brain and the rest of the body, such as a message from the brain to cause muscles to move or a message from the skin to the brain to feel touch.

Overview of Brain and Spinal Cord Tumors[2]

Tumors of the brain and spinal cord are abnormal growths of tissue found inside the skull or the bony spinal column. The brain and spinal cord are the primary components of the CNS. Benign tumors are noncancerous, and malignant tumors are cancerous. The CNS is housed within rigid, bony quarters (i.e., the skull and spinal column), so any abnormal growth, whether benign or malignant, can place pressure on sensitive tissues and impair function. Tumors that originate in the brain or spinal cord are called "primary tumors." Most primary tumors are caused by out-of-control growth among cells that surround and support neuron, specific genetic disease (such as neurofibromatosis type 1 and tuberous sclerosis), or from exposure to radiation or cancer-causing chemicals. Metastatic, or secondary, tumors in the CNS are caused by cancer cells that break away from a primary tumor located in another region of the body. Tumors can place pressure on sensitive tissues and impair function.

About Childhood Brain and Spinal Cord Tumors[1]

A childhood brain or spinal cord tumor is a disease in which abnormal cells form in the tissues of the brain or spinal cord. There are many types of childhood brain and spinal cord tumors. The tumors are formed by the abnormal growth of cells and may begin in different areas of the brain or spinal cord.

The tumors may be benign (not cancer) or malignant (cancer). Benign brain tumors grow and press on nearby areas of the brain. They rarely spread into other tissues. Malignant brain tumors are likely to grow quickly and spread into other brain tissue. When a tumor grows into or presses on an area of the brain, it may stop that part of the brain from working the way it should. Both benign and malignant brain tumors can cause signs or symptoms and need treatment.

Brain and spinal cord tumors are a common type of childhood cancer. Although cancer is rare in children, brain and spinal cord tumors are the second most common type of childhood cancer, after leukemia. Brain tumors can occur in both children and adults. Treatment for children is usually different than treatment for adults.

This chapter describes the treatment of primary brain and spinal cord tumors (tumors that begin in the brain and spinal cord).

Signs and Symptoms of Childhood Brain and Spinal Cord Tumors[1]

The cause of most childhood brain and spinal cord tumors is unknown. The signs and symptoms of childhood brain and spinal cord tumors are not the same in every child.

Signs and symptoms depend on the following:

- Where the tumor forms in the brain or spinal cord
- The size of the tumor
- How fast the tumor grows
- The child's age and development

Signs and symptoms may be caused by childhood brain and spinal cord tumors or by other conditions, including cancer that has spread to the brain. Check with your child's doctor if your child has any of the following:

The brain tumor signs and symptoms include:

- Morning headache or headache that goes away after vomiting
- Frequent nausea and vomiting
- Vision, hearing, and speech problems
- Loss of balance and trouble walking
- Unusual sleepiness or change in activity level
- Unusual changes in personality or behavior
- Seizures
- Increase in head size (in infants)

The signs and symptoms of spinal cord tumor include:

- Back pain or pain that spreads from the back towards the arms or legs
- A change in bowel habits or trouble urinating
- Weakness in the legs
- Trouble walking

In addition to these signs and symptoms of brain and spinal cord tumors, some children are unable to reach certain growth and development milestones, such as sitting up, walking, and talking in sentences.

Diagnosis of Spinal Cord Tumor[1]

Tests that examine the brain and spinal cord are used to detect (find) childhood brain and spinal cord tumors.

The following tests and procedures may be used:

- **Physical exam and history**. An exam of the body to check general signs of health, including checking for signs of disease, such as lumps or anything else that seems unusual. A history of the patient's health habits and past illnesses and treatments will also be taken.
- **Neurological exam**. A series of questions and tests to check the brain, spinal cord, and nerve function. The exam checks a person's mental status, coordination, and ability to walk normally, and how well the muscles, senses, and reflexes work. This may also be called a "neuro exam" or a "neurologic exam."
- **Magnetic resonance imaging (MRI) with gadolinium**. A procedure that uses a magnet, radio waves, and a computer to make a series of detailed pictures of the brain and spinal cord. A substance called "gadolinium" is injected into a vein. The gadolinium collects around the cancer cells so they show up brighter in the picture. This procedure is also called "nuclear magnetic resonance imaging" (NMRI).
- **Serum tumor marker test**. A procedure in which a sample of blood is examined to measure the amounts of certain substances released into the blood by organs, tissues, or tumor cells in the body. Certain substances are linked to specific types of cancer when found in increased levels in the blood. These are called "tumor markers."

- **Immunohistochemistry**. A test that uses antibodies to check for certain antigens in a sample of tissue. The antibody is usually linked to a radioactive substance or a dye that causes the tissue to light up under a microscope. This type of test may be used to tell the difference between different types of cancer.

Certain Factors Affect Prognosis

The prognosis (chance of recovery) depends on the following:

- Whether there are any cancer cells left after surgery
- The type of tumor
- Where the tumor is in the body
- The child's age
- Whether the tumor has just been diagnosed or has recurred (come back)

Staging Childhood Brain and Spinal Cord Tumors[1]

In childhood brain and spinal cord tumors, treatment options are based on several factors.

Staging is the process used to find how much cancer there is and if cancer has spread within the brain, spinal cord, or to other parts of the body. It is important to know the stage in order to plan cancer treatment.

In childhood brain and spinal cord tumors, there is no standard staging system. Instead, the plan for cancer treatment depends on several factors:

The type of tumor and where the tumor formed in the brain:

- **Whether the tumor is newly diagnosed or recurrent.** A newly diagnosed brain or spinal cord tumor is one that has never been treated. A recurrent childhood brain or spinal cord tumor is one that has recurred after it has been treated. Childhood brain and spinal cord tumors may come back in the same place or in another part of the brain or spinal cord. Sometimes they come back in another part of the body. The tumor may come back many years after first being treated. Tests and procedures, including biopsy, that were done to diagnose and stage the tumor may be done to find out if the tumor has recurred.

- **The grade of the tumor.** The grade of the tumor is based on how abnormal the cancer cells look under a microscope and how quickly the tumor is likely to grow and spread. It is important to know the grade of the tumor and if there were any cancer cells remaining after surgery in order to plan treatment. The grade of the tumor is not used to plan treatment for all types of brain and spinal cord tumors.
- **The tumor risk group.** Risk groups are either average risk and poor risk or low, intermediate, and high risk. The risk groups are based on the amount of tumor remaining after surgery; the spread of cancer cells within the brain, spinal cord, or other parts of the body, where the tumor has formed; and the age of the child. The risk group is not used to plan treatment for all types of brain and spinal cord tumors.

The information from tests and procedures done to detect childhood brain and spinal cord tumors is used to determine the tumor risk group.

After the tumor is removed in surgery, some of the tests used to detect childhood brain and spinal cord tumors are repeated to help determine the tumor risk group. This is to find out how much tumor remains after surgery.

Other tests and procedures may be done to find out if cancer has spread:

- **Lumbar puncture.** A procedure used to collect cerebrospinal fluid (CSF) from the spinal column. This is done by placing a needle between two bones in the spine and into the CSF around the spinal cord and removing a sample of the fluid. The sample of CSF is checked under a microscope for signs that the tumor has spread to the CSF. The sample may also be checked for the amounts of protein and glucose. A higher than normal amount of protein or lower than normal amount of glucose may be a sign of a tumor. This procedure is also called an "LP" or "spinal tap." A lumbar puncture is usually not used to stage childhood spinal cord tumors.
- **Bone scan.** A procedure to check if there are rapidly dividing cells, such as cancer cells, in the bone. A very small amount of radioactive material is injected into a vein and travels through the bloodstream. The radioactive material collects in the bones with cancer and is detected by a scanner.

- **Bone marrow aspiration and biopsy.** The removal of bone marrow, blood, and a small piece of bone by inserting a hollow needle into the hipbone or breastbone. A pathologist views the bone marrow, blood, and bone under a microscope to look for signs of cancer.

Treatment Options Overview[1]

Different types of treatment are available for children with brain and spinal cord tumors. Some treatments are standard (the currently used treatment), and some are being tested in clinical trials. A treatment clinical trial is a research study meant to help improve current treatments or obtain information on new treatments for patients with cancer. When clinical trials show that a new treatment is better than the standard treatment, the new treatment may become the standard treatment.

Because cancer in children is rare, taking part in a clinical trial should be considered. Clinical trials are taking place in many parts of the country. Some clinical trials are open only to patients who have not started treatment.

Children with brain or spinal cord tumors should have their treatment planned by a team of healthcare providers who are experts in treating childhood brain and spinal cord tumors.

Treatment will be overseen by a pediatric oncologist, a doctor who specializes in treating children with cancer. The pediatric oncologist works with other healthcare providers who are experts in treating children with brain tumors and who specialize in certain areas of medicine. These may include the following specialists:

- Pediatrician
- Neurosurgeon
- Neurologist
- Neuro-oncologist
- Neuropathologist
- Neuroradiologist
- Radiation oncologist
- Endocrinologist
- Psychologist
- Ophthalmologist

- Rehabilitation specialist
- Social worker
- Nurse specialist

Treatment for Childhood Brain and Spinal Cord Tumors May Cause Side Effects

Side effects from cancer treatment that begin after treatment and continue for months or years are called "late effects." Late effects of cancer treatment may include the following:

- Physical problems
- Changes in mood, feelings, thinking, learning, or memory
- Second cancers (new types of cancer)

Some late effects may be treated or controlled. It is important to talk with your child's doctors about the effects cancer treatment can have on your child.

Types of Treatment

Three types of standard treatment are used:

Surgery

Surgery may be used to diagnose and treat childhood brain and spinal cord tumors.

Radiation Therapy

Radiation therapy is a cancer treatment that uses high-energy X-rays or other types of radiation to kill cancer cells or keep them from growing. There are two types of radiation therapy:

- **External radiation therapy** uses a machine outside the body to send radiation toward the cancer.
- **Internal radiation therapy** uses a radioactive substance sealed in needles, seeds, wires, or catheters that are placed directly into or near the cancer.

The way the radiation therapy is given depends on the type of cancer being treated. External radiation therapy is used to treat childhood brain and spinal cord tumors.

Chemotherapy

Chemotherapy is a cancer treatment that uses drugs to stop the growth of cancer cells, either by killing the cells or by stopping them from dividing. When chemotherapy is taken by mouth or injected into a vein or muscle, the drugs enter the bloodstream and can reach cancer cells throughout the body (systemic chemotherapy). When chemotherapy is placed directly in the cerebrospinal fluid; an organ; or a body cavity, such as the abdomen, the drugs mainly affect cancer cells in those areas (regional chemotherapy). The way the chemotherapy is given depends on the type and stage of the cancer being treated.

Anticancer drugs given by mouth or vein to treat brain and spinal cord tumors cannot cross the blood-brain barrier and enter the fluid that surrounds the brain and spinal cord. Instead, an anticancer drug is injected into the fluid-filled space to kill cancer cells there. This is called "intrathecal chemotherapy."

High-Dose Chemotherapy with Stem Cell Transplant

High doses of chemotherapy are given to kill cancer cells. Healthy cells, including blood-forming cells, are also destroyed by the cancer treatment. Stem cell transplant is a treatment to replace the blood-forming cells. Stem cells (immature blood cells) are removed from the blood or bone marrow of the patient or a donor and are frozen and stored. After the patient completes chemotherapy, the stored stem cells are thawed and given back to the patient through an infusion. These reinfused stem cells grow into (and restore) the body's blood cells.

Follow-Up Tests May Be Needed

Some of the tests that were done to diagnose the cancer or to find out the stage of the cancer may be repeated. Some tests will be repeated in order to see how well the treatment is working. Decisions about whether to continue, change, or stop treatment may be based on the results of these tests.

Some of the tests will continue to be done from time to time after treatment has ended. The results of these tests can show if your child's condition has changed or if the cancer has recurred. These tests are sometimes called "follow-up tests" or "checkups."

Chapter 57

Metastatic Squamous Neck Cancer

Metastatic squamous neck cancer with occult primary is a disease in which squamous cell cancer spreads to lymph nodes in the neck, and it is not known where the cancer first formed in the body.

Squamous cells are thin, flat cells found in tissues that form the surface of the skin and the lining of body cavities, such as the mouth; hollow organs, such as the uterus and blood vessels; and the lining of the respiratory (breathing) and digestive tracts. Some organs with squamous cells are the esophagus, lungs, kidneys, and uterus. Cancer can begin in squamous cells anywhere in the body and metastasize (spread) through the blood or lymph system to other parts of the body.

When squamous cell cancer spreads to lymph nodes in the neck or around the collarbone, it is called "metastatic squamous neck cancer." The doctor will try to find the primary tumor (the cancer that first formed in the body) because treatment for metastatic cancer is the same as treatment for the primary tumor. For example, when lung cancer spreads to the neck, the cancer cells in the neck are lung cancer cells, and they are treated the same as the cancer in the lung. Sometimes, doctors cannot find where in the body the cancer first began to grow. When tests cannot find a primary tumor, it is called an "occult

---

This chapter includes text excerpted from "Metastatic Squamous Neck Cancer with Occult Primary Treatment (Adult) (PDQ®)—Patient Version," National Cancer Institute (NCI), May 2, 2018.

(hidden) primary tumor." In many cases, the primary tumor is never found.

Signs and Symptoms of Metastatic Squamous Neck Cancer with Occult Primary

Signs and symptoms of metastatic squamous neck cancer with occult primary include a lump or pain in the neck or throat.

Check with your doctor if you have a lump or pain in your neck or throat that does not go away. These and other signs and symptoms may be caused by metastatic squamous neck cancer with occult primary. Other conditions may cause the same signs and symptoms.

Diagnosis of Metastatic Squamous Neck Cancer with Occult Primary

Tests that examine the tissues of the neck, respiratory tract, and upper part of the digestive tract are used to detect (find) and diagnose metastatic squamous neck cancer and the primary tumor.

Tests will include checking for a primary tumor in the organs and tissues of the respiratory tract (part of the trachea), the upper part of the digestive tract (including the lips, mouth, tongue, nose, throat, vocal cords, and part of the esophagus), and the genitourinary system.

The following procedures may be used:

- **Physical exam and history**. An exam of the body, especially the head and neck, to check general signs of health. This includes checking for signs of disease, such as lumps or anything else that seems unusual. A history of the patient's health habits and past illnesses and treatments will also be taken.
- **Biopsy**. The removal of cells or tissues so they can be viewed under a microscope by a pathologist or tested in the laboratory to check for signs of cancer. Three types of biopsy may be done:
    - **Fine-needle aspiration (FNA) biopsy**. The removal of tissue or fluid with the use of a thin needle.
    - **Core needle biopsy**. The removal of tissue with the use of a wide needle.
    - **Excisional biopsy**. The removal of an entire lump of tissue.

The following procedures are used to remove samples of cells or tissue:

- **Tonsillectomy**. Surgery to remove both tonsils.
- **Endoscopy**. A procedure to look at organs and tissues inside the body to check for abnormal areas. An endoscope is inserted through an incision (cut) in the skin or opening in the body, such as the mouth or nose. An endoscope is a thin, tube-like instrument with a light and a lens for viewing. It may also have a tool to remove abnormal tissue or lymph node samples, which are checked under a microscope for signs of disease. The nose, throat, back of the tongue, esophagus, stomach, voice box, windpipe, and large airways will be checked.

One or more of the following laboratory tests may be done to study the tissue samples:

- **Immunohistochemistry (IHC)**. A test that uses antibodies to check for certain antigens in a sample of blood or bone marrow. The antibody is usually linked to a radioactive substance or a dye that causes the tissue to light up under a microscope. This type of test may be used to tell the difference between different types of cancer.
- **Light and electron microscopy**. A test in which cells in a sample of tissue are viewed under regular and high-powered microscopes to look for certain changes in the cells.
- **Epstein-Barr virus (EBV) and human papillomavirus (HPV) test**. A test that checks the cells in a sample of tissue for EBV and HPV deoxyribonucleic acid (DNA).

- **Magnetic resonance imaging (MRI)**. A procedure that uses a magnet, radio waves, and a computer to make a series of detailed pictures of areas inside the body. This procedure is also called "nuclear magnetic resonance imaging" (NMRI).
- **Computed tomography (CT)/computed axial tomography (CAT) scan**. A procedure that makes a series of detailed pictures of areas inside the body, taken from different angles. The pictures are made by a computer linked to an X-ray machine. A dye may be injected into a vein or swallowed to help the organs or tissues show up more clearly. This procedure is also called "computed tomography," "computerized tomography," or "computerized axial tomography."
- **Positron emission tomography (PET) scan**. A procedure to find malignant tumor cells in the body. A small amount of

radioactive glucose (sugar) is injected into a vein. The PET scanner rotates around the body and makes a picture of where glucose is being used in the body. Malignant tumor cells show up brighter in the picture because they are more active and take up more glucose than normal cells do. A whole-body PET scan and a CT scan are done at the same time to look for where the cancer first formed. If there is any cancer, this increases the chance that it will be found.

A diagnosis of the occult primary tumor is made if the primary tumor is not found during testing or treatment.

Certain Factors Affect Prognosis

The prognosis and treatment options depend on the following:

- The number and size of lymph nodes that have cancer in them
- Whether the cancer has responded to treatment or has recurred
- How abnormal the cancer cells look under a microscope
- The patient's age and general health

Treatment options also depend on the following:

- Which part of the neck the cancer is in
- Whether certain tumor markers are found

Stages of Metastatic Squamous Neck Cancer with Occult Primary

After metastatic squamous neck cancer with occult primary has been diagnosed, tests are done to find out if cancer cells have spread to other parts of the body.

The process used to find out if cancer has spread to other parts of the body is called "staging." The results from tests and procedures used to detect and diagnose the primary tumor are also used to find out if cancer has spread to other parts of the body.

There is no standard staging system for metastatic squamous neck cancer with occult primary. The tumors are described as "untreated" or "recurrent." Untreated metastatic squamous neck cancer with occult primary is cancer that is newly diagnosed and has not been treated, except to relieve signs and symptoms caused by the cancer.

There are three ways that cancer spreads in the body.

Cancer can spread through tissue, the lymph system, and the blood:

- **Tissue.** The cancer spreads from where it began by growing into nearby areas.
- **Lymph system.** The cancer spreads from where it began by getting into the lymph system. The cancer travels through the lymph vessels to other parts of the body.
- **Blood.** The cancer spreads from where it began by getting into the blood. The cancer travels through the blood vessels to other parts of the body.

Treatment Options Overview for Metastatic Squamous Neck Cancer

There are different types of treatment for patients with metastatic squamous neck cancer with occult primary.

Different types of treatment are available for patients with metastatic squamous neck cancer with occult primary. Some treatments are standard (the currently used treatment), and some are being tested in clinical trials. A treatment clinical trial is a research study meant to help improve current treatments or obtain information on new treatments for patients with cancer. When clinical trials show that a new treatment is better than the standard treatment, the new treatment may become the standard treatment. Patients may want to think about taking part in a clinical trial. Some clinical trials are open only to patients who have not started treatment.

Two types of standard treatment are used:

Surgery

Surgery may include neck dissection. There are different types of neck dissection, based on the amount of tissue that is removed.

- **Radical neck dissection:** Surgery to remove tissues in one or both sides of the neck between the jawbone and the collarbone, including the following:
  - All lymph nodes
  - The jugular vein

- Muscles and nerves that are used for face, neck, and shoulder movement; speech; and swallowing

The patient may need physical therapy of the throat, neck, shoulder, and/or arm after radical neck dissection. Radical neck dissection may be used when cancer has spread widely in the neck.

- **Modified radical neck dissection:** Surgery to remove all the lymph nodes in one or both sides of the neck without removing the neck muscles. The nerves and/or the jugular vein may be removed.
- **Partial neck dissection:** Surgery to remove some of the lymph nodes in the neck. This is also called "selective neck dissection."

After the doctor removes all the cancer that can be seen at the time of surgery, some patients may be given radiation therapy (RT) after surgery to kill any cancer cells that are left. Treatment given after surgery, to lower the risk that the cancer will come back, is called "adjuvant therapy."

Radiation Therapy

Radiation therapy is a cancer treatment that uses high-energy X-rays or other types of radiation to kill cancer cells or keep them from growing. There are two types of radiation therapy:

- **External radiation therapy** uses a machine outside the body to send radiation toward the cancer.

Certain ways of giving radiation therapy can help keep radiation from damaging nearby healthy tissue. This type of radiation therapy may include the following:

- **Intensity-modulated radiation therapy (IMRT).** IMRT is a type of three-dimensional (3-D) radiation therapy that uses a computer to make pictures of the size and shape of the tumor. Thin beams of radiation of different intensities (strengths) are aimed at the tumor from many angles. This type of radiation therapy is less likely to cause dry mouth, trouble swallowing, and damage to the skin.
- **Internal radiation therapy** uses a radioactive substance sealed in needles, seeds, wires, or catheters that are placed directly into or near the cancer.

The way the radiation therapy is given depends on the type of cancer being treated. External radiation therapy is used to treat metastatic squamous neck cancer with occult primary.

Radiation therapy to the neck may change the way the thyroid gland works. Blood tests may be done to check the thyroid hormone level in the body before treatment and at regular checkups after treatment.

Chemotherapy

Chemotherapy is a cancer treatment that uses drugs to stop the growth of cancer cells, either by killing the cells or by stopping them from dividing. When chemotherapy is taken by mouth or injected into a vein or muscle, the drugs enter the bloodstream and can reach cancer cells throughout the body (systemic chemotherapy). When chemotherapy is placed directly into the cerebrospinal fluid; an organ; or a body cavity, such as the abdomen, the drugs mainly affect cancer cells in those areas (regional chemotherapy).

Hyperfractionated Radiation Therapy

Hyperfractionated radiation therapy is a type of external radiation treatment in which a smaller than usual total daily dose of radiation is divided into two doses, and the treatments are given twice a day. Hyperfractionated radiation therapy is given over the same period of time (days or weeks) as standard radiation therapy.

Treatment for metastatic squamous neck cancer with occult primary may cause side effects.

Follow-Up Tests May Be Needed

Some of the tests that were done to diagnose the cancer or to find out the stage of the cancer may be repeated. Some tests will be repeated in order to see how well the treatment is working. Decisions about whether to continue, change, or stop treatment may be based on the results of these tests.

Some of the tests will continue to be done from time to time after treatment has ended. The results of these tests can show if your condition has changed or if the cancer has recurred. These tests are sometimes called "follow-up tests" or "checkups."

Treatment Options for Metastatic Squamous Neck Cancer with Occult Primary

Untreated Metastatic Squamous Neck Cancer with Occult Primary

Treatment of untreated metastatic squamous neck cancer with occult primary may include the following:

- Radiation therapy
- Surgery
- Radiation therapy, followed by surgery
- A clinical trial of chemotherapy, followed by radiation therapy
- A clinical trial of chemotherapy given at the same time as hyperfractionated radiation therapy
- Clinical trials of new treatments

Chapter 58

Nasopharyngeal Cancer

Nasopharyngeal cancer is a disease in which malignant (cancer) cells form in the nasopharynx. The nasopharynx is made of the nasal cavity (inside of the nose) and the top part of the throat. Nasopharyngeal cancer is rare in children younger than 10 years of age and more common in adolescents.

Risks of Nasopharyngeal Cancer

Anything that increases your chance of getting a disease is called a "risk factor." Having a risk factor does not mean that you will get cancer; not having risk factors does not mean that you will not get cancer. Talk with your child's doctor if you think your child may be at risk.

Being infected with the Epstein-Barr virus (EBV) is strongly linked to having nasopharyngeal cancer.

Signs and Symptoms of Nasopharyngeal Cancer

Signs and symptoms of nasopharyngeal cancer include painless lumps in the neck and headache. These and other signs and symptoms may be caused by nasopharyngeal cancer or by other conditions.

Check with your child's doctor if your child has any of the following:

- Painless lumps in the neck

This chapter includes text excerpted from "Childhood Nasopharyngeal Cancer Treatment (PDQ®)—Patient Version," National Cancer Institute (NCI), April 12, 2019.

- Headache
- Blocked or stuffy nose
- Nosebleeds
- Pain in the ear
- Ear infection
- Problems moving the jaw
- Hearing loss
- Double vision or droopy eyelid

Tests and Diagnosis of Nasopharyngeal Cancer

The following tests and procedures may be used:

- **Physical exam and history**. An exam of the body to check general signs of health, including checking for signs of disease, such as lumps or anything else that seems unusual. A history of the patient's health habits and past illnesses and treatments will also be taken.
- **Magnetic resonance imaging (MRI).** A procedure that uses a magnet, radio waves, and a computer to make a series of detailed pictures of areas of the body, such as the nasopharynx and neck. This procedure is also called "nuclear magnetic resonance imaging" (NMRI).
- **Computed tomography (CT)/computerized axial tomography (CAT) scan**. A procedure that makes a series of detailed pictures of areas inside the body, such as the nasopharynx or lymph nodes, taken from different angles. The pictures are made by a computer linked to an X-ray machine. A dye may be injected into a vein or swallowed to help the organs or tissues show up more clearly. This procedure is also called "computed tomography," "computerized tomography," or "computerized axial tomography."
- **Positron emission tomography (PET) scan**. A procedure to find malignant tumor cells in the body. A small amount of radioactive glucose (sugar) is injected into a vein. The PET scanner rotates around the body and makes a picture of where glucose is being used in the body. Malignant tumor cells show up

brighter in the picture because they are more active and take up more glucose than normal cells do.

- **Positron emission tomography-computed tomography (PET-CT) scan**. A procedure that combines the pictures from a PET scan and a CT scan. The PET and CT scans are done at the same time on the same machine. The pictures from both scans are combined to make a more detailed picture than either test would make by itself.
- **Endoscopy**. A procedure to look at organs and tissues inside the body to check for abnormal areas. A flexible or rigid endoscope is inserted through the nose. An endoscope is a thin, tube-like instrument with a light and a lens for viewing. It may also have a tool to remove tissue samples, which are checked under a microscope by a pathologist for signs of disease.
- **Epstein-Barr virus (EBV) tests**. Blood tests to check for antibodies to the EBV and DNA markers of the EBV. These are found in the blood of patients who have been infected with EBV.

Stages of Nasopharyngeal Cancer

After nasopharyngeal cancer has been diagnosed, tests are done to find out if cancer cells have spread within the nasal cavity, throat, or to other parts of the body.

To plan treatment, it is important to know whether cancer cells have spread within the nasal cavity or to other parts of the body. The process used to find out if cancer has spread is called "staging." Most children with nasopharyngeal cancer are at an advanced stage at the time of diagnosis. Nasopharyngeal cancer spreads most often to the bone, lung, and liver.

The following tests and procedures may be used to find out if cancer has spread:

- **Neurological exam**. A series of questions and tests to check the brain, spinal cord, and nerve function. The exam checks a person's mental status, coordination, and ability to walk normally, and how well the muscles, senses, and reflexes work. This may also be called a "neuro exam" or a "neurologic exam."
- **Chest X-ray**. An X-ray of the organs and bones inside the chest. An X-ray is a type of energy beam that can go through the body and onto film, making a picture of areas inside the body.

- **Computed tomography (CT)/computerized axial tomography (CAT) scan.** A procedure that makes a series of detailed pictures of areas inside the body, such as the chest or abdomen, taken from different angles. The pictures are made by a computer linked to an X-ray machine. A dye may be injected into a vein or swallowed to help the organs or tissues show up more clearly.
- **Bone scan**. A procedure to check if there are rapidly dividing cells, such as cancer cells, in the bone. A very small amount of radioactive material is injected into a vein and travels through the bloodstream. The radioactive material collects in the bones with cancer and is detected by a scanner.

There Are Three Ways through Which Cancer Is Spread

Cancer can spread through tissue, the lymph system, and the blood:

- **Tissue**. The cancer spreads from where it began by growing into nearby areas.
- **Lymph system**. The cancer spreads from where it began by getting into the lymph system. The cancer travels through the lymph vessels to other parts of the body.
- **Blood**. The cancer spreads from where it began by getting into the blood. The cancer travels through the blood vessels to other parts of the body.

Cancer may spread from where it began to other parts of the body. When cancer spreads to another part of the body, it is called "metastasis." Cancer cells break away from where they began (the primary tumor) and travel through the lymph system or blood.

- **Lymph system**. The cancer gets into the lymph system, travels through the lymph vessels, and forms a tumor (metastatic tumor) in another part of the body.
- **Blood**. The cancer gets into the blood, travels through the blood vessels, and forms a tumor (metastatic tumor) in another part of the body.

The metastatic tumor is the same type of cancer as the primary tumor. For example, if nasopharyngeal cancer spreads to the lung, the cancer cells in the lung are actually nasopharyngeal cancer cells. The disease is metastatic nasopharyngeal cancer, not lung cancer.

Treatment Options for Nasopharyngeal Cancer

There are different types of treatment for children with nasopharyngeal cancer.

Some treatments are standard (the currently used treatment), and some are being tested in clinical trials. A treatment clinical trial is a research study meant to help improve current treatments or obtain information on new treatments for patients with cancer. When clinical trials show that a new treatment is better than the standard treatment, the new treatment may become the standard treatment.

Because cancer in children is rare, taking part in a clinical trial should be considered. Some clinical trials are open only to patients who have not started treatment.

Children with nasopharyngeal cancer should have their treatment planned by a team of doctors who are experts in treating childhood cancer.

Treatment will be overseen by a pediatric oncologist, a doctor who specializes in treating children with cancer. The pediatric oncologist works with other pediatric health professionals who are experts in treating children with cancer and who specialize in certain areas of medicine. This may include the following specialists and others:

- Pediatrician
- Pediatric surgeon
- Radiation oncologist
- Pathologist
- Pediatric nurse specialist
- Social worker
- Rehabilitation specialist
- Psychologist
- Child-life specialist

Treatment for childhood nasopharyngeal cancer may cause side effects.

Side effects from cancer treatment that begin after treatment and continue for months or years are called "late effects." Late effects of cancer treatment may include:

- Physical problems, including problems with the thyroid gland, hearing, fully opening the mouth, dental cavities, and chronic sinusitis or ear infections

- Changes in mood, feelings, thinking, learning, or memory
- Second cancers (new types of cancer) or other conditions

Some late effects may be treated or controlled. It is important to talk with your child's doctors about the possible late effects caused by some treatments.

Types of Standard Treatment for Nasopharyngeal Cancer

Chemotherapy

Chemotherapy is a cancer treatment that uses drugs to stop the growth of cancer cells, either by killing the cells or by stopping them from dividing. When chemotherapy is taken by mouth or injected into a vein or muscle, the drugs enter the bloodstream and can reach cancer cells throughout the body (systemic chemotherapy).

Radiation therapy

Radiation therapy is a cancer treatment that uses high-energy X-rays or other types of radiation to kill cancer cells or keep them from growing. There are two types of radiation therapy:

- **External radiation therapy** uses a machine outside the body to send radiation toward the cancer.
- **Internal radiation therapy** uses a radioactive substance sealed in needles, seeds, wires, or catheters that are placed directly into or near the cancer.

Surgery

Surgery to remove the tumor is done if the tumor has not spread throughout the nasal cavity and throat at the time of diagnosis.

Immunotherapy

Immunotherapy is a treatment that uses the patient's immune system to fight cancer. Substances made by the body or made in a laboratory are used to boost, direct, or restore the body's natural defenses against cancer.

Several types of immunotherapy are being used or studied to treat children with nasopharyngeal cancer:

- Interferon affects the division of cancer cells and can slow tumor growth. Interferon is used to treat newly diagnosed nasopharyngeal cancer.
- EBV-specific cytotoxic T-lymphocytes are a type of immune cell that can kill certain cells, including foreign cells, cancer cells, and cells infected with the Epstein-Barr virus. Cytotoxic T-lymphocytes can be separated from other blood cells, grown in the laboratory, and then given to the patient to kill cancer cells. EBV-specific cytotoxic T-lymphocytes are being studied to treat refractory or recurrent nasopharyngeal cancer.
- Immune checkpoint inhibitor therapy blocks certain proteins. PD-1 is a protein on the surface of T cells that helps keep the body's immune responses in check. When PD-1 attaches to another protein called "PDL-1" on a cancer cell, it stops the T cell from killing the cancer cell. PD-1 inhibitors attach to PDL-1 and allow the T cells to kill cancer cells. Pembrolizumab and nivolumab have been used to treat adults with refractory soft tissue sarcoma and may be considered to treat children.

Treatment Options for Childhood Nasopharyngeal Cancer

Newly Diagnosed Childhood Nasopharyngeal Cancer

Treatment of newly diagnosed nasopharyngeal cancer in children may include the following:

- Chemotherapy given before or at the same time as external radiation therapy
- Chemotherapy and external radiation therapy, followed by interferon
- Surgery to remove the tumor

Refractory or Recurrent Childhood Nasopharyngeal Cancer

Treatment of refractory or recurrent nasopharyngeal cancer may include the following:

- Immunotherapy with EBV-specific cytotoxic T-lymphocytes

- Immunotherapy with an immune checkpoint inhibitor (pembrolizumab or nivolumab)
- A clinical trial that checks a sample of the patient's tumor for certain gene changes. The type of treatment that will be given to the patient depends on the type of gene change.

Chapter 59

Hypopharyngeal Cancer

Hypopharyngeal cancer is a disease in which malignant (cancer) cells form in the tissues of the hypopharynx.

The hypopharynx is the bottom part of the pharynx (throat). The pharynx is a hollow tube, about five inches long, that starts behind the nose, goes down the neck, and ends at the top of the trachea (windpipe) and esophagus (the tube that goes from the throat to the stomach). Air and food pass through the pharynx on the way to the trachea or the esophagus.

Most hypopharyngeal cancers form in squamous cells—the thin, flat cells lining the inside of the hypopharynx. The hypopharynx has three different areas. Cancer may be found in one or more of these areas.

Hypopharyngeal cancer is a type of head and neck cancer.

Risk of Hypopharyngeal Cancer

Use of tobacco products and heavy drinking can affect the risk of developing hypopharyngeal cancer.

Anything that increases your risk of getting a disease is called a "risk factor." Having a risk factor does not mean that you will get cancer; not having risk factors does not mean that you will not get cancer. Talk with your doctor if you think you may be at risk. Risk factors include the following:

- Smoking tobacco

This chapter includes text excerpted from "Hypopharyngeal Cancer Treatment (Adult) (PDQ®)—Patient Version," National Cancer Institute (NCI), May 1, 2018.

- Chewing tobacco
- Heavy alcohol use
- Eating a diet without enough nutrients
- Having Plummer-Vinson syndrome

Signs and Symptoms of Hypopharyngeal Cancer

These and other signs and symptoms may be caused by hypopharyngeal cancer or by other conditions. Check with your doctor if you have any of the following:

- A sore throat that does not go away
- Ear pain
- A lump in the neck
- Painful or difficult swallowing
- A change in voice

Diagnosing Hypopharyngeal Cancer

Tests that examine the throat and neck are used to help detect (find) and diagnose hypopharyngeal cancer.

The following tests and procedures may be used.

- **Physical exam of the throat.** An exam in which the doctor feels for swollen lymph nodes in the neck and looks down the throat with a small, long-handled mirror to check for abnormal areas.
- **Computed tomography (CT) scan.** A procedure that makes a series of detailed pictures of areas inside the body, taken from different angles. The pictures are made by a computer linked to an X-ray machine. A dye may be injected into a vein or swallowed to help the organs or tissues show up more clearly. This procedure is also called "computed tomography," "computerized tomography," or "computerized axial tomography."
- **Positron emission tomography (PET) scan.** A procedure to find malignant tumor cells in the body. A small amount of radioactive glucose (sugar) is injected into a vein. The PET scanner rotates around the body and makes a picture of where

glucose is being used in the body. Malignant tumor cells show up brighter in the picture because they are more active and take up more glucose than normal cells do. A PET scan and CT scan may be done at the same time. This is called a "PET-CT."

- **Magnetic resonance imaging (MRI) scan.** A procedure that uses a magnet, radio waves, and a computer to make a series of detailed pictures of areas inside the body. This procedure is also called "nuclear magnetic resonance imaging" (NMRI).
- **Bone scan.** A procedure to check if there are rapidly dividing cells, such as cancer cells, in the bone. A very small amount of radioactive material is injected into a vein and travels through the bloodstream. The radioactive material collects in the bones with cancer and is detected by a scanner.
- **Barium esophagogram.** An X-ray of the esophagus. The patient drinks a liquid that contains barium (a silver-white metallic compound). The liquid coats the esophagus and X-rays are taken.
- **Endoscopy.** A procedure used to look at areas in the throat that cannot be seen with a mirror during the physical exam of the throat. An endoscope (a thin, lighted tube) is inserted through the nose or mouth to check the throat for anything that seems unusual. Tissue samples may be taken for biopsy.
- **Esophagoscopy.** A procedure to look inside the esophagus to check for abnormal areas. An esophagoscope (a thin, lighted tube) is inserted through the mouth or nose and down the throat into the esophagus. Tissue samples may be taken for biopsy.
- **Bronchoscopy.** A procedure to look inside the trachea and large airways in the lung for abnormal areas. A bronchoscope (a thin, lighted tube) is inserted through the nose or mouth into the trachea and lungs. Tissue samples may be taken for biopsy.
- **Biopsy.** The removal of cells or tissues so they can be viewed under a microscope to check for signs of cancer.

Stages of Hypopharyngeal Cancer

After hypopharyngeal cancer has been diagnosed, tests are done to find out if cancer cells have spread within the hypopharynx or to other parts of the body.

The process used to find out if cancer has spread within the hypopharynx or to other parts of the body is called "staging." The information gathered from the staging process determines the stage of the disease. It is important to know the stage of the disease in order to plan treatment. The results of some of the tests used to diagnose hypopharyngeal cancer are often also used to stage the disease.

The following stages are used for hypopharyngeal cancer.

Stage 0 (Carcinoma in Situ)

In stage 0, abnormal cells are found in the lining of the hypopharynx. These abnormal cells may become cancer and spread into nearby normal tissue. Stage 0 is also called "carcinoma in situ."

Stage I

In stage I, cancer has formed in one area of the hypopharynx only, and/or the tumor is two centimeters or smaller.

Stage II

In stage II, the tumor is either:

- Larger than two centimeters but not larger than four centimeters and has not spread to the Larynx (voice box)
- Found in more than one area of the hypopharynx or in nearby tissues

Stage III

In stage III, the tumor:

- Is larger than four centimeters or has spread to the larynx (voice box) or esophagus. Cancer may have spread to one lymph node on the same side of the neck as the tumor, and the lymph node is three centimeters or smaller.
- Has spread to one lymph node on the same side of the neck as the tumor, and the lymph node is three centimeters or smaller. The cancer is found:
    - In one area of the hypopharynx and/or is two centimeters or smaller

- In more than one area of the hypopharynx or in nearby tissues, or is larger than two centimeters but not larger than four centimeters and has not spread to the larynx

Stage IV

Stage IV is divided into stage IVA, IVB, and IVC as follows:
In stage IVA, cancer:

- Has spread to cartilage around the thyroid or trachea, the bone under the tongue, the thyroid, or nearby soft tissue. Cancer may have spread to one lymph node on the same side of the neck as the tumor, and the lymph node is three centimeters or smaller.
- Has spread to one lymph node on the same side of the neck as the tumor (the lymph node is larger than three centimeters but not larger than six centimeters) or to lymph nodes anywhere in the neck (affected lymph nodes are six centimeters or smaller), and one of the following is true:
    - Cancer is found in one area of the hypopharynx and/or is two centimeters or smaller.
    - Cancer is found in more than one area of the hypopharynx or in nearby tissues, or is larger than two centimeters but not larger than four centimeters and has not spread to the larynx (voice box).
    - Cancer has spread to the larynx or esophagus and is larger than four centimeters.
    - Cancer has spread to cartilage around the thyroid or trachea, the bone under the tongue, the thyroid, or nearby soft tissue.
- In stage IVB, the tumor:
    - Has spread to muscles around the upper part of the spinal column, the carotid artery, or the lining of the chest cavity and may have spread to lymph nodes, which can be any size
    - May be any size and has spread to one or more lymph nodes that are larger than six centimeters.
- In stage IVC, the tumor may be any size and has spread beyond the hypopharynx to other parts of the body.

Treatment for Patients with Hypopharyngeal Cancer

There are different types of treatment for patients with hypopharyngeal cancer:

Different types of treatment are available for patients with hypopharyngeal cancer. Some treatments are standard (the currently used treatment), and some are being tested in clinical trials. A treatment clinical trial is a research study meant to help improve current treatments or obtain information on new treatments for patients with cancer. When clinical trials show that a new treatment is better than the standard treatment, the new treatment may become the standard treatment. Patients may want to think about taking part in a clinical trial. Some clinical trials are open only to patients who have not started treatment.

Surgery

Surgery (removing the cancer in an operation) is a common treatment for all stages of hypopharyngeal cancer. The following surgical procedures may be used:

Laryngopharyngectomy: Surgery to remove the larynx (voice box) and part of the pharynx (throat).

Partial laryngopharyngectomy: Surgery to remove part of the larynx and part of the pharynx. A partial laryngopharyngectomy prevents loss of the voice.

Neck dissection: Surgery to remove lymph nodes and other tissues in the neck.

After the doctor removes all the cancer that can be seen at the time of the surgery, some patients may be given chemotherapy or radiation therapy after surgery to kill any cancer cells that are left. Treatment given after the surgery, to lower the risk that the cancer will come back, is called "adjuvant therapy."

Radiation Therapy

Radiation therapy is a cancer treatment that uses high-energy X-rays or other types of radiation to kill cancer cells or keep them from growing. There are two types of radiation therapy:

- **External radiation therapy** uses a machine outside the body to send radiation toward the cancer.

- **Internal radiation therapy** uses a radioactive substance sealed in needles, seeds, wires, or catheters that are placed directly into or near the cancer.

The way the radiation therapy is given depends on the type and stage of the cancer being treated. External radiation therapy is used to treat hypopharyngeal cancer.

Radiation therapy may work better in patients who have stopped smoking before beginning treatment. External radiation therapy to the thyroid or the pituitary gland may change the way the thyroid gland works. A blood test to check the thyroid hormone level in the body may be done before and after therapy to make sure the thyroid gland is working properly.

Chemotherapy

Chemotherapy is a cancer treatment that uses drugs to stop the growth of cancer cells, either by killing the cells or by stopping the cells from dividing. When chemotherapy is taken by mouth or injected into a vein or muscle, the drugs enter the bloodstream and can reach cancer cells throughout the body (systemic chemotherapy). When chemotherapy is placed directly into the cerebrospinal fluid; an organ; or a body cavity, such as the abdomen, the drugs mainly affect cancer cells in those areas (regional chemotherapy). The way the chemotherapy is given depends on the type and stage of the cancer being treated.

Chemotherapy may be used to shrink the tumor before surgery or radiation therapy. This is called “neoadjuvant chemotherapy.”

Follow-Up Tests May Be Needed

Some of the tests that were done to diagnose the cancer or to find out the stage of the cancer may be repeated. Some tests will be repeated in order to see how well the treatment is working. Decisions about whether to continue, change, or stop treatment may be based on the results of these tests.

Some of the tests will continue to be done from time to time after treatment has ended. The results of these tests can show if your condition has changed or if the cancer has recurred (come back). These tests are sometimes called “follow-up tests” or “checkups.”

For hypopharyngeal cancer, follow-ups to check for recurrence should include careful head and neck exams once a month in the first year after treatment ends, every two months in the second year, every three months in the third year, and every six months thereafter.

Chapter 60

Oropharyngeal Cancer

Oropharyngeal cancer is a disease in which malignant (cancer) cells form in the tissues of the oropharynx. The oropharynx is the middle part of the pharynx (throat), behind the mouth. The pharynx is a hollow tube, about five inches long, that starts behind the nose and ends where the trachea (windpipe) and esophagus (the tube from the throat to the stomach) begin. Air and food pass through the pharynx on the way to the trachea or the esophagus.

The oropharynx includes the following:

- Soft palate
- Side and back walls of the throat
- Tonsils
- Back one-third of the tongue

Oropharyngeal cancer is a type of head and neck cancer. Sometimes, more than one cancer can occur in the oropharynx and in other parts of the oral cavity, nose, pharynx, larynx (voice box), trachea, or esophagus at the same time.

Most oropharyngeal cancers are squamous cell carcinomas (SCC). Squamous cells are the thin, flat cells that line the inside of the oropharynx.

This chapter includes text excerpted from "Oropharyngeal Cancer Treatment (Adult) (PDQ®)—Patient Version," National Cancer Institute (NCI), March 28, 2019.

Risks of Oropharyngeal Cancer

Smoking or being infected with human papillomavirus (HPV) can increase the risk of oropharyngeal cancer. Anything that increases your risk of getting a disease is called a "risk factor." Having a risk factor does not mean that you will get cancer; not having risk factors does not mean that you will not get cancer. Talk with your doctor if you think you may be at risk.

The most common risk factors for oropharyngeal cancer include the following:

- A history of smoking cigarettes for more than 10 years and other tobacco use
- Personal history of head and neck cancer
- Heavy alcohol use
- Being infected with HPV, especially HPV type 16. The number of cases of oropharyngeal cancers linked to HPV infection is increasing.
- Chewing betel quid, a stimulant commonly used in parts of Asia

Signs and Symptoms of Oropharyngeal Cancer

Signs and symptoms of oropharyngeal cancer include a lump in the neck and a sore throat.

These and other signs and symptoms may be caused by oropharyngeal cancer or by other conditions. Check with your doctor if you have any of the following:

- A sore throat that does not go away
- Trouble swallowing
- Trouble opening the mouth fully
- Trouble moving the tongue
- Weight loss for no known reason
- Ear pain
- A lump in the back of the mouth, throat, or neck
- A white patch on the tongue or lining of the mouth that does not go away
- Coughing up blood

Sometimes, oropharyngeal cancer does not cause early signs or symptoms.

Diagnosing Oropharyngeal Cancer

The following tests and procedures may be used:

- **Physical exam and history.** An exam of the body to check general signs of health, including checking for signs of disease, such as swollen lymph nodes in the neck or anything else that seems unusual. The medical doctor or dentist does a complete exam of the mouth and neck and looks under the tongue and down the throat with a small, long-handled mirror to check for abnormal areas. An exam of the eyes may be done to check for vision problems that are caused by nerves in the head and neck. A history of the patient's health habits and past illnesses and treatments will also be taken.
- **Positron emission tomography-computed technology (PET-CT) scan.** A procedure that combines the pictures from a positron emission tomography (PET) scan and a computed tomography (CT) scan. The PET and CT scans are done at the same time with the same machine. The combined scans give more detailed pictures of areas inside the body than either scan gives by itself. A PET-CT scan may be used to help diagnose disease, such as cancer; plan treatment; or find out how well treatment is working.
    - **Computed tomography (CT)/computed axial tomography (CAT) scan.** A procedure that makes a series of detailed pictures of areas inside the body, such as the head and neck, taken from different angles. The pictures are made by a computer linked to an X-ray machine. A dye is injected into a vein or swallowed to help the organs or tissues show up more clearly. This procedure is also called "computed tomography," "computerized tomography," or "computerized axial tomography."
    - **Positron emission tomography (PET) scan.** A procedure to find malignant tumor cells in the body. A small amount of radioactive glucose (sugar) is injected into a vein. The PET scanner rotates around the body and makes a picture of where glucose is being used in the body. Malignant tumor cells show up brighter in the picture because they are more active and take up more glucose than normal cells do.

- **Magnetic resonance imaging (MRI).** A procedure that uses a magnet, radio waves, and a computer to make a series of detailed pictures of areas inside the body. This procedure is also called "nuclear magnetic resonance imaging" (NMRI).
- **Biopsy.** The removal of cells or tissues so they can be viewed under a microscope by a pathologist to check for signs of cancer. A fine-needle aspiration (FNA) biopsy is usually done to remove a sample of tissue using a thin needle.

The following procedures may be used to remove samples of cells or tissue:

- **Endoscopy.** A procedure to look at organs and tissues inside the body to check for abnormal areas. An endoscope is inserted through an incision (cut) in the skin or opening in the body, such as the mouth or nose. An endoscope is a thin, tube-like instrument with a light and a lens for viewing. It may also have a tool to remove abnormal tissue or lymph node samples, which are checked under a microscope for signs of disease. The nose, throat, back of the tongue, esophagus, stomach, larynx, windpipe, and large airways will be checked. The type of endoscopy is named for the part of the body that is being examined. For example, pharyngoscopy is an exam to check the pharynx.
- **Laryngoscopy.** A procedure in which the doctor checks the larynx with a mirror or with a laryngoscope. A laryngoscope is a thin, tube-like instrument with a light, and a lens for viewing. It may also have a tool to remove abnormal tissue or lymph node samples, which are checked under a microscope for signs of disease.

If cancer is found, the following test may be done to study the cancer cells:

- **Human papillomavirus (HPV) test.** A laboratory test used to check the sample of tissue for certain types of HPV infection. This test is done because oropharyngeal cancer can be caused by HPV.

Certain factors affect the prognosis (chance of recovery) and treatment options.

The prognosis depends on the following:

- Whether the patient has HPV infection of the oropharynx

- Whether the patient has a history of smoking cigarettes for 10 years or more
- The stage of cancer
- The number and size of lymph nodes with cancer

Oropharyngeal tumors related to HPV infection have a better prognosis and are less likely to recur than tumors not linked to HPV infection.

Treatment options depend on the following:

- The stage of the cancer
- Keeping the patient's ability to speak and swallow as normal as possible
- The patient's general health

Patients with oropharyngeal cancer have an increased risk of another cancer in the head or neck. This risk is increased in patients who continue to smoke or drink alcohol after treatment.

Stages of Oropharyngeal Cancer

After oropharyngeal cancer has been diagnosed, tests are done to find out if cancer cells have spread within the oropharynx or to other parts of the body.

The process used to find out if cancer has spread within the oropharynx or to other parts of the body is called "staging." The information gathered from the staging process determines the stage of the disease. It is important to know the stage in order to plan treatment. The results of some of the tests used to diagnose oropharyngeal cancer are often used to stage the disease.

There are three ways that cancer spreads in the body.

Cancer can spread through tissue, the lymph system, and the blood:

- **Tissue.** The cancer spreads from where it began by growing into nearby areas.
- **Lymph system.** The cancer spreads from where it began by getting into the lymph system. The cancer travels through the lymph vessels to other parts of the body.
- **Blood.** The cancer spreads from where it began by getting into the blood. The cancer travels through the blood vessels to other parts of the body.

Cancer may spread from where it began to other parts of the body.

When cancer spreads to another part of the body, it is called "metastasis." Cancer cells break away from where they began (the primary tumor) and travel through the lymph system or blood.

- **Lymph system.** The cancer gets into the lymph system, travels through the lymph vessels, and forms a tumor (metastatic tumor) in another part of the body.
- **Blood.** The cancer gets into the blood, travels through the blood vessels, and forms a tumor (metastatic tumor) in another part of the body.

The metastatic tumor is the same type of cancer as the primary tumor. For example, if oropharyngeal cancer spreads to the lung, the cancer cells in the lung are actually oropharyngeal cancer cells. The disease is metastatic oropharyngeal cancer, not lung cancer.

The following stages are used for oropharyngeal cancer:

Stage 0 (Carcinoma in Situ)

In stage 0, abnormal cells are found in the lining of the oropharynx. These abnormal cells may become cancer and spread into nearby normal tissue. Stage 0 is also called "carcinoma in situ."

Stage I

In stage I, cancer has formed and is two centimeters or smaller and is found in the oropharynx only.

Stage II

In stage II, the cancer is larger than two centimeters but not larger than four centimeters and is found in the oropharynx only.

Stage III

In stage III, the cancer is either:

- Four centimeters or smaller; cancer has spread to one lymph node on the same side of the neck as the tumor, and the lymph node is three centimeters or smaller.

- Larger than four centimeters or has spread to the epiglottis (the flap that covers the trachea during swallowing). Cancer may have spread to one lymph node on the same side of the neck as the tumor, and the lymph node is three centimeters or smaller.

Stage IV

Stage IV is divided into stage IVA, IVB, and IVC.

- **In stage IVA, cancer:**
  - Has spread to the larynx, front part of the roof of the mouth, lower jaw, or muscles that move the tongue or are used for chewing. Cancer may have spread to one lymph node on the same side of the neck as the tumor, and the lymph node is three centimeters or smaller.
  - Has spread to one lymph node on the same side of the neck as the tumor (the lymph node is larger than three centimeters but not larger than six centimeters) or to more than one lymph node anywhere in the neck (the lymph nodes are six centimeters or smaller), and one of the following is true:
    - Tumor in the oropharynx is any size and may have spread to the epiglottis (the flap that covers the trachea during swallowing).
    - Tumor has spread to the larynx, front part of the roof of the mouth, lower jaw, or muscles that move the tongue or are used for chewing.
- **In stage IVB, the tumor:**
  - Surrounds the carotid artery or has spread to the muscle that opens the jaw, the bone attached to the muscles that move the jaw, nasopharynx, or base of the skull. Cancer may have spread to one or more lymph nodes, which can be any size.
  - Maybe any size and has spread to one or more lymph nodes that are larger than six centimeters.
- **In stage IVC**, the tumor may be any size and has spread beyond the oropharynx to other parts of the body, such as the lung, bone, or liver.

Treatment Options Overview for Oropharyngeal Cancer

There are different types of treatment for patients with oropharyngeal cancer.

Different types of treatment are available for patients with oropharyngeal cancer. Some treatments are standard (the currently used treatment), and some are being tested in clinical trials. A treatment clinical trial is a research study meant to help improve current treatments or obtain information on new treatments for patients with cancer. When clinical trials show that a new treatment is better than the standard treatment, the new treatment may become the standard treatment. Patients may want to think about taking part in a clinical trial. Some clinical trials are open only to patients who have not started treatment.

Patients with oropharyngeal cancer should have their treatment planned by a team of doctors with expertise in treating head and neck cancer.

The patient's treatment will be overseen by a medical oncologist, a doctor who specializes in treating people with cancer. Because the oropharynx helps in breathing, eating, and talking, patients may need special help adjusting to the side effects of cancer and its treatment. The medical oncologist may refer the patient to other health professionals with special training in the treatment of patients with head and neck cancer. These may include the following specialists:

- Head and neck surgeon
- Radiation oncologist
- Plastic surgeon
- Dentist
- Dietitian
- Psychologist
- Rehabilitation specialist
- Speech therapist

Four types of standard treatment are used:

Surgery

Surgery (removing the cancer in an operation) is a common treatment of all stages of oropharyngeal cancer. A surgeon may remove the cancer and some of the healthy tissue around the cancer. After the surgeon removes all the cancer that can be seen at the time of the surgery, some patients may be given chemotherapy or radiation therapy after surgery to kill any cancer cells that are left. Treatment given after the surgery, to lower the risk that the cancer will come back, is called "adjuvant therapy."

New types of surgery, including transoral robotic surgery, are being studied for the treatment of oropharyngeal cancer. Transoral robotic surgery may be used to remove cancer from hard-to-reach areas of the mouth and throat. Cameras attached to a robot give a three-dimensional (3-D) image that a surgeon can see. Using a computer, the surgeon guides very small tools at the ends of the robot arms to remove the cancer. This procedure may also be done using an endoscope.

Radiation Therapy

Radiation therapy is a cancer treatment that uses high-energy X-rays or other types of radiation to kill cancer cells or keep them from growing. There are two types of radiation therapy:

- **External radiation therapy** uses a machine outside the body to send radiation toward the cancer. Certain ways of giving radiation therapy can help keep radiation from damaging nearby healthy tissue. These types of radiation therapy include the following:
    - **Intensity-modulated radiation therapy (IMRT).** IMRT is a type of 3-D radiation therapy that uses a computer to make pictures of the size and shape of the tumor. Thin beams of radiation of different intensities (strengths) are aimed at the tumor from many angles.
    - **Stereotactic body radiation therapy (SBRT).** Stereotactic body radiation therapy is a type of external radiation therapy. Special equipment is used to place the patient in the same position for each radiation treatment. Once a day for several days, a radiation machine aims a larger than usual dose of radiation directly at the tumor. By having the patient in the same position for each treatment, there is less damage to nearby healthy tissue. This procedure is also called "stereotactic external-beam radiation therapy" and "stereotaxic radiation therapy."

- **Internal radiation therapy** uses a radioactive substance sealed in needles, seeds, wires, or catheters that are placed directly into or near cancer.

In advanced oropharyngeal cancer, dividing the daily dose of radiation into smaller-dose treatments improves the way the tumor responds to treatment. This is called "hyperfractionated radiation therapy." The way the radiation therapy is given depends on the type and stage of the cancer being treated. External radiation therapy is used to treat oropharyngeal cancer. Radiation therapy may work better in patients who have stopped smoking before beginning treatment. If the thyroid or pituitary gland is part of the radiation treatment area, the patient has an increased risk of hypothyroidism (too little thyroid hormone). A blood test to check the thyroid hormone level in the body should be done before and after treatment.

Chemotherapy

Chemotherapy is a cancer treatment that uses drugs to stop the growth of cancer cells, either by killing the cells or by stopping them from dividing. When chemotherapy is taken by mouth or injected into a vein or muscle, the drugs enter the bloodstream and can reach cancer cells throughout the body (systemic chemotherapy). When chemotherapy is placed directly into the cerebrospinal fluid; an organ; or a body cavity, such as the abdomen, the drugs mainly affect cancer cells in those areas (regional chemotherapy). The way the chemotherapy is given depends on the type and stage of the cancer being treated. Systemic chemotherapy is used to treat oropharyngeal cancer.

Targeted Therapy

Targeted therapy is a type of treatment that uses drugs or other substances to attack specific cancer cells. Targeted therapies usually cause less harm to normal cells than chemotherapy or radiation therapy do. Monoclonal antibodies are a type of targeted therapy being used in the treatment of oropharyngeal cancer.

Monoclonal antibody therapy is a cancer treatment that uses antibodies made in the laboratory from a single type of immune system cell. These antibodies can identify substances on cancer cells or normal substances in the blood or tissues that may help cancer cells grow. The antibodies attach to the substances and kill the cancer cells, block their growth, or keep them from spreading. Monoclonal antibodies are given by infusion. They may be used alone or to carry drugs, toxins, or radioactive material directly to cancer cells.

Cetuximab is a type of monoclonal antibody that works by binding to a protein on the surface of the cancer cells and stops the cells from growing and dividing. It is used in the treatment of recurrent oropharyngeal cancer.

Other types of monoclonal antibody therapy are being studied in the treatment of oropharyngeal cancer. Nivolumab is being studied in the treatment of stage III and IV oropharyngeal cancer.

Follow-Up Tests May Be Needed

Some of the tests that were done to diagnose the cancer or to find out the stage of the cancer may be repeated. Some tests will be repeated in order to see how well the treatment is working. Decisions about whether to continue, change, or stop treatment may be based on the results of these tests.

Some of the tests will continue to be done from time to time after treatment has ended. The results of these tests can show if your condition has changed or if the cancer has recurred. These tests are sometimes called "follow-up tests" or "checkups."

Following treatment, it is important to have careful head and neck exams to look for signs that the cancer has come back. Checkups will be done every 6 to 12 weeks in the first year, every 3 months in the second year, every 3 to 4 months in the third year, and every 6 months thereafter.

Part Eight

Clinical Trials and Research Studies

Chapter 61

Understanding Clinical Trials and Observational Studies

What Are Clinical Trials and Observational Studies?

Clinical research is medical research that involves people. There are two types: observational studies and clinical trials.

Observational studies observe people in normal settings. Researchers gather information, group volunteers according to broad characteristics, and compare changes over time. For example, researchers may collect data through medical exams, tests, or questionnaires about a group of older adults over time to learn more about the effects of different lifestyles on cognitive health. These studies may help identify new possibilities for clinical trials.

Clinical trials are research studies performed on people and are aimed at evaluating medical, surgical, or behavioral intervention. They are the primary way that researchers find out if a new treatment, such as a new drug, diet, medical device (for example, a pacemaker), is safe and effective for conventional use. Often, a clinical trial is used to learn if a new treatment is more effective and/or has less harmful side effects than the standard treatment.

This chapter includes text excerpted from "What Are Clinical Trials and Studies?" National Institute on Aging (NIA), National Institutes of Health (NIH), May 17, 2017.

Some clinical trials test ways to find a disease early, sometimes even before an individual experiences symptoms, while others test ways to prevent a health problem. A clinical trial may also look at how to make life better for people living with a life-threatening disease or a chronic health problem. Clinical trials also sometimes study the role of caregivers or support groups.

Before the U.S. Food and Drug Administration (FDA) allows a clinical trial to begin, scientists perform laboratory tests and studies in animals to test a potential therapy's safety and efficacy. If these studies show favorable results, the FDA gives approval for the intervention to be tested among humans.

Phases of Clinical Trials

Clinical trials advance through four phases to test a treatment, find the appropriate dosage, and look for side effects. If, after the first three phases, researchers find a drug or other intervention to be safe and effective, the FDA approves it for clinical use and continues to monitor its effects.

Clinical trials of drugs are usually described based on their phase. The FDA typically requires Phase I, II, and III trials in order to determine if the drug can be approved for use.

- A **phase I** trial tests an experimental treatment on a small group of often healthy people (20 to 80) to judge its safety and side effects and to find the correct drug dosage.
- A **phase II** trial requires an increase of participants (100 to 300). While the emphasis in Phase I is on safety, the emphasis in Phase II is on effectiveness. This phase aims to obtain preliminary data on whether the drug works in people who have a certain disease or condition. These trials also continue to study safety, including short-term side effects. This phase can last for several years.
- A **phase III** trial gathers more information about safety and effectiveness, while studying different populations and different dosages and using the drug in combination with other drugs. The number of subjects usually ranges from several hundred to about 3,000 people. If the FDA agrees that the trial results are positive, it will approve the experimental drug or device.
- A **phase IV** trial for drugs or devices takes place after the FDA approves their use. A device or drug's effectiveness and safety

are monitored in large, diverse populations. Sometimes, the side effects of a drug may not become clear until more people have taken it over a longer period of time.

Chapter 62

Ongoing Clinical Trials for Back and Neck Related Problems

Chapter Contents

Section 62.1—Change of Lumbar Symptom after Surgical Treatment for Patients with Cervical Stenosis (LBP) 466

Section 62.2—Behavior of the Upper Cervical Spine in Rugby Players (Cervistab) 467

Section 62.3—Dosing of Methadone for Spine Surgery 468

Section 62.4—Postoperative Pain Management Following Spine Surgery (EXPAREL) 469

Section 62.5—Outcome Analysis for Minimally Invasive Spine Surgery 471

Section 62.6—The Effects of Thoracic Spine Mobilizations in Individuals with Neck Pain 473

Section 62.1

Change of Lumbar Symptom after Surgical Treatment for Patients with Cervical Stenosis (LBP)

This section includes text excerpted from "Change of Lumbar Symptom after Surgical Treatment for Patients with Cervical Stenosis (LBP)," ClinicalTrials.gov, National Institutes of Health (NIH), February 6, 2018.

Study Description

Brief summary: Low back pain may be reduced after cervical spinal surgery.

Detailed description: The improved back pain score after cervical spinal surgery would be higher than that after nonsurgical treatment.

Eligibility Criteria

Ages eligible for study: 18 to 90 years of age (adult, older adult)
Sexes eligible for study: All
Accepts healthy volunteers: No
Sampling method: Nonprobability sample

Study Population

Patients with cervical myelopathy and low back pain

Criteria

Inclusion Criteria

- All patients with cervical myelopathy and low back pain

Exclusion Criteria

- Previous surgery on the lumbar spine
- Malignancy
- Previous surgery on the cervical spine

Section 62.2

Behavior of the Upper Cervical Spine in Rugby Players (Cervistab)

This section includes text excerpted from "Behavior of the Upper Cervical Spine in Rugby Players (Cervistab)," ClinicalTrials.gov, National Institutes of Health (NIH), February 8, 2019.

Study Description

Brief summary: Rugby players are often exposed to destabilization of the upper cervical spine. This kind of trauma may lead to dramatic injuries due to lesion of spinal cord.

CerviStab© is a device which evaluates the biomechanical and neuromuscular behavior of the upper cervical spine.

The aim of this study is to evaluate the dynamic stabilization of the upper cervical spine in reaction to the unexpected impact.

Eligibility Criteria

Ages eligible for study: 18 to 40 years of age (adult)
Sexes eligible for study: Male
Accepts healthy volunteers: Yes

Criteria

Inclusion Criteria

- Rugby players (has been playing for at least five years)
- Amateurs or professionals players
- Able to play in rugby competition

Exclusion Criteria

- Medical history of cervical spine injury that required surgical intervention
- Active cervical symptomatology
- Medical history of migraine or epilepsy

Section 62.3

Dosing of Methadone for Spine Surgery

This section includes text excerpted from "Dosing of Methadone for Spine Surgery," ClinicalTrials.gov, National Institutes of Health (NIH), April 4, 2019.

Study Description

Brief summary: This study compares two methods of dosing methadone for complex spine cases.

Detailed description: Patients with spine surgery experience a significant amount of pain that can interfere with healing and rehabilitation, which can contribute to morbidity in the post-operative period. This study will compare postoperative opioid requirement at 24 and 48 hours to determine if methadone given in small aliquots, until respiratory depression, can act as a self-control in order to determine the correct dose required.

Eligibility Criteria

Ages eligible for study: 18 to 65 years of age (adult, older adult)
Sexes eligible for study: All
Accepts healthy volunteers: No

Criteria

Inclusion Criteria

- Patients must consent to participate and sign the Institutional Review Board (IRB)-approved informed consent prior to beginning any study specific procedures.
- Undergoing multiple thoracolumbar spine surgeries with instrumentation and fusion

Exclusion Criteria

- History of methadone use
- Morbid obesity with a body mass index (BMI) >40 Kg/m2.
- Chronic renal failure with creatinine >2.0 mg/dL
- Liver failure, as determined by cirrhosis or a history of fulminant hepatic failure

- History of alcohol abuse
- History of drug abuse
- History of myocardial infarction or heart failure.
- Patients with American Society of Anesthesiologists (ASA) status IV or V

Section 62.4

Postoperative Pain Management Following Spine Surgery (EXPAREL)

This section includes text excerpted from "Post-Operative Pain Management Following Spine Surgery (EXPAREL)," ClinicalTrials.gov, National Institutes of Health (NIH), December 14, 2018.

Study Description

Brief summary: The primary objective of this pilot study is to assess the feasibility of comparing two standardized approaches to manage postoperative pain following spine surgery: one approach using patient-controlled analgesia (PCA) devices to deliver opioid analgesics, and the other approach using EXPAREL® infiltration at the site of surgery and nurse-administered opioid analgesics.

Detailed description: The study will assess the feasibility of the methods proposed, including recruitment, eligibility, standardization of both postoperative pain management approaches, clinical efficiency, hospital efficiency, medication use, health-services use, and economic outcomes.

Eligibility Criteria

Ages eligible for study: 18 to 65 years of age (adult, older adult)
Sexes eligible for study: All
Accepts healthy volunteers: Yes
Sampling method: Nonprobability sample

Study Population

Patients undergoing primary, single level, lumbar fusion surgical procedures.

Criteria

Inclusion Criteria

- Between the ages of 18 and 65
- Ability to speak, read, and write in English or Spanish
- Primary indication is low back pain, radiculopathy, disc degeneration, disc herniation, foraminal stenosis, or mild 1-level spondylolisthesis or deformity
- Scheduled to undergo primary, single level, lumbar fusion surgical procedure at the study center in the next 30 days
- Willing to provide informed consent, participate in the study, and comply with study protocol

Exclusion Criteria

- A body mass index (BMI) >35
- Pregnant or contemplating pregnancy prior to surgery
- Current or previous psychiatric, behavioral, or emotional disorder that may interfere with postsurgical pain, analgesia, or opioid use as according to treating surgeon
- Prior treatment for alcohol, recreational drug, or opioid abuse
- Chronic inflammatory conditions (e.g., Crohn, lupus, and rheumatoid arthritis)
- Chronic neurologic conditions (e.g., multiple sclerosis and Parkinson)
- Serious spinal conditions (e.g., cauda equina syndrome, infection, tumor, and fracture)
- Hypersensitivity or allergy to local anesthetics
- Previous surgery in lumbar spine (i.e., other than microdiscectomy)
- Continuous (e.g., daily) opioid consumption for more than 30 days prior to surgery

Section 62.5

Outcome Analysis for Minimally Invasive Spine Surgery

This section includes text excerpted from "Outcome Analysis for Minimally Invasive Spine Surgery," ClinicalTrials.gov, National Institutes of Health (NIH), January 30, 2018.

Study Description

Brief summary: Prospective/retrospective data analysis, chart reviews, and clinical outcomes of minimally invasive spine surgery

Detailed description: Study rationale and primary objective/hypothesis: To assess the clinical and radiographic outcome of spinal fusion procedures by using silicate-substituted calcium phosphate (Si-CaP), a newer-generation of synthetic ceramics designed to maximize osteoinduction and osteoconduction.

Study design: Retrospective study

Purpose of the study: Providing compelling evidence for the efficacy of Si-CaP in terms of resulting in satisfactory fusion.

Summary of methods: A prospectively collected database will be reviewed retrospectively to retrieve data of 200 patients who have undergone different spinal fusion procedures using Si-CaP. An average follow-up duration of at least 12 months will be considered. Clinical outcomes will be assessed using the visual analog scale (VAS), Oswestry Disability Index (ODI), and Neck Disability Index (NDI). Preoperative scores will be compared to the latest follow-up scores. A board-certified neuroradiologist will assess the fusion rate. Fusion will be determined by the presence of bony bridging on two consecutive sections in at least two planes on computed tomographic imaging.

Secondary endpoints and expected results: The purpose of this study is to evaluate the level of clinical and radiographic improvement in patients implanted with Si-CaP as a bone-graft substitute material for spinal fusions. More comprehensive long-term studies will be able to provide compelling evidence for the efficacy of Si-CaP in terms of resulting in satisfactory fusion. They can more strongly support the previously published data implying that Si-CaP can be utilized as an alternative to autogenous bone graft in spinal arthrodesis procedures.

Eligibility Criteria

Ages eligible for study: Child, adult, older adult
Sexes eligible for study: All
Accepts healthy volunteers: No
Sampling method: Probability sample

Study Population

Our prospectively collected institutional database will be reviewed to identify all consecutive patients with spinal fusion procedures using Si-CaP (Actifuse®, Baxter, Deerfield, IL) as a bone graft substitute. Surgeries have been performed at the hospital between 2007 and 2011. The estimated number of patients enrolled in the study is 200 patients. Patient demographics will be extracted using the database. The study population are from different age, gender, and ethnicity groups. The indications for surgery will be recorded for each patient as well. Institutional research board approval has been granted. All patients have provided informed consent for data collection regarding their treatment and outcomes.

Criteria

Inclusion Criteria

Patients with different spinal fusion procedures (including axial lumbar interbody fusion (AxiaLIF), transforaminal lumbar interbody fusion (TLIF), extreme lateral interbody fusion (ELIF), posterior cervical fusion (PCF), and anterior discectomy and fusion (ACDF)) using silicate-substituted calcium phosphate (Actifuse®, Baxter, Deerfield, IL) as a bone graft substitute.

Exclusion Criteria

Utilization of any other bone extenders in addition to Si-CaP as a bone graft substitute.

Section 62.6

The Effects of Thoracic Spine Mobilizations in Individuals with Neck Pain

This section includes text excerpted from "The Effects of Thoracic Spine Mobilizations in Individuals with Neck Pain. (THSPMOBS)," ClinicalTrials.gov, National Institutes of Health (NIH), October 27, 2017.

Study Description

Brief summary: To determine the effects of physical therapists's clinical reasoning in using thoracic spine mobilization for neck pain rather than a standard protocol.

Detailed description: The purpose of this research is to compare the effects of two commonly used, safe, thoracic spine treatments: grade one to four, as performed by Cleland et. al., and grade one to four mobilization to the thoracic spine, as selected by the physical therapist (PT) for cervical spine pain. The immediate effects of thoracic spine mobilization have been shown to facilitate a greater range of motion, increases in the cervical spine, and greater pain decreases within a treatment session and on follow-up visits. There is no research utilizing pain threshold perception as an objective outcome of these treatments. Only one study compared the two treatment techniques and concluded that future research should be completed, which includes manual therapy for the thoracic spine. If the PT identifies an appropriate patient, they will ask if they are interested in being a research subject. The physical therapist that are recruiting subjects all have completed their doctor of physical therapy degree and have advanced training in manual physical therapy. The techniques employed are considered standard practice and are defined as "entry level skills" by the Commission of Accreditation (CoA) of Physical Therapy Programs. These techniques are typically taught in physical therapy or physiotherapy doctorate programs.

Eligibility Criteria

Ages eligible for study: 18 to 60 years of age (adult)
Sexes eligible for study: All
Accepts healthy volunteers: Yes

Criteria

Inclusion Criteria

- Patients with neck pain
- Between the ages of 18 and 60

Exclusion Criteria

- **Red flags:** leg weakness, night pain, history of cancer, upper motor neuron signs, infection, tumors, osteoporosis, fracture, cervical stenosis, central nervous system (CNS) involvement, signs consistent with nerve-root compression, previous surgery, pending legal action

The inclusion and exclusion criteria above represent a conservative approach based on combining criteria of recent studies in published review articles.

Chapter 63

Research Studies on Spinal Cord Injuries

Scientists continue to investigate new ways to better understand and treat spinal cord injuries (SCIs).

Much of this research is supported by the National Institute of Neurological Disorders and Stroke (NINDS), a part of the National Institutes of Health (NIH). Other NIH components, as well as the U.S. Department of Veterans Affairs (VA), other federal agencies, research institutions, and voluntary health organizations, also fund and conduct basic to clinical research related to improvement of function in paralyzed individuals.

Many hospitals have developed specialized centers for spinal cord injury care. Many of these bring together spinal cord injury researchers from a variety of disciplines for partnerships regarding basic and clinical research, clinical care, and knowledge translation.

Current research is focused on advancing our understanding of four key principles of spinal cord repair:

- Neuroprotection—protecting surviving nerve cells from further damage
- Regeneration—stimulating the regrowth of axons and targeting their connections appropriately

---

This chapter includes text excerpted from "Spinal Cord Injury: Hope through Research," National Institute of Neurological Disorders and Stroke (NINDS), August 8, 2018.

- Cell replacement—replacing damaged nerve or glial cells
- Retraining CNS circuits and plasticity to restore body functions

A spinal cord injury is complex. Repairing it has to take into account all of the different kinds of damage that occur during and after the injury. Because the molecular and cellular environment of the spinal cord is constantly changing from the moment of injury until several weeks or even months later, combination therapies will have to be designed to address specific types of damage at different stages of the injury.

Neuroprotection

Strategies involving neuroprotection are aimed at preventing cell death, limiting or reducing inflammation, and stopping overexcitability of certain cells and their functions. Investigators are looking at ways to reduce inflammation within or near the injured spinal cord, which can restrict blood flow, affect nerve signal transmission, and increase cell death. One approach is using steroid drugs to reduce nerve cell damage and suppress activities of immune cells. One clinical trial identified slight improvement in motor function among some individuals who were given a steroid within eight hours after injury. However, other trials showed the drug's modest benefit did not outweigh serious side effects. Steroid therapy has not been approved by the U.S. Food and Drug Administration (FDA) for the treatment of acute spinal cord injury.

Antibiotics, which can cross the protective blood-brain barrier, have been shown to improve motor function, restoration, decrease lesion size, and reduce cell death in animal models of SCI.

The kidney hormone erythropoietin promotes the growth of new red blood cells and increases oxygen levels in the blood. Studies in animal models have shown that erythropoietin can reduce inflammation in the brain, improve blood flow to the brain, and reduce nerve cell death following brain injury. It also aids in the recovery of motor function. However, other trials in animal models show conflicting results regarding the drug's usefulness in preventing inflammation and cell death. Researchers continue to study the drug in preclinical models.

Therapeutic hypothermia (controlled lowering of the body's core temperature) can protect cells from damage following cardiac arrest, stroke, and traumatic brain injury. Therapeutic hypothermia has been shown to reduce the swelling and inflammation that presses on the spinal cord following injury in animal models and in small, limited human studies. It also can reduce damage to susceptible neurons following the primary injury, reduce damage to spinal cord microvasculature, and improve functional outcome. Researchers are studying the safety and effectiveness of different durations of hypothermia following spinal cord injury.

Researchers are trying to manipulate macrophages—a type of white blood cell that travels to the injury site during the inflammatory response—to promote nerve cell growth without causing further tissue damage. Following a spinal cord injury, macrophages at the site of injury begin to remove cellular debris and receive signals that help them promote the growth of axons. But, within a few days postinjury, the collection of macrophages increases inflammation, scarring, and toxicity, which can worsen the damage. Scientists hope to learn how to signal macrophages to continue their restorative function, while turning off their damaging consequences.

The buildup of sodium and glutamate in cells following a spinal cord injury can lead to cell damage and impaired or blocked cell signaling. The drug riluzole, which slows the progression of the disease amyotrophic lateral sclerosis, has shown in animal models to improve motor function and reduce cell death loss caused by decreased blood flow following spinal cord injury. The experimental drug HP 184 blocks the entry of sodium into cells (which can impair nerve function) and may enhance cell signaling in surviving axons that have had their protective myelin cover either destroyed or damaged following spinal cord injury. Other scientists are examining drugs that target glutamate, whose release is greatly increased following a spinal injury. Excess glutamate leads to cell death and blocked transmission of signals across nerve synapses. Researchers are studying different drugs that may reduce glutamate binding among cells following spinal cord injury, which could reduce secondary cell death, improve motor function outcome, and reduce long-term hypersensitive pain postinjury.

Regeneration

Neurons have a limited capacity to regenerate. As nerve cells are either damaged or destroyed by injury, and as others die naturally during development, the number of chemical interactions between adjacent nerve cells (synapses) decreases. Nerve cells can die when they do not make enough synapses, leaving large numbers of supporting glial cells in the area of damage. Glial cells are thought to support tissue after an injury to the spinal cord but also inhibit the growth of axons.

Some anti-inflammatory drugs have been shown to encourage axonal regeneration by stimulating CNS nerve axons to grow and by inhibiting amino acid toxicity and cell death that occurs after the initial injury. Two such nonsteroidal anti-inflammatory drugs are ibuprofen and indomethacin. The drug rolipram was shown to encourage axonal regeneration in an animal model of spinal cord injury. Preclinical studies are examining the effectiveness of rolipram in combination with other drugs given at different delivery times postinjury.

Antibodies are proteins made by immune cells and are designed to attach themselves to specific foreign proteins (called "antigens") and disable them. Therapeutically, antibodies can be made that target specific proteins that inhibit repair of the body after injury. Monoclonal antibodies, produced in a laboratory, may promote nerve fiber regeneration by blocking proteins in the myelin debris that inhibit regeneration after spinal cord injury. Scientists are testing monoclonal antibodies at the site of the spinal cord injury in animal models in an attempt to block antiregeneration activity of cells in the damaged central nervous system and improve nerve function and recovery. For example, researchers are using a Nogo-A monoclonal antibody to block proteins that inhibit the sprouting and regeneration of axons following a spinal injury. Other antibodies, called "anti-MAG" (myelin-associated glycoproteins), are designed to counteract protein-sugar molecules on myelin-forming debris at the site of injury.

A number of other targets are being tested to overcome inhibition to regeneration. Cethrin, a recombinant protein that blocks activation of Rho (a protein that inhibits axon regeneration), has been tested clinically. A drug that targets Nogo-receptors is being developed to promote regeneration after spinal cord injury and stroke. Some animal studies showing that inhibition of the tumor-suppressing gene PTEN can promote growth of upper motor neurons has led to active research into strategies to promote regeneration after spinal cord and optic nerve injuries. Finally, the histone deacetylases (HDAC) are a class of compounds that are involved in the regulation of gene expression and negatively affect cell structure following a traumatic spinal cord injury. Preclinical studies are examining ways to inhibit HDAC activity as a way to protect and allow axons to overcome inhibition in regions of a spinal injury.

To get past the glial scar that forms after a spinal cord injury and be able to transmit signals from the cell body, an axon has to advance between the tangles of long, branching molecules made up of inhibitory proteins and sugars that surround the cells. Experiments have successfully used a bacterial enzyme, chondroitinase ABC, to clear away the tangles so that axons could grow in animal models of injury. Researchers are looking at ways to combine chondroitinase ABC with other treatments, such as cell transplants, to increase functional recovery.

Other researchers are using a tissue-engineered highway-like matrix that is implanted onto the spinal cord to help axons "bridge" the lesion that forms at the injury site and to rebuild neural circuits. They also will look at using the matrix as a way of delivering growth factors that can promote nerve cell survival and inhibit proteins associated with the glial scar.

Cell Replacement

Controversy exists over potential benefits and possible harmful consequences of cell replacement and cell transplants. The potential of several cell types, including stem cells and glial cells, to treat spinal cord injury is being investigated eagerly, but there are many things about stem cells that researchers still need to understand. For example, researchers know there are many different kinds of chemical signals that tell a stem cell what to do. Some of these are internal to the stem cell, but many others are external—within the cellular environment—and will have to be recreated in the transplant region to encourage proper growth and differentiation. Because of the complexities involved in stem cell treatment, researchers expect these kinds of therapies to be possible only after much more research is done. Preclinical research results are limited but show that cell transplants can regenerate neuronal growth and create new connections between neurons.

Scientists are experimenting with a variety of cells for effectiveness and safety in increasing connectivity and restoring function following a spinal cord injury:

- Human oligodendrocyte progenitor cells have been shown to reduce secondary damage following a spinal cord injury and promote functional recovery and remyelination. Researchers are expanding trials to better determine optimal cell delivery windows and evaluate potential risks of transplants, such as the formation of tumors and inflammatory reactions.
- Schwann cells surround and insulate peripheral nerves, and often grow into the spinal cord after injury. Schwann cells that have been transplanted at the site of the spinal cord injury

can produce growth factors and reinsulate damaged nerve axons. They are not stem cells in that their fate as Schwann cells is determined before transplantation. Schwann cells can be taken from the individual's own body, which reduces the need for immune-suppressing drugs and the risk of tumor formation, but this requires several weeks after injury before grafting can be done. Preclinical studies are examining their potential in safely treating both acute and chronic spinal cord injury.

- Bone marrow stromal cells, taken from the tissue found inside bones, have been shown in some studies to increase recovery from an injury to the spinal cord. Scientists are studying the injection of these cells into the cerebrospinal fluid (fluid that bathes the brain and spinal cord) to promote proteins needed to grow and maintain nerves and increase nerve signaling across the glial scarring that forms postinjury.
- Nasal olfactory ensheathing cells, taken from the lining of the nose, are special types of glial cells that have been shown to promote axon regeneration and remyelination at the injury site. The transplanted cells have been shown to permit regrowth of axons in both the peripheral and central nervous systems, and improve functional outcome in animal models of spinal cord injury. Early-stage trials in humans are being conducted overseas.

Retraining Central Nervous System Circuits and Plasticity

Recovery from a spinal cord injury may occur for quite some time after the initial injury, as part of the brain's ability to reorganize or form new nerve connections and pathways following injury or cell death (called "neuroplasticity").

Active Rehabilitation and Exercise

Specific training can improve function, coordination of fine muscle movements, and overall strength and health. Scientists are comparing the relative effectiveness of an intensive task-specific motor training program added to standard rehabilitation compared with standard rehabilitation alone for improving hand function and clinical outcomes in people with recent tetraplegia.

Much as in the general population, cardiovascular disease (CVD) is a leading cause of death in persons with spinal cord injury. After the injury, the opportunity to actively exercise large muscles affected by paralysis is limited or may require assistive technologies. Researchers have recently shown that such injuries increase the risk of CVD, along with other muscle atrophy and effects of deconditioning. Since CVD occurs earlier in life for those with a spinal cord injury, researchers are assessing the impact of acute exercise, conditioning, and dietary supplementation on measures of fitness, function, and CVD risk factors/modifiers in individuals with tetraplegia. Other scientists are examining an add-on group exercise program to the usual physical therapy delivered in the hospital to see if it improves the participant's overall outlook on exercise and recovery, and to promote physical activity as part of a healthy lifestyle.

Epidural Stimulation

In May 2011, scientists funded in part by the National Institutes of Health reported that after intensive physical therapy and electrical stimulation to the spine, a man with a paralyzing spinal cord injury from the chest down had recovered the ability to stand and move paralyzed muscles at will when the stimulator is active. The man participated in a pilot study that combined epidermal stimulation and locomotor training—involving his being suspended for hours a day in a harness, walking on a treadmill while physical therapists moved his legs in stepping motions. Two years of locomotor training following his injury did not improve his ability to walk or stand. But he did improve after December 2009, when electrodes were surgically implanted over the paralyzed area of his spinal cord and began sending rhythmic electrical bursts to neurons in the spinal cord during the locomotor training sessions. This epidural simulation imitates the brain's sending signals to the spinal cord to begin movement. He gradually became able to stand and fully bear his own weight for a few minutes at a time. Although he cannot walk without assistance, he can bend one leg at the knee and flex his ankle when the stimulator is active. Locomotor training without any epidural stimulation is routinely used as a rehabilitative technique for people with spinal cord injuries—which allows some individuals to retain the ability to move and feel below the injury. Meanwhile, a form of epidural stimulation is used to relieve pain for some individuals. The researchers and NIH scientists caution that this finding was in only one person, and further study is required to confirm these early, promising results and to understand exactly how the stimulation is working.

Functional Electrical Stimulation

Exciting and promising results in restoring or assisting function in individuals with chronic spinal cord injury have been shown in studies using functional electrical stimulation (FES). FES devices use a computer system and electrodes to deliver small bursts of a low-level electrical current to paralyzed muscles, to generate muscle contractions. Researchers are working to improve the electrode and computer interfaces so they can produce more natural yet complex movements. FES is being used to restore breathing without a ventilator, help with unassisted coughing, enhance bladder and bowel control, increase hand movement and grasping, and improve blood flow to the skin.

Several studies continue to investigate the use of FES in restoring or improving function following a spinal cord injury. Researchers are using FES to help individuals with tetraplegia move paralyzed muscles to restore voluntary grasping function. Others are attempting to stimulate recovery with the goal of being able to grasp objects without stimulation once the treatment program is completed. This approach has been shown to be useful for people who have had a stroke.

An NINDS-supported clinical trial demonstrated that FES of the diaphragm and intercostal muscles (muscles between adjacent ribs that help move the chest wall) can produce effective cough in persons with high tetraplegia. The ability to cough at will eliminates the need for assistance in suctioning secretions and reduces the risk of lung disease. These researchers are now working to improve electrode design to allow for a less invasive surgical implantation.

One study is using a surgically implanted FES to facilitate exercise, standing, stepping, and/or balance in people with various degrees of paralysis. A related study is using a surgically implanted FES to facilitate stability of the trunk and hips, and to evaluate how stabilizing and stiffening the trunk can change the way spinal cord injured volunteers sit, breathe, reach, push a wheelchair, or roll in bed.

Transcranial direct current stimulation (tDCS) is another form of electric stimulation that is being tested experimentally to improve patient outcomes after a spinal cord injury. tDCS is a noninvasive procedure that delivers continuous low electrical current to areas of the brain involved with movement via small electrodes placed on the scalp. Researchers are investigating if combining tDCS with exercise therapy for the affected hand will increase performance over exercise therapy alone. Other researchers hope to determine if tDCS can decrease chronic pain in people with spinal cord injury.

Robotic-Assisted Therapy

Most recovery following SCI takes place within 6 months after injury. Substantial recovery after 12 months is unusual, but researchers continue to test ways to restore function in persons with chronic paralysis. In one very small study involving patients one year after injury, scientists are testing the safety and efficacy of a type of robotic therapy device known as the "AMES device." The aim of this study is to investigate the use of assisted movement and enhanced sensation (AMES) technology in the rehabilitation of the legs of participants with incomplete spinal cord injury. The AMES device rotates the ankle over a range of 30 degrees while vibrators stimulate the tendons attached to muscles that move the leg. The subject's task is to assist the motion of the device.

In another study, researchers will determine the effect of using body-weight supported treadmill training and a robotic gait trainer on functional movement from place to place (ambulation) in people with an incomplete spinal cord injury. The person is suspended in a harness and onto a treadmill, and the robotic legs are strapped to the person. A computer controls the pace of the walking. The effect of the therapy will be evaluated by analyzing changes in ambulation and gait patterns during walking.

Brain-Computer Interfaces

The goal of brain-computer interface (BCI) technology is to bypass the damaged nerve circuits in the spinal cord and establish a direct link between the brain and an assistive implanted device, which may restore an individual's control of voluntary muscle movement and coordination of paralyzed muscles.

Most individuals with tetraplegia have intact brain function but are unable to move due to injury or disease affecting the spinal cord. Brain-computer interface technology is based on the finding that with intact brain function, neural signals for movement are generated in the brain and can be used to control computer-assisted devices. By implanting electrodes in the brain, individuals can be trained to practice thoughts and thereby generate neural signals that are interpreted by a computer and translated to movement which can then be used to control a variety of devices or computer displays.

Researchers are working to develop BCI technology to offer individuals with upper limb paralysis a natural and rich control signal for prosthetic arms or FES device to re-animate paralyzed arms. The study uses electrocorticographic (ECoG) electrodes that interface with neurons in the brain's cortex (the part of the brain that is responsible for higher thought and motor control) to measure brain activity. Participants will learn to control computer cursors; virtual reality environments; and assistive devices, such as hand orthotics and FES devices, using neural activity recorded with the ECoG sensor.

Another preliminary study is assessing the safety and effectiveness of a brain-computer interface to give people with tetraplegia the ability to control a computer cursor and other assistive devices with their thoughts. A small electrode array is inserted into the part of the brain's surface that controls movements. Using the very precise signals this device records, researchers are working to improve the computer's ability to interpret the person's intent and transfer that to the display screen.

How Can I Help with Research?

Clinical trials offer hope for many people and an opportunity to help researchers find better ways to safely detect, treat, or prevent disease, but trials can be done only if people volunteer to participate. Many neurological disorders do not have good treatment options. By participating in a clinical trial, you—as a healthy individual or someone with an illness or disease—can greatly affect the lives of people affected by a neurological disorder.

Part Nine

Additional Help and Information

Chapter 64

Glossary of Terms Related to Back and Neck Care

absorption: The process of taking in. For a person or an animal, absorption is the process of a substance getting into the body through the eyes, skin, stomach, intestines, or lungs.

addiction: A chronic, relapsing disease characterized by compulsive drug seeking and use despite serious adverse consequences, and by long-lasting changes in the brain.

alcohol: A chemical substance found in drinks such as beer, wine, and liquor. It is also found in some medicines, mouthwashes, household products, and essential oils (scented liquid taken from certain plants). It is made by a chemical process called "fermentation" that uses sugars and yeast.

amenorrhea: The abnormal absence of menstrual periods. Early amenorrhea caused by overtraining can cause bones to become brittle and break.

amino acid: One of several molecules that join together to form proteins. There are 20 common amino acids found in proteins.

anesthetic: A drug that causes insensitivity to pain and is used for surgeries and other medical procedures.

This glossary contains terms excerpted from documents produced by several sources deemed reliable.

antibiotic: A drug used to treat infections caused by bacteria and other microorganisms.

antibody: A protein made by plasma cells (a type of white blood cell) in response to an antigen (a substance that causes the body to make a specific immune response). Each antibody can bind to only one specific antigen.

antigen: Any substance that causes the body to make an immune response against that substance. Antigens include toxins, chemicals, bacteria, viruses, or other substances that come from outside the body.

anxiety: Feelings of fear, dread, and uneasiness that may occur as a reaction to stress. A person with anxiety may sweat, feel restless, and tense, and have a rapid heartbeat.

arthritis: A term used to describe more than 100 rheumatic diseases and conditions that affect joints, the tissues which surround the joint and other connective tissue.

aspiration: The removal of fluid or tissue through a needle. Also, the accidental breathing in of food or fluid into the lungs.

assessment: The process of gathering evidence and documentation of a student's learning.

assistive device: Tools that enable individuals with disabilities to perform essential job functions, e.g., telephone headsets, adapted computer keyboards, and enhanced computer monitors.

assistive technology: Products, devices, or equipment that help maintain, increase, or improve the functional capabilities of people with disabilities.

asthma: A chronic disease in which the bronchial airways in the lungs become narrowed and swollen, making it difficult to breathe.

axon: A nerve fiber in the peripheral nervous system that conducts impulses away from the cell body.

biomechanics: Application of scientific principles, such as force and power, in the study of human movement.

bladder: The organ in the human body that stores urine. It is found in the lower part of the abdomen.

blood: A tissue with red blood cells (RBCs), white blood cells (WBCs), platelets, and other substances suspended in fluid called plasma. Blood takes oxygen and nutrients to the tissues, and carries away wastes.

body mass index (BMI): A measure of body weight relative to height. The BMI tool uses a formula that produces a score often used to determine if a person is underweight, at a normal weight, overweight, or obese.

bone: A living, growing tissue made mostly of collagen.

brain tumor: The growth of abnormal cells in the tissues of the brain. Brain tumors can be benign (not cancer) or malignant (cancer).

calcium: A mineral that is an essential nutrient for bone health. It is also needed for the heart, muscles, and nerves to function properly and for blood to clot.

calorie: A unit of energy in food. Carbohydrates, fats, protein, and alcohol in the foods and drinks we eat provide food energy or "calories."

cancer: A term for diseases in which abnormal cells in the body divide without control. Cancer cells can invade nearby tissues and can spread to other parts of the body through the blood and lymphatic system, which is a network of tissues that clears infections and keeps body fluids in balance.

cauda equina syndrome (CES): A group of symptoms that occur when nerves in the cauda equina (a collection of nerve roots that spread out from the bottom of the spinal cord) become compressed or damaged. These nerve roots connect the central nervous system and peripheral nervous system.

central nervous system (CNS): Comprised of the nerves in the brain and spinal cord. These nerves are used to send electrical impulses throughout the body, resulting in voluntary and reflexive movement. Information about the environment is received by the senses and sent to the central nervous system, which causes the body to respond appropriately.

cetuximab: A drug used to treat certain types of head and neck cancer, and a certain type of colorectal cancer that has spread to other parts of the body. It is also being studied in the treatment of other types of cancer. Cetuximab binds to a protein called epidermal growth factor receptor (EGFR), which is on the surface of some types of cancer cells. This may stop cancer cells from growing. Cetuximab is a type of monoclonal antibody. Also called "Erbitux."

chemotherapy: Treatment with anticancer drugs.

chronic disease: A disease that has one or more of the following characteristics: is permanent; leaves residual disability; is caused by nonreversible pathological alteration; requires special training of the patient for rehabilitation; or may be expected to require a long period of supervision, observation, or care.

chronic pain: Pain that can range from mild to severe, and persists or progresses over a long period of time.

cigarette: A tube-shaped tobacco product that is made of finely cut, cured tobacco leaves wrapped in thin paper. It may also have other ingredients, including substances to add different flavors.

clinical trial: A research study in which one or more human subjects are prospectively assigned to one or more interventions (which may include placebo or other control) to evaluate the effects of those interventions on health-related biomedical or behavioral outcomes.

computed tomography (CT): A procedure for taking X-ray images from many different angles and then assembling them into a cross-section of the body. This technique is generally used to visualize bone.

constipation: A decrease in frequency of stools or bowel movements with hardening of the stool. Some forms of osteogenesis imperfecta are associated with increased risk for constipation caused by increased perspiration, growth impairment, pelvic malformation, and diminished physical activity.

corticosteroids: Steroid-type hormones that have antitumor activity in lymphomas and lymphoid leukemias. In addition, corticosteroids may be used for hormone replacement and for the management of some of the complications of cancer and its treatment.

deoxyribonucleic acid (DNA): The double-helix molecule that provides the basis of genetic heredity, about two nanometers in diameter but often several millimeters in length.

diabetes: A disease in which blood glucose (blood sugar) levels are above normal. There are two main types of diabetes. Type 1 diabetes is caused by a problem with the body's defense system, called the "immune system."

diet: What a person eats and drinks. Any type of eating plan.

endocrinologist: A physician who specializes in diagnosing and treating disorders of the body's glands and hormones.

enzyme: A protein that speeds up chemical reactions in the body.

ergonomics: It is the science of designing the job and the workplace to suit the capabilities of the workers. Simply stated, ergonomics means "fitting the task to the worker." The aim of ergonomics is the evaluation and design of facilities, workstations, jobs, training methods, and equipment to match the capabilities of users and workers, and thereby reduce stress and eliminate injuries and disorders associated with the overuse of muscles, bad posture, and repeated tasks.

estrogen: A group of female hormones that are responsible for the development of breasts and other secondary sex characteristics in women. Estrogen is produced by the ovaries and other body tissues. Estrogen, along with progesterone, is important in preparing a woman's body for pregnancy.

exercise: A type of physical activity that involves planned, structured, and repetitive bodily movement done to maintain or improve one or more components of physical fitness.

exposure: Swallowing, breathing, or touching a substance through the skin or eyes. Exposure duration may be immediate, short term (14 days or less), intermediate, or long term (more than 1 year).

fetus: A developing unborn offspring in the uterus (womb). This stage of pregnancy begins eight weeks after conception and lasts until birth.

fracture: Broken bone. People with osteoporosis, osteogenesis imperfecta, and Paget disease are at greater risk for bone fracture.

genetics: The study of particular genes, deoxyribonucleic acid (DNA), and heredity.

gynecologist: A doctor who diagnoses and treats conditions of the female reproductive system and associated disorders.

hormone: Substance produced by one tissue and conveyed by the bloodstream to another to affect a function of the body, such as growth or metabolism.

human immunodeficiency virus (HIV): A virus that infects and destroys the body's immune cells and causes a disease called "acquired immunodeficiency syndrome" (AIDS).

hypertension: Also called high blood pressure, it is having blood pressure greater than 140 over 90 mmHg (millimeters of mercury). Long-term high blood pressure can damage blood vessels and organs, including the heart, kidneys, eyes, and brain.

hypopharyngeal cancer: Cancer that forms in tissues of the hypopharynx (the bottom part of the throat). The most common type is squamous cell carcinoma (cancer that begins in flat cells lining the hypopharynx).

immune system: A complex system of cellular and molecular components having the primary function of distinguishing self from not self and defense against foreign organisms or substances.

laryngoscopy: Procedure used to see, directly or indirectly, the vocal folds (formerly known as vocal cords), and neighboring tissue in the larynx (voice box) or other parts of the throat.

larynx: The area of the throat containing the vocal cords and used for breathing, swallowing, and talking. Also called voice box.

lesion: An area of abnormal tissue. A lesion may be benign (not cancer) or malignant (cancer).

lupus: A chronic inflammatory disease that occurs when the body's immune system attacks its own tissues and organs. Also, called "systemic lupus erythematosus" (SLE). Inflammation caused by lupus can affect many different body systems including joints, skin, kidneys, blood cells, heart, and lungs. People with lupus are at increased risk for osteoporosis.

magnetic resonance imaging (MRI): A noninvasive procedure that uses magnetic fields and radio waves to produce three-dimensional computerized images of areas inside the body.

meningitis: Inflammation of the meninges, the membranes that envelop the brain and the spinal cord; may cause hearing loss or deafness.

menopause: The cessation of menstruation in women. Bone health in women often deteriorates after menopause due to a decrease in the female hormone estrogen.

metabolism: The chemical changes that take place in a cell or an organism. These changes make energy and the materials cells and organisms need to grow, reproduce, and stay healthy. Metabolism also helps get rid of toxic substances.

migraine: A medical condition that usually involves a very painful headache, usually felt on one side of the head. Besides intense pain, migraine also can cause nausea and vomiting and sensitivity to light and sound. Some people also may see spots or flashing lights or have a temporary loss of vision.

mutation: A change in a DNA sequence that can result from DNA copying mistakes made during cell division, exposure to ionizing radiation, exposure to chemical mutagens, or infection by viruses.

nasopharyngeal cancer: Cancer that forms in tissues of the nasopharynx (upper part of the throat behind the nose). Most nasopharyngeal cancers are squamous cell carcinomas (cancer that begins in flat cells lining the nasopharynx).

neurotransmitter: A chemical produced by neurons that carry messages from one nerve cell to another.

nivolumab: A drug used alone or with ipilimumab to treat a certain type of colorectal cancer that has mutations (changes) in genes involved in DNA repair.

nutrition: The taking in and use of food and other nourishing material by the body. Nutrition is a 3-part process. First, food or drink is consumed. Second, the body breaks down the food or drink into nutrients.

obesity: Refers to excess body fat. Because body fat is usually not measured directly, a ratio of body weight to height is often used instead.

organ: A part of the body that performs a specific function. For example, the heart is an organ.

oropharyngeal cancer: Cancer that forms in tissues of the oropharynx (the part of the throat at the back of the mouth, including the soft palate, the base of the tongue, and the tonsils). Most oropharyngeal cancers are squamous cell carcinomas (cancer that begins in flat cells lining the oropharynx).

osteoporosis: Literally means "porous bone." This disease is characterized by too little bone formation, excessive bone loss, or a combination of both, leading to bone fragility and an increased risk of fractures of the hip, spine, and wrist.

over-the-counter (OTC): Diseases, including ulcerative colitis (UC) and Crohn disease, that cause swelling in the intestine and/or digestive tract, which may result in diarrhea, abdominal pain, fever, and weight loss. People with inflammatory bowel disease (IBD) are at an increased risk for osteoporosis.

overweight: Refers to an excessive amount of body weight that includes muscle, bone, fat, and water. A person who has a body mass index (BMI) of 25 to 29.9 is considered overweight.

papillomavirus: Group of viruses that can cause noncancerous wart-like tumors to grow on the surface of skin and internal organs, such as the respiratory tract; can be life-threatening.

perception (hearing): Process of knowing or being aware of information through the ear.

physical activity: Any bodily movement that is produced by the contraction of skeletal muscle and that substantially increases energy expenditure.

placebo: A pill or liquid that looks like the new treatment but does not have any treatment value from active ingredients.

pregnancy: The condition between conception (fertilization of an egg by a sperm) and birth, during which the fertilized egg develops in the uterus. In humans, pregnancy lasts about 288 days.

prevention: Actions that reduce exposure or other risks, keep people from getting sick, or keep disease from getting worse.

prognosis: The likely outcome or course of a disease; the chance of recovery or recurrence.

protein: A molecule made up of amino acids. Proteins are needed for the body to function properly. They are the basis of body structures, such as skin and hair, and of other substances such as enzymes, cytokines, and antibodies.

puberty: Time when the body is changing from the body of a child to the body of an adult. This process begins earlier in girls than in boys, usually between ages 8 and 13, and lasts 2 to 4 years.

radiation: Energy moving in the form of particles or waves. Familiar radiations are heat, light, radio, and microwaves.

rheumatoid arthritis (RA): An inflammatory disease that causes pain, swelling, stiffness, and loss of function in the joints. It occurs when the immune system, which normally defends the body from invading organisms, attacks the membrane lining the joints. Studies have found an increased risk of bone loss and fracture in individuals with RA.

smell: To perceive odor or scent through stimuli affecting the olfactory nerves.

sodium: A mineral and an essential nutrient needed by the human body in relatively small amounts (provided that substantial sweating does not occur).

spina bifida: A condition that affects the spine and is usually apparent at birth. It is a type of neural tube defect (NTD).

steroid: Any of a group of lipids (fats) that have a certain chemical structure. Steroids occur naturally in plants and animals or they may be made in the laboratory.

stroke: Also known as a "cerebrovascular accident" (CVA); caused by a lack of blood to the brain, resulting in the sudden loss of speech, language, or the ability to move a body part, and, if severe enough, death.

tai chi: A form of traditional Chinese mind/body exercise and meditation that uses slow sets of body movements and controlled breathing. Tai chi is done to improve balance, flexibility, muscle strength, and overall health.

tobacco: A plant with leaves that have high levels of the addictive chemical nicotine. After harvesting, tobacco leaves are cured, aged, and processed in various ways. The resulting products may be smoked (in cigarettes, cigars, and pipes), applied to the gums (as dipping and chewing tobacco), or inhaled (as snuff).

tongue: Large muscle on the floor of the mouth that manipulates food for chewing and swallowing. It is the main organ of taste, and assists in forming speech sounds.

transcutaneous electrical nerve stimulation (TENS): A technique in which a special device transmits low-voltage electrical impulses through electrodes on the skin to the area of the body that is in pain.

urinary tract infection (UTI): An infection anywhere in the urinary tract, or organs that collect and store urine and release it from your body (the kidneys, ureters, bladder, and urethra).

virus: A small organism that can infect a person and cause illness or disease.

vitamin D: A nutrient that the body needs to absorb calcium.

X-ray: A type of high-energy radiation. In low doses, X-rays are used to diagnose diseases by making pictures of the inside of the body.

yoga: A mind and body practice with origins in ancient Indian philosophy. The various styles of yoga typically combine physical postures, breathing techniques, and meditation or relaxation.

Chapter 65

Directory of Back and Neck Organizations and Resources

Government Agencies and Organizations

Agency for Healthcare Research and Quality (AHRQ)
Office of Communications and Knowledge Transfer (OCKT)
5600 Fishers Ln.
Seventh Fl.
Rockville, MD 20857
Phone: 301-427-1104
Website: www.ahrq.gov

The Brain Research through Advancing Innovative Neurotechnologies (BRAIN) Initiative®
National Institutes of Health (NIH)
P.O. Box 5801
Bethesda, MD 20892
Website: www.braininitiative.nih.gov

Resources in this chapter were compiled from several sources deemed reliable; all contact information was verified and updated in April 2019.

Centers for Disease Control and Prevention (CDC)
1600 Clifton Rd.
Atlanta, GA 30329-4027
Toll-Free: 800-CDC-INFO
(800-232-4636)
Toll-Free TTY: 888-232-6348
Website: www.cdc.gov

Healthfinder.gov
U.S. Department of Health and Human Services (HHS)
1101 Wootton Pkwy
Rockville, MD 20852
Website: www.healthfinder.gov
E-mail: healthfinder@hhs.gov

National Center for Complementary and Integrative Health (NCCIH)
9000 Rockville Pike
Bethesda, MD 20892
Toll-Free: 888-644-6226
Toll-Free TTY: 866-464-3615
Website: www.nccih.nih.gov
E-mail: info@nccih.nih.gov

National Institute of Arthritis and Musculoskeletal and Skin Diseases (NIAMS)
1 AMS Cir.
Bethesda, MD 20892-3675
Toll-Free: 877-22-NIAMS
(877-226-4267)
TTY: 301-565-2966
Fax: 301-718-6366
Website: www.niams.nih.gov
E-mail: niamsinfo@mail.nih.gov

National Institute of Neurological Disorders and Stroke (NINDS)
National Institutes of Health (NIH) Neurological Institute
P.O. Box 5801
Bethesda, MD 20824
Toll-Free: 800-352-9424
Website: www.ninds.nih.gov

National Institute on Aging (NIA)
Bldg. 31 Rm. 5C27
31 Center Dr. MSC 2292
Bethesda, MD 20892
Toll-Free: 800-222-2225
Phone: 301-496-1752
Toll-Free TTY: 800-222-4225
Website: www.nia.nih.gov
E-mail: niaic@nia.nih.gov

National Institutes of Health (NIH)
9000 Rockville Pike
Bethesda, MD 20892
Toll-Free: 888-346-3656
Phone: 301-496-4000
TTY: 301-402-9612
Website: www.nih.gov

U.S. Food and Drug Administration (FDA)
10903 New Hampshire Ave.
Silver Spring, MD 20993
Toll-Free: 888-INFO-FDA
(888-463-6332)
Website: www.fda.gov

U.S. National Library of Medicine (NLM)
8600 Rockville Pike
Bethesda, MD 20894
Website: www.nlm.nih.gov

Private and Nonprofit Organizations

American Academy of Neurology (AAN)
201 Chicago Ave.
Minneapolis, MN 55415
Toll-Free: 800-879-1960
Fax: 612-454-2746
Website: www.aan.com
E-mail: memberservices@aan.com

American Academy of Orthopaedic Surgeons (AAOS)
9400 W. Higgins Rd.
Rosemont, IL 60018
Toll-Free: 800-346-AAOS (800-346-2267)
Phone: 847-823-7186
Fax: 847-823-8125
Website: www.aaos.org
E-mail: custserv@aaos.org

American Academy of Pain Medicine (AAPM)
8735 W. Higgins Rd., Ste. 300
Chicago, IL 60631-2738
Phone: 847-375-4731
Fax: 209-533-9750
Website: www.painmed.org
E-mail: info@painmed.org

American Academy of Physical Medicine and Rehabilitation (AAPM&R)
9700 W. Bryn Mawr Ave.
Ste. 200
Rosemont, IL 60018-5701
Toll-Free: 877-227-6799
Phone: 847-737-6000
Website: www.aapmr.org
E-mail: info@aapmr.org

American Academy of Spine Physicians (AASP)
1795 Grandstand Place
Elgin, IL 60123-4980
Phone: 847-697-4660
Fax: 847-931-7975
Website: www.spinephysicians.org
E-mail: aasp@spinephysicians.org

American Association of Neurological Surgeons (AANS)
5550 Meadowbrook Dr.
Rolling Meadows, IL 60008-3852
Toll-Free: 888-566-AANS (888-566-2267)
Phone: 847-378-0500
Fax: 847-378-0600
Website: www.aans.org
E-mail: info@aans.org

American Chiropractic Association (ACA)
1701 Clarendon Blvd.
Arlington, VA 22209
Phone: 703-276-8800
Fax: 703-243-2593
Website: www.acatoday.org
E-mail: memberinfo@acatoday.org

American Chronic Pain Association (ACPA)
P.O. Box 850
Rocklin, CA 95677
Toll-Free: 800-533-3231
Fax: 916-652-8190
Website: www.theacpa.org
E-mail: ACPA@theacpa.org

American College of Rheumatology (ACR)
2200 Lake Blvd. N.E.
Atlanta, GA 30319
Phone: 404-633-3777
Fax: 404-633-1870
Website: www.rheumatology.org

American Medical Association (AMA)
330 N. Wabash Ave.
Ste. 39300
Chicago, IL 60611-5885
Website: www.ama-assn.org

American Occupational Therapy Association (AOTA)
4720 Montgomery Ln.
Ste. 200
Bethesda, MD 20814
Toll-Free: 800-SAY-AOTA (800-729-2682)
Phone: 301-652-6611
Website: www.aota.org

American Osteopathic Association (AOA)
142 E. Ontario St.
Chicago, IL 60611-2864
Toll-Free: 888-62-MYAOA (888-626-9262)
Website: www.osteopathic.org

American Pain Society (APS)
8735 W. Higgins Rd.
Chicago, IL 60631
Phone: 847-375-4715
Website: www.ampainsoc.org
E-mail: info@americanpainsociety.org

American Physical Therapy Association (APTA)
1111 N. Fairfax St.
Alexandria, VA 22314-1488
Toll-Free: 800-999-APTA (800-999-2782)
Phone: 703-684-APTA (703-684-2782)
TDD: 703-683-6748
Fax: 703-684-7343
Website: www.apta.org

American Podiatric Medical Association (APMA)
9312 Old Georgetown Rd.
Bethesda, MD 20814-1621
Phone: 301-581-9200
Website: www.apma.org

Arthritis Foundation
1355 Peachtree St. N.E.
Ste. 600
Atlanta, GA 30309
Toll-Free: 844-571-4357
Phone: 404-872-7100
Website: www.arthritis.org

Cleveland Clinic
9500 Euclid Ave.
Cleveland, OH 44195
Toll-Free: 800-223-2273
Phone: 216-444-2200
TTY: 216-444-0261
Website: my.clevelandclinic.org

Dynamic Chiropractic
13950 Milton Ave.
Ste. 200A
Westminster, CA 92683
Phone: 714-230-3150
Website: www.chiroweb.com

Dystonia Medical Research Foundation (DMRF)
One E. Wacker Dr.
Ste. 1730
Chicago, IL 60601-1980
Toll-Free: 800-377-DYST
(800-377-3978)
Phone: 312-755-0198
Fax: 312-803-0138
Website: dystonia-foundation.org
E-mail: dystonia@
dystoniafoundation.org

Federation of Chiropractic Licensing Boards (FCLB)
5401 W. 10th St., Ste. 101
Greeley, CO 80634-4400
Phone: 970-356-3500
Fax: 970-356-3599
Website: www.fclb.org
E-mail: info@fclb.org

Hospital for Special Surgery (HSS)
Rheumatology Division
535 E. 70th St.
New York, NY 10021
Toll-Free: 877-477-1543
Phone: 212-606-1000
Website: www.hss.edu/
rheumatology.asp

International Chiropractors Association (ICA)
6400 Arlington Blvd.
Ste. 800
Falls Church, VA 22042
Toll-Free: 800-423-4690
Phone: 703-528-5000
Fax: 703-528-5023
Website: www.chiropractic.org
E-mail: info@chiropractic.org

International Intradiscal Therapy Society (IITS)
1635 E. Myrtle Ave.
Ste. 400
Phoenix, AZ 85020
Phone: 310-279-3159
Fax: 602-944-0064
Website:
endoscopicspinetherapy.org

National Osteoporosis Foundation (NOF)
251 18th St. S.
Ste. 630
Arlington, VA 22202
Toll-Free: 800-231-4222
Website: www.nof.org
E-mail: info@nof.org

National Scoliosis Foundation (NSF)
5 Cabot Place
Stoughton, MA 02072
Toll-Free: 800-NSF-MYBACK
(800-673-6922)
Fax: 781-341-8333
Website: www.scoliosis.org
E-mail: NSF@scoliosis.org

Nemours Foundation Center for Children's Health Media
The Nemours Foundation/
KidsHealth®
1600 Rockland Rd.
Wilmington, DE 19803
Phone: 302-651-4046
Website: www.kidshealth.org
E-mail: info@KidsHealth.org

North American Spine Society (NASS)
7075 Veterans Blvd.
Burr Ridge, IL 60527
Phone: 630-230-3600
Website: www.spine.org
E-mail: info@spine.org

Pain Connection
U.S. Pain Foundation (USPF)
6105 E. Grant Rd.
Tucson, AZ 85712
Toll-Free: 800-910-0664
Website: www.painconnection.org
E-mail: info@painconnection.org

Scoliosis Research Society (SRS)
555 E. Wells St.
Ste. 1100
Milwaukee, WI 53202-3823
Phone: 414-289-9107
Fax: 414-276-3349
Website: www.srs.org
E-mail: info@srs.org

Spina Bifida Association of America (SBAA)
1600 Wilson Blvd.
Ste. 800
Arlington, VA 22209
Toll-Free: 800-621-3141
Website: www.spinabifidaassociation.org
E-mail: sbaa@sbaa.org

SPINE-health.com
Veritashealth.com
Website: www.spine-health.com
E-mail: admin@spinehealth.com

Spine Intervention Society (SIS)
120 E. Ogden Ave.
Ste. 202
Hinsdale, IL 60521
Toll-Free: 888-255-0005
Phone: 630-203-2252
Website: www.spinalinjection.com/ISIS

SpineSource, Inc.
17826 Edison Ave.
Chesterfield, MO 63005
Phone: 636-532-9300
Fax: 636-532-9829
Website: www.spinesource.com

SpineUniverse
Vertical Health, LLC.
7 N. Willow St.
Ste. 7A
Montclair, NJ 07042
Phone: 973-783-7009
Website: www.spineuniverse.com

Spondylitis Association of America (SAA)
16360 Roscoe Blvd.
Ste. 100
Van Nuys, CA 91406
Toll-Free: 800-777-8189
Phone: 818-892-1616
Fax: 818-892-1611
Website: www.spondylitis.org
E-mail: info@spondylitis.org

Spinal Cord Injury Resources

American Paraplegia Society (APS)
Academy of Spinal Cord Injury Professionals, Inc. (ASCIP)
206 S. 6th St.
Springfield, IL 62701
Phone: 217-321-2488
Fax: 217-525-1271
Website: www.academyscipro.org/about-aps

American Spinal Injury Association (ASIA)
2209 Dickens Rd.
Richmond, VA 23230-2005
Phone: 804-565-6396
Fax: 804-282-0090
Website: www.asia-spinalinjury.org
E-mail: asia.office@asia-spinalinjury.org

Christopher & Dana Reeve Foundation
Paralysis Resource Center (PRC)
636 Morris Tpke, Ste. 3A
Short Hills, NJ 07078
Toll-Free: 800-225-0292
Phone: 973-467-8270
Website: www.christopherreeve.org/living-with-paralysis/about-the-paralysis-resource-center
E-mail: InfoSpecialist@ChristopherReeve.org

Darrell Gwynn Foundation
P.O. Box 291318
Davie, FL 33329-1318
Website: www.darrellgwynn.com
E-mail: dgrc@darrellgwynn.com

Miami Project to Cure Paralysis / Buoniconti Fund
1095 N.W. 14th Terr.
Lois Pope LIFE Center
Miami, FL 33136
Toll-Free: 800-STAND-UP (800-782-6387)
Phone: 305-243-6001
Fax: 305-243-6017
Website: www.themiamiproject.org
E-mail: miamiproject@med.miami.edu

Spinal Cord Injury Model System (SCIMS) Information Network
University of Alabama at Birmingham (UAB)
1717 Sixth Ave. S.
529 Spain Rehabilitation Center
Birmingham, AL 35249-7330
Phone: 205-934-3283
Website: www.uab.edu/medicine/sci

Spinal Cord Society (SCS)
19051 County Hwy 1
Fergus Falls, MN 56537
Phone: 218-739-5252
Fax: 218-739-5262
Website: www.scsus.org

United Spinal Association
120-34 Queens Blvd.
Ste. 320
Kew Gardens, NY 11415
Phone: 718-803-3782
Fax: 718-803-0414
Website: www.unitedspinal.org

Organizations That Provide Information and Assistance for People Disabled by Back and Neck Disorders

Americans with Disabilities Act (ADA)
U.S. Department of Justice (DOJ)
950 Pennsylvania Ave. N.W.
Civil Rights Division Disability Rights Section New York Ave.
Washington, DC 20530
Toll-Free: 800-514-0301
Phone: 202-307-0663
Toll-Free TTY: 800-514-0383
Fax: 202-307-1197
Website: www.ada.gov

Center for Assistive Technology & Environmental Access (CATEA)
512 Means St. N.W.
Ste. 300
Atlanta, GA 30318
Phone: 404-894-4960
Fax: 404-894-9320
Website: catea.gatech.edu
E-mail: catea@design.gatech.edu

Job Accommodation Network (JAN)
P.O. Box 6080
Morgantown, WV 26506-6080
Toll-Free: 800-526-7234
Phone: 304-293-7186
Toll-Free TTY: 877-781-9403
Fax: 304-293-5407
Website: askjan.org
E-mail: jan@askjan.org

Medicare Rights Center
266 W. 37th St.
Third Fl.
New York, NY 10018
Toll-Free: 800-333-4114
Phone: 212-869-3850
Fax: 212-869-3532
Website: www.medicarerights.org
E-mail: info@medicarerights.org

National Center on Health, Physical Activity and Disability (NCHPAD)
4000 Ridgeway Dr.
Birmingham, AL 35209
Toll-Free: 800-900-8086
Fax: 205-313-7475
Website: www.nchpad.org
E-mail: email@nchpad.org

National Organization of Social Security Claimants' Representatives (NOSSCR)
560 Sylvan Ave.
Ste. 2200
Englewood Cliffs, NJ 07632
Toll-Free: 800-431-2804
Phone: 201-567-4228
Fax: 201-567-1542
Website: www.nosscr.org
E-mail: nosser@nosser.org

National Organization on Disability (NOD)
77 Water St.
Ste. 204
New York, NY 10005
Phone: 646-505-1191
Fax: 646-505-1184
Website: www.nod.org
E-mail: info@nod.org

Office of Disability Employment Policy (ODEP)
U.S. Department of Labor (DOL)
200 Constitution Ave. N.W.
Washington, DC 20210
Toll-Free: 866-4-USA-DOL
(866-487-2365)
Website: www.dol.gov/odep

Rehabilitation Services Administration (RSA)
U.S. Department of Education
(ED)
Website: rsa.ed.gov/index.cfm

Index

Index

Page numbers followed by 'n' indicate a footnote. Page numbers in *italics* indicate a table or illustration.

A

"A Guide to Safe Use of Pain Medicine" (FDA) 327n
AANS *see* American Association of Neurological Surgeons
AAOS *see* American Academy of Orthopaedic Surgeons
AAPM&R *see* American Academy of Physical Medicine and Rehabilitation
abdominal aortic aneurysms (AAAs), defined 36
abdominal belts, injury prevention 116
absorption, defined 487
"Accelerating Adoption of Assistive Technology to Reduce Physical Strain among Family Caregivers of the Chronically Disabled Elderly Living at Home." (ASPE) 101n
ACDF *see* anterior cervical discectomy and fusion
acetaminophen
  analgesic medications 51
  chronic pain 324
  defined 17
acetaminophen, *continued*
  osteoarthritis (OA) 214
  osteoporosis 167
  spina bifida 250
  spinal stenosis 238
acetylcholine, acupuncture 52
achondroplasia
  lordosis 193
  spinal stenosis 234
acupressure, back pain 25
acupuncture
  back pain 52
  complementary and alternative medicine (CAM) 227
  described 17
  needle procedures 314
  osteoarthritis (OA) 215
  overview 370–4
  spinal stenosis 239
"Acupuncture: In Depth" (NCCIH) 373n
acute pain
  defined 12
  low back pain 129
  neck pain 41
  opioids 324
  physical therapy 342
  sacroiliac joint syndrome 302
  spinal stenosis 239

addiction, defined 487
adjustments
  driving 112
  pain treatment 362
adolescents
  nasopharyngeal cancer 431
  osteoporosis 152
  Scheuermann kyphosis 191
  spina bifida 264
  spinal cord injury (SCI) 182
aerobic exercise
  back pain 27
  described 108
  physical therapy 343
aerobic walking program, spine fractures 148
Agency for Healthcare Research and Quality (AHRQ)
  contact 497
  publication
    questions to doctor before your surgery 383n
aging
  cervical disc disease 297
  disc herniation 224
  intervertebral discs 6
  osteoporosis 156
  spinal cord injury (SCI) 183
  spine 29
  work-related back injuries 84
alcohol
  central nervous system (CNS) tumors 277
  defined 487
  nonsteroidal anti-inflammatory medications 334
  osteoporosis 171
  vitamin D deficiency 159
alignment
  spinal stenosis 240
  spine 72
  sterno-occipital mandibular immobilization device (SOMI) 346
allograft, anterior cervical discectomy and fusion (ACDF) 392
amenorrhea, defined 487
American Academy of Neurology (AAN), contact 499
American Academy of Orthopaedic Surgeons (AAOS), contact 499
American Academy of Pain Medicine (AAPM), contact 499
American Academy of Physical Medicine and Rehabilitation (AAPM&R), contact 499
American Academy of Spine Physicians (AASP), contact 499
American Association of Neurological Surgeons (AANS), contact 499
American Chiropractic Association (ACA), contact 499
American Chronic Pain Association (ACPA), contact 499
American College of Rheumatology (ACR), contact 500
American Medical Association (AMA), contact 500
American Occupational Therapy Association (AOTA), contact 500
American Osteopathic Association (AOA), contact 500
American Pain Society (APS), contact 500
American Paraplegia Society (APS), contact 503
American Physical Therapy Association (APTA), contact 500
American Podiatric Medical Association (APMA), contact 500
American Spinal Injury Association (ASIA), contact 503
Americans with Disabilities Act (ADA), contact 504
amino acid, defined 487
analgesics
  pain management 331
  spinal pain 327
"Anatomy and Functions of the Spine" (Omnigraphics) 3n
anesthesia
  neurosurgery 284
  surgical procedures 241
anesthetic, defined 487
ankylosing spondylitis, overview 203–8
"Ankylosing Spondylitis" (NIAMS) 203n

annulus fibrosus, intervertebral discs 7
anterior cervical discectomy and fusion (ACDF)
 cervical disc disease 299
 defined 44
antibiotic, defined 488
antibody, defined 488
antigens
 defined 488
 immunohistochemistry 417
anxiety, defined 488
APMA *see* American Podiatric Medical Association
APS *see* American Paraplegia Society
arachnoiditis, syringomyelia 289
"Are There Disorders or Conditions Associated with Spina Bifida?" (NICHD) 248n
arthritis
 back pain 22
 defined 488
 described 81
 genetics 37
 overview 200–3
 spinal stenosis 235
"Arthritis" (NIAMS) 200n
Arthritis Foundation, contact 500
arthroscopic debridement, osteoarthritis (OA) 214
artificial cervical disc replacement (ACDR), surgical treatment 44
artificial disc replacement
 back pain 54
 defined 399
AS *see* ankylosing spondylitis
ASIA Impairment Scale, described 179
aspiration, defined 488
aspirin
 ibuprofen 191
 kyphosis 191
 nonsteroidal anti-inflammatory drugs (NSAIDs) 335
 spinal fusion surgery 404
assessment, defined 488
assistive device, defined 488
assistive technology (AT)
 defined 488
 504 plan 261
asthma, defined 488
athletes
 Pilates 199
 warming up 107
autonomic dysreflexia (or hyperreflexia), spinal cord injury (SCI) 181
axons
 defined 488
 spinal cord injuries 173

B

"Back and Neck Braces" (Omnigraphics) 345n
back belts, overview 115–20
"Back Belts Do They Prevent Injury?" (CDC) 115n
"Back Disorders and Injuries" (OSHA) 84n
"Back Exercise 2" (*Go4Life*) 129n
back exercises, low back pain 129
back extension, low back pain 352
"Back Health" (DOHS) 88n
backbone *see* spinal column
backpack safety, kids 121
"Backpack Safety" (OWH) 121n
backpacks
 childhood back injury 121
 low back pain 58
back pain
 ankylosing spondylitis 205
 back exercises 108
 diagnosis 49
 kyphosis 189
 lumbar spine 145
 overview 21–8
 pregnancy 125
 traumatic injury 35
 workplace 89
"Back Pain" (NIAMS) 21n, 396n
"Back Pain during Pregnancy" (Omnigraphics) 125n
"Back Pain Information Page" (NINDS) 396n
back problems
 ankylosing spondylitis 205
 lumbar spinal surgery 396
back supports, injury prevention 116

barium esophagogram, defined 441
BCI *see* brain-computer interface
bed rest
  back pain 50
  nonsurgical treatment 226
"Behavior of the Upper Cervical Spine in Rugby Players (Cervistab)" (NIH) 467n
behavioral modification, back pain 24
"The Benefits and Risks of Pain Relievers: Q and A on NSAIDs with Sharon Hertz, M.D." (FDA) 333n
benign tumors, spinal cord 414
Bextra (valdecoxib), COX-2 selective inhibitors 335
biofeedback
  back pain 52
  described 18
biomechanics, defined 488
biopsy, tumors 278
bladder, defined 488
bleeding
  neurosurgery 284
  nonsteroidal anti-inflammatory drugs (NSAIDs) 329
  spinal injections 340
blood, defined 488
blood-brain barrier, chemotherapy 421
blood clots
  spinal cord injury (SCI) 178
  spinal surgery 406
blood flow
  low back pain 39
  spinal cord injury (SCI) 176
  spinal tumors 281
blood tests
  back pain 49
  neck cancer 429
  osteoarthritis (OA) 213
BMP *see* bone morphogenetic proteins
body mass index (BMI)
  defined 489
  methadone usage 468
body mechanics
  back pain 38
  described 89
bone, defined 489
bone disease, osteoporosis 36
bone grafts
  anterior cervical discectomy and fusion (ACDF) 392
  cervical disc disease 299
"Bone Graft" (NIH) 407n
bone morphogenetic proteins (BMPs), bone graft 405
bone scans
  hypopharyngeal cancer 441
  low back pain 49
  spinal cord tumors 418
bone spurs
  anterior cervical corpectomy 393
  depicted *212*
  osteoarthritis (OA) 213
  spinal stenosis 234
  X-rays 298
botulinum toxin, nerve block therapies 52
braces
  neck injuries 143
  overview 345–8
  personal protective equipment (PPE) 83
  Scheuermann kyphosis 191
  spina bifida 253
  spinal fusion surgery 405
  spinal stenosis 31
"Brain and Spinal Cord Tumors: Hope through Research" (NINDS) 274n
"Brain and Spinal Tumors Information Page" (NINDS) 413n
brain–computer interface (BCI), described 483
The Brain Research through Advancing Innovative Neurotechnologies (BRAIN) Initiative®, contact 497
brain tumors
  central nervous system (CNS) tumors 277
  defined 489
broken neck *see* cervical fracture
bronchoscopy, defined 441
bulging discs, low back pain 48

C

C-reactive protein, blood tests 49

calcium
defined 489
diagnostic imaging 280
osteoporosis 153
spinal stenosis 234
calorie
back pain 21
defined 489
osteoporosis 154
cancer
brain and spinal cord 282
defined 489
hypopharynx 439
kyphosis 189
nasopharynx 431
oropharynx 447
squamous cells 423
cardiovascular disease (CVD)
nonsteroidal anti-inflammatory drugs (NSAIDs) 51
rehabilitation 481
spinal injection 339
caregivers, back injury 101
carmustine, chemotherapy 287
carpal tunnel syndrome (CTS)
pinched nerve 244
work-related musculoskeletal disorders 79
cartilage
arthroscopic debridement 214
depicted *200*
cauda equina syndrome (CES)
defined 489
low back pain 36
overview 245–6
"Cauda Equina Syndrome," (GARD) 245n
CBT *see* cognitive behavioral therapy
CDC *see* Centers for Disease Control and Prevention
Celebrex (celecoxib), nonsteroidal anti-inflammatory drugs (NSAIDs) 334
cell replacement, spinal cord injuries research 476
Center for Assistive Technology & Environmental Access (CATEA), contact 504
Centers for Disease Control and Prevention (CDC)
contact 498
publications
back belts 115n
backpacks 121n
bone allografts 407n
ergonomics for computer workstations 92n
osteoarthritis (OA) 211n
spina bifida 248n, 254n
what you should know before your surgery 379n
work-related musculoskeletal disorders (WMSDs) and ergonomics 78n
central nervous system (CNS)
cauda equina syndrome (CES) 245
chronic pain 16
defined 489
Klippel-Feil syndrome (KFS) 316
central sensitization, pain 14
ceramics, anterior cervical discectomy and fusion (ACDF) 392
cerebellum
brain 274
defined 413
cerebrospinal fluid (CSF)
cell replacement 480
chemotherapy 421
Chiari II malformation
spinal tumors 279
Tarlov cysts 293
cerebrum, brain 274
cervical brace
described 345
neck pain 43
rehabilitation 143
cervical collars, Klippel-Feil syndrome (KFS) 318
cervical corpectomy, defined 393
cervical disc disease, overview 297–300
"Cervical Disc Disease" (Omnigraphics) 297n
"Cervical Fracture" (Omnigraphics) 141n
cervical fractures, overview 141–4
cervical spine *see* neck

cervical vertebrae
cervical disc disease 297
depicted *4*
Klippel-Feil syndrome (KFS) 316
spinal cord injury (SCI) 173
spine 4
CES *see* cauda equina syndrome
cetuximab
defined 489
targeted therapy 457
"Change of Lumbar Symptom after Surgical Treatment for Patients with Cervical Stenosis (LBP)" (NIH) 466n
chemotherapy
childhood brain tumors 421
defined 489
hypopharyngeal cancer 445
metastatic squamous neck cancer 429
nasopharyngeal cancer 437
oropharyngeal cancer 456
tumors 278
"Childhood Brain and Spinal Cord Tumors Treatment Overview (PDQ®)—Patient Version" (NCI) 413n
"Childhood Nasopharyngeal Cancer Treatment (PDQ®)—Patient Version" (NCI) 431n
children
arthritis 201
back pain
backpacks 121
Chiari II malformation 251
Klippel-Feil syndrome (KFS) 317
kyphosis 191
low back pain 37
nasopharyngeal cancer 433
neck injuries 143
nonsteroidal anti-inflammatory drugs (NSAIDs) 330
osteoporosis 170
spinal tumors 288
Chinese medicine, acupuncture 17
chiropractic care
back pain 51
described 18
overview 356–63
spinal stenosis 239
"Chiropractic: In Depth" (NCCIH) 356n
chiropractic treatment
back pain 357
scoliosis 198
spinal stenosis 239
chiropractors
osteoarthritis (OA) 216
spinal manipulation 350
spinal stenosis 239
Christopher & Dana Reeve Foundation, contact 503
chronic back pain
chiropractic care 18
low back 34
osteoporosis 152
chronic disease
chronic pain 12
defined 489
osteoarthritis (OA) 216
chronic myofascial pain, overview 312–5
"Chronic Myofascial Pain" (Omnigraphics) 312n
chronic pain
aging 30
cauda equina syndrome (CES) 246
defined 490
described 12
intervertebral disc disease (IVDD) 219
management 325
nerve block therapies 52
sacroiliac joint syndrome 302
slipped disc 227
cigarette
defined 490
low back pain 22
oropharyngeal cancer 448
Cleveland Clinic, contact 500
clinical trials
alternative therapies 163
back and neck 466–74
defined 490
spinal manipulation 351
CMP *see* chronic myofascial pain
CNS *see* central nervous system
coccygeal, spine 145
coccygeal vertebrae, depicted *4*

coccyx
lumbar spine 145
spine 3
codeine
acetaminophen 17
analgesic medications 51
opioids 328
cognitive behavioral therapy (CBT), pain management 365
cold therapy
cervical disc disease 299
slipped disc 227
collagens, intervertebral disc disease (IVDD) 220
complementary and alternative treatments, back pain 24
compresses
cauda equina syndrome (CES) 36
lower back 224
see also RICE
compression fracture
neck 143
vertebroplasty and kyphoplasty 397
computed tomography (CAT scan; CT scan)
central nervous system (CNS) tumors 280
defined 490
low back pain diagnosis 48
lumbar fracture 146
metastatic squamous neck cancer 425
slipped disc 226
spina bifida 251
spinal cord injury (SCI) 178
spinal deformities 190
spinal fusion surgery 404
computer workstation, ergonomics 92
"Computer Workstations eTool" (OSHA) 92n
congenital defects, work-related back injuries 84
congenital torticollis, overview 309–12
constipation
analgesic medications 51
defined 490
pain medications 331
conventional medicine, alternative therapies 239
corsets, back braces 346
cortex
brain-computer interfaces 484
pain 12
corticosteroids
ankylosing spondylitis 207
defined 490
nonsteroidal anti-inflammatory drugs (NSAIDs) 334
osteoarthritis (OA) 214
pinched nerve 244
cortisone
osteoporosis 168
spinal injections 337
counseling
back pain 357
mental health 266
osteoporosis 166
pain 19
spinal tumors 288
COX-2 inhibitors
back pain 51
nonsteroidal anti-inflammatory drugs (NSAIDs) 334
CSF *see* cerebrospinal fluid
CT scan *see* computed tomography
CTS *see* carpal tunnel syndrome
curvature *see* lordosis; scoliosis
CVD *see* cardiovascular disease
cyclooxygenase-1 (COX-1)
nonsteroidal anti-inflammatory drugs (NSAIDs) 334
see also COX-2 inhibitors
cyclooxygenase-2 (COX-2), nonsteroidal anti-inflammatory drugs (NSAIDs) 334
cysts
cervical fracture 142
tethered spinal cord syndrome 271
cytokines
inflammation 15
spinal cord injury (SCI) 177

D

Darrell Gwynn Foundation, contact 503
DBM *see* demineralized bone matrices
DDD *see* degenerative disc disease

deep brain stimulation, pain management 19
deep breathing exercise, chronic myofascial pain 314
degeneration
  intervertebral disc disease (IVDD) 219
  lower back pain 34
  spinal stenosis 238
degenerative disc disease (DDD)
  back pain 26
  spinal fusion surgery 403
demineralized bone matrices (DBM), bone grafts 405
deoxyribonucleic acid (DNA), defined 490
depression
  back pain 50
  brain and spinal cord tumors 282
  opioids 331
  osteoporosis 166
  spina bifida 266
  spinal cord injury (SCI) 183
  whiplash 140
dexamethasone, osteoporosis 168
diabetes
  defined 490
  osteoarthritis (OA) 216
  pain 12
  spinal cord injury (SCI) 181
  spinal injections 339
diclofenac, spinal pain 329
diet
  back pain 21
  brain and spinal cord tumors 288
  chiropractic care 357
  defined 490
  minimally invasive spinal surgery 390
  osteoarthritis (OA) 215
  osteoporosis 154
discectomy
  back pain 25
  intervertebral disc disease (IVDD) 221
  lumbar spinal surgery 397
  neck surgery 392
discitis
  lordosis 193
  lower back pain 35
discography
  back pain 48
  spinal injections 339
disc degeneration
  intervertebral disc disease (IVDD) 221
  kyphosis 289
  low back pain 400
  spinal stenosis 235
disc replacement, back pain 26
discs
  aging and spine 29
  low back surgery 400
  neck surgery 391
  slipped (herniated) disc 223
  spine 6
disease-modifying antirheumatic drugs (DMARDs), ankylosing spondylitis 207
distraction test, sacroiliac joint syndrome 303
Division of Occupational Health and Safety (DOHS)
  publications
    back health 88n
    exercises and stretches 105n
DMARDs *see* disease-modifying antirheumatic drugs
dorsal horn, pain 12
"Dosing of Methadone for Spine Surgery" (NIH) 468n
driving
  ergonomics 111
  spinal cord injury (SCI) 175
"Driving Ergonomics" (USDA) 111n
dura mater, spinal tumors 275
Dynamic Chiropractic, contact 500
dynamic posture, guide to good posture 61
Dystonia Medical Research Foundation (DMRF), contact 501

E

EBV *see* Epstein-Barr virus
education programs, spinal pain at work 82

"The Effects of Thoracic Spine Mobilizations in Individuals with Neck Pain (THSPMOBS)" (NIH) 473n
electrical stimulation
chiropractic care 357
pain 19
physical therapy for back and neck 342
scoliosis 198
spinal cord injury (SCI) 181
electromyography (EMG)
cervical disc disease 298
low back pain 48
EMG *see* electromyography
endocrinologist, defined 490
endorphins, pain management 14, 52
endoscopy
metastatic squamous neck cancer 425
minimally invasive spinal surgery 388
nasopharyngeal cancer 433
neck surgery 392
oropharyngeal cancer 450
enkephalins, pain management 14
environmental stressors, pain 12
enzyme, defined 490
epidural steroid injection (ESI)
back pain 53
spondylolisthesis 308
Epstein-Barr virus (EBV)
metastatic squamous neck cancer 425
nasopharyngeal cancer 431
erector spinae, spine 8
ergonomic awareness programs, low back pain 38
ergonomic principles, physical therapy 341
ergonomic workplace redesign, work-related musculoskeletal disorders (WMSDs) 80
ergonomically designed furniture, back pain 38
ergonomics, defined 490
"Ergonomics—Positioning Your Body for Whole Health" (VA) 71n
ESI *see* epidural steroid injection
esophagoscopy, hypopharyngeal cancer 441
estrogen
defined 491
osteoporosis 154
Eunice Kennedy Shriver National Institute of Child Health and Human Development (NICHD)
publications
spina bifida 248n
spinal cord injury (SCI) 173n
excitotoxicity, spinal cord injury (SCI) 177
exercises
ankylosing spondylitis 208
back pain 27
back pain during pregnancy 127
defined 491
kyphosis 191
low back pain 129
neck pain 353
osteoporosis 160
physical therapy 343
sacroiliac joint syndrome 304
spina bifida 258
spinal stenosis 232
torticollis 311
workplace 105
see also Pilates; yoga
"Exercises and Stretches" (DOHS) 105n
"Exercising with Pain" (*Go4Life*) 129n
exposure, defined 491
extension fracture, thoracic and lumbar spine 147

F

facet joint injections, spinal injections 338
facet joints
depicted *6*
neck surgery 393
spinal stenosis 234
spondylolisthesis 306
fall prevention, osteoporosis 160
FDA *see* U.S. Food and Drug Administration
Federation of Chiropractic Licensing Boards (FCLB), contact 501

fentanyl, spinal pain 328
FES *see* functional electrical stimulation
fetus, defined 491
fibromyalgia (FM)
  acupuncture 372
  back pain 23
  chiropractic care 358
  low back pain 36
fitness level
  back pain 21
  low back pain 37
  Pilates 134
504 plan, spina bifida 261
flexibility
  ankylosing spondylitis 205
  cervical disc disease 298
  chronic myofascial pain 312
  low back pain 37
  lumbar spinal surgery 399
  neck pain 44
  neck surgery 394
  Pilates 134
  spina bifida 265
flexion fracture, thoracic and lumbar spine 147
fluoroscopy, spinal injections 338
FM *see* fibromyalgia
fMRI *see* functional magnetic resonance imaging
folic acid, spina bifida 250
foramen, neck surgery 391
foramina, neck surgery 391
foraminotomy, low back pain 53
fractures
  aging and spine 29
  defined 491
  minimally invasive spinal surgery 388
  osteoporosis 153
  spinal fusion surgery 403
  spondylolisthesis 306
"Fractures of the Thoracic and Lumbar Spine" (Omnigraphics) 145n
"Frequently Asked Questions—Bone Allografts" (CDC) 407n
functional electrical stimulation (FES), spinal cord injury (SCI) 181
functional magnetic resonance imaging (fMRI), central nervous system (CNS) tumors 281
fusion
  ankylosing spondylitis 208
  Klippel-Feil syndrome (KFS) 316
  spinal stenosis 240
  see also spinal fusion

G

gamma-aminobutyric acid (GABA), pain 14
gamma knife, spinal tumors and cysts 286
Genetic and Rare Diseases Information Center (GARD) publications
    cauda equina syndrome (CES) 245n
    intervertebral disc disease (IVDD) 219n
    Klippel Feil syndrome (KFS) 315n
    Tarlov cysts 293n
genetics, defined 491
Genetics Home Reference (GHR) publication
    intervertebral disc disease (IVDD) 219n
"Getting It Straight: Improve Your Posture for Better Health" (*NIH News in Health*) 58n
glutamate
  pain 13
  spinal cord injury (SCI) research 477
Go4Life
  publication
    lower back exercises 129n
good posture
  ankylosing spondylitis 209
  driving ergonomics 113
  neck pain 44
  overview 61–5
  safe lifting techniques 88
gout, arthritis 201
"Guide to Good Posture" (NIH) 61n
gynecologist, defined 491

H

halo ring, back and neck braces 346
hamstrings, physical therapy 343
hand massage, workplace exercises 107
headaches
  central nervous system (CNS) tumors 279
  childhood brain and spinal cord tumors 415
  neck pain 42
  pain 18
  spinal injections 340
  spinal pain 330
  syringomyelia 289
  whiplash 140
  see also migraine headache
Healthfinder.gov, contact 498
health history *see* medical history
"Healthy Movements" (NIH) 67n
heart problems
  spinal cord injury (SCI) 181
  spinal stenosis 238
heat therapy, slipped (herniated) disc 227
heredity
  back pain 22
  spondylolisthesis 306
herniated discs
  chiropractic care 358
  depicted *235*
  intervertebral disc disease (IVDD) 219
  lumbar spinal surgery 398
  minimally invasive spinal surgery 389
  overview 223–7
  sacroiliac joint syndrome 302
hips
  arthritis 201
  bone graft 407
  computer workstations 93
  good posture 64
  spina bifida 252
HLA-B27 gene
  ankylosing spondylitis 205
  back pain 49
home modifications (HM), back injury among caregivers 103
homeopathy, chiropractic care 359
hormone, defined 491
hormone therapy, osteoporosis 163
horse's tail *see* cauda equina syndrome (CES)
Hospital for Special Surgery (HSS), contact 501
hot or cold packs, back pain 24
housework, cervical disc disease 299
HPV *see* human papillomavirus
human immunodeficiency virus (HIV)
  bone allografts 408
  defined 491
human papillomavirus (HPV)
  metastatic squamous neck cancer 425
  oropharyngeal cancer 448
hunchback, kyphosis 188
hunched posture, osteoporosis 153
hyaluronic acid, osteoarthritis (OA) 214
hydrocephalus
  central nervous system (CNS) tumors 279
  spina bifida 251
  syringomyelia 289
hydrocodone
  back pain 51
  spinal pain 328
hyperextension braces, back and neck braces 347
hyperlordosis, lordosis 192
hypertension
  chiropractic care 358
  defined 491
  Pilates 135
  spinal injections 339
hypopharyngeal cancer
  defined 491
  overview 439–45
"Hypopharyngeal Cancer Treatment (Adult) (PDQ®)—Patient Version" (NCI) 439n
hypothermia, spinal cord injuries (SCIs) research 476

I

ibuprofen
  ankylosing spondylitis 206

ibuprofen, *continued*
back pain 24
nonsteroidal anti-inflammatory drugs (NSAIDs) 334
opioids 324
pain management 18
sacroiliac joint syndrome 304
IDET *see* intradiscal electrothermal therapy
imaging techniques
back pain 47
central nervous system (CNS) tumors 280
spinal cord injury (SCI) 179
torticollis 311
immune system
central nervous system (CNS) tumors 277
defined 492
inflammation and pain 15
oropharyngeal cancer 456
spinal cord injury (SCI) 177
immunotherapy, nasopharyngeal cancer 436
incontinence
spina bifida 253
spinal cord injury (SCI) 175
indomethacin
spinal cord injuries research 478
spinal stenosis 238
infections
arthritis 202
EXPAREL 470
low back pain 35
nasopharyngeal cancer 432
neck injuries 143
neurosurgery 284
oropharyngeal cancer 450
spina bifida 259
spinal cord injury (SCI) 177
spinal fusion surgery 404
spinal injections 339
spinal stenosis 241
surgery 379
understanding pain 15
inflammation
low back pain 34
lumbar spinal surgery 396
magnetic resonance imaging (MRI) 48
inflammation, *continued*
neuroprotection 476
nonsteroidal anti-inflammatory drugs (NSAIDs) 333
osteoarthritis (OA) 214
rheumatoid arthritis (RA) 236
sacroiliac joint syndrome 303
skeletal deformities 193
spinal cord injury (SCI) 177
spinal tumors 274
understanding pain 12
inhibitory neurotransmitter
neurochemistry of pain 14
regeneration 478
insurance coverage, chiropractic care 359
International Chiropractors Association (ICA), contact 501
International Intradiscal Therapy Society (IITS), contact 501
intervertebral disc degeneration, low back pain 34
"Intervertebral Disc Disease" (GARD) 219n
"Intervertebral Disc Disease" (GHR) 219n
intervertebral discs
anatomy of spine 3
depicted *7*
disc regeneration 400
low back pain 33
overview 219–21
skeletal deformities 193
spinal injections 339
spondylolisthesis 308
intradiscal electrothermal therapy (IDET)
surgical procedures 398
treatment of back pain 26
IVDD *see* intervertebral disc disease

J

Job Accommodation Network (JAN), contact 504
job-related risk factors, back pain 22
joint diseases
bone scans 49
osteoarthritis (OA) 215
see also inflammatory joint disease

joint resurfacing, osteoarthritis (OA) 214
joints
anatomy and functions of spine 3
arthritis 200
body mechanics 68
bone graft 407
musculoskeletal conditions 302
neck surgery 393
nonsurgical treatment 43
pregnancy 126
spinal cord injury (SCI) 176
spinal injections 338
spinal manipulation 354
spinal stenosis 231
understanding pain 20
whiplash 140

K

ketoprofen
back pain 51
nonsteroidal anti-inflammatory drugs (NSAIDs) 24, 334
KFS *see* Klippel-Feil syndrome
Klippel-Feil syndrome (KFS), overview 315–9
"Klippel Feil Syndrome" (GARD) 315n
knees
acupuncture 370
back exercises 108
body maintenance 70
bone graft 407
epidural stimulation 481
low back pain 39
osteoarthritis (OA) 211
posture 58
pregnancy 127, 200
sacroiliac joint syndrome 303
kyphoplasty
low back surgery 397
treatment of back pain 26
kyphosis
osteoporosis 166
overview 188–92
"Kyphosis" (Omnigraphics) 188n
kyphotic curve, anatomy of spine 4

L

laminae, described 5
laminectomy
decompressive surgery 388
herniated discs treatment 25
laptop workstation, components arrangement 95
laryngoscopy, defined 492
larynx, defined 492
laser surgery
herniated discs treatment 25
nucleoplasty 398
latex allergy, spina bifida 252
LBP *see* low back pain
lesion, defined 492
lidocaine
sacroiliac joint injection 303
therapeutic spinal injections 337
lifting belts, described 337
lifting techniques
overview 88–91
see also back belts
ligaments
ankylosing spondylitis 204
described 9
intervertebral disc disease (IVDD) 220
physical therapy 341
sacroiliac joints 302
spinal cord injury (SCI) 176
spine 118
whiplash 140
LINAC *see* linear-accelerated radiosurgery
linear-accelerated radiosurgery, stereotactic radiosurgery procedure 286
lomustine, CNS chemotherapeutics 287
lordosis
overview 192–5
raney flexion jacket 347
skeletal irregularities 35
spondylolisthesis 307
"Lordosis" (Omnigraphics) 192n
lordotic curve, spine 4
low back *see* lumbar spine

low back pain (LBP)
acupuncture 370
exercises 129
meditation 365
spinal manipulation 349
"Low Back Pain Fact Sheet" (NINDS) 33n, 47n, 121n, 396n, 399n
"Lower Back Exercise" (*Go4Life*) 129n
low-impact exercises, recommendations for healthy back 38
lumbar puncture (spinal tap), described 418
lumbar spinal surgery,overview 396–9
lumbar spine, fracture 145
lumbar vertebrae, depicted *4*
lupus
arthritis 202
defined 492

M

macrophage, research 477
magnetic resonance imaging (MRI)
ankylosing spondylitis diagnosis 206
cauda equina syndrome (CES) diagnosis 245
cervical disc disease diagnosis 298
defined 492
described 48
hypopharyngeal cancer diagnosis 440
imaging tests 226
nasopharyngeal cancer diagnosis 432
neck injury diagnosis 143
neck pain diagnosis 43
osteoarthritis (OA) 213
spina bifida diagnosis 251
spinal cord syndrome, diagnosis 271
spinal cord tumor, diagnosis 416
spinal stenosis diagnosis 237
syringomyelia diagnosis 290
Tarlov cyst diagnosis 293
magnetoencephalography (MEG), laboratory tests 281
malignant tumors, brain and spinal cord tumors 282
"Managing Pain" (NIH) 323n
manual materials handling, back injuries risk factor 85
massage, alternative therapies for osteoarthritis (OA) 215
massage therapists, healthcare professionals 216
MBSR *see* mindfulness-based stress reduction
mechanical assist device, engineering controls 82
mechanical stresses, tendons 9
medical history
ankylosing spondylitis 205
arthritis 202
central nervous system (CNS) tumors 280
congenital torticollis 311
herniated disc 225
kyphosis 190
low back pain 47
neck pain 43
osteoarthritis (OA) 213
sacroiliac joint syndrome 303
scoliosis 197
spinal stenosis 236
syringomyelia 290
see also physical examination
Medicare Rights Center, contact 504
medications
abuse of pain medications 330
bone-building medications 162
bone density loss 172
chronic back pain 24
chronic low back pain 50
chronic myofascial pain 313
nonsteroidal anti-inflammatory medications 333
osteoarthritis (OA) 214
osteoporosis risk 154
prescription opioid medications 328
sacroiliac joint syndrome 304
Scheuermann kyphosis 191
spinal fusion surgery 405
spinal injections 337
spinal pain 327
therapeutic spinal injections 337
"Meditation and Cognitive-Behavioral Therapy Ease Low Back Pain" (NIH) 365n

MEG *see* magnetoencephalography
meningitis
  defined 492
  syringomyelia 289
menopause
  calcitonin 163
  defined 492
  osteoporosis 154
  smoking 171
mental-health factors, low back pain 37
metabolism, defined 492
metastatic squamous neck cancer, overview 423–30
"Metastatic Squamous Neck Cancer with Occult Primary Treatment (Adult) (PDQ®)—Patient Version" (NCI) 423n
methotrexate
  ankylosing spondylitis 207
  CNS chemotherapeutics 287
  osteoporosis 155
methylprednisolone (Medrol), acute injury treatment 180
Miami Project to Cure Paralysis/Buoniconti Fund, contact 503
microdiscectomy, herniated (ruptured) discs 25
migraine headache
  defined 492
  placebos 20
mindfulness-based stress reduction (MBSR), cognitive-behavioral therapy (CBT) 365
"Minimally Invasive Spinal Surgery" (Omnigraphics) 387n
minimally invasive spine surgery (MISS), overview 387–90
MISS *see* minimally invasive spine surgery
mobilization, spinal mobilization 52
molded jackets, back braces 347
monoclonal antibodies, targeted therapy 456
morphine
  analgesic medications 51
  opioid receptors 14
  prescription opioid medications 328
Motrin (ibuprofen)
  chronic myofascial pain
    medications 313
  OTC ibuprofen 334
MRI *see* magnetic resonance imaging
"M6-C™ Artificial Cervical Disc—P170036" (FDA) 375n
muscle fatigue, low back pain 121
muscle pain
  fibromyalgia 23
  lordosis 193
muscle relaxants
  chronic back pain 24
  whiplash 141
muscles, function 8
musculoskeletal disorders (MSDs)
  heat/ice packs 342
  hot or cold packs 27
  over-the-counter (OTC)
    medications 226
  scoliosis 197
musculoskeletal exercises, examples 105
mutation, defined 493
myelograms, imaging tests 48

N

naproxen sodium, nonsteroidal anti-inflammatory drugs (NSAIDs) 51
nasal olfactory ensheathing cells, spinal cord injury (SCI) 480
nasopharyngeal cancer
  defined 493
  overview 431–8
National Cancer Institute (NCI)
  publications
    childhood brain and spinal cord tumors 413n
    childhood nasopharyngeal cancer 431n
    hypopharyngeal cancer 439n
    metastatic squamous neck cancer 423n
National Center for Complementary and Integrative Health (NCCIH)
  contact 498
  publications
    acupuncture 373n

National Center for Complementary and Integrative Health (NCCIH)
publications, *continued*
chiropractic 356n
spinal manipulation and home exercise for acute neck pain 353n
spinal manipulation for low back pain 349n
National Center on Health, Physical Activity and Disability (NCHPAD), contact 504
National Institute of Arthritis and Musculoskeletal and Skin Diseases (NIAMS)
contact 498
publications
aging and spine 29n
ankylosing spondylitis 203n
arthritis 200n
back pain 21n, 396n
osteoarthritis (OA) 211n
osteoporosis 151n
scoliosis in children and adolescents 196n
spinal stenosis 229n
National Institute of Neurological Disorders and Stroke (NINDS)
contact 498
publications
back pain 396n
brain and spinal tumors 413n
low back pain 33n, 47n, 121n, 396n, 399n
pain 11n
spinal cord injury (SCI) 475n
syringomyelia 288n
tethered spinal cord syndrome 271n
whiplash 140n
National Institute on Aging (NIA)
contact 498
publication
clinical trials and studies 461n
National Institutes of Health (NIH)
contact 498
publications
behavior of the upper cervical spine in rugby players (Cervistab) 467n
National Institutes of Health (NIH)
publications, *continued*
bone graft 407n
change of lumbar symptom after surgical treatment for patients with cervical stenosis (LBP) 466n
exercising with pain 129n
guide to good posture 61n
healthy movements 67n
managing pain 323n
meditation and cognitive-behavioral therapy for low back pain 365n
methadone and spine surgery 468n
minimally invasive spine surgery 471n
postoperative pain management following spine surgery (EXPAREL) 469n
spinal stenosis 29n
thoracic spine mobilizations in individuals with neck pain (THSPMOBS) 473n
National Library of Medicine (NLM) *see* U.S. National Library of Medicine
National Organization of Social Security Claimants' Representatives (NOSSCR), contact 504
National Organization on Disability (NOD), contact 505
National Osteoporosis Foundation (NOF), contact 501
National Scoliosis Foundation (NSF), contact 501
nausea
brain and spinal cord tumors symptoms 279
chemotherapy side effects 287
spinal injections side effects 340
NCS *see* nerve conduction studies
neck
braces 345
cancer 423
pain 41
spinal manipulation 353
surgery 391

neck, *continued*
thoracic spine mobilizations 473
whiplash 140
see also cervical spine
neck braces, described 345
neck pain
overview 41–5
physical therapy 341
spinal manipulation 353
whiplash 140
"Neck Pain" (Omnigraphics) 41n
neck surgery, overview 391–4
"Neck Surgery" (Omnigraphics) 391n
needle procedure, chronic myofascial pain 314
Nemours Foundation Center for Children's Health Media, contact 501
nerve blocks, spinal stenosis 239
nerve cell self-destruction, described 177
nerve conduction studies (NCS)
cervical disc disease 298
low back pain 48
nerve damage
intervertebral disc disease (IVDD) 220
lordosis 194
low back pain 49
minimally invasive spine surgery 389
rotation fractures 147
spina bifida 265, 269
nerve fibers, transcutaneous electrical stimulation (TENS) 19
nerve roots
cauda equina syndrome (CES) 36
cervical disc disease 381
spinal decompression 388
nervous systems *see* central nervous system (CNS); peripheral nervous system (PNS)
neural tube defects, pregnancy 250
neuronal plasticity, inflammation and pain 16
neurons
brain and spinal cord tumors 414
neurochemistry of pain 13
spinal tumors and cysts 275
neurons, *continued*
thoracic spine mobilizations 474
neurosurgeons
childhood brain and spinal cord tumors 419
spinal stenosis 241
syringomyelia 291
neurosurgery, spinal tumors and cysts 283
neurotransmitters
defined 493
managing chronic pain 325
pain 13
spinal cord injury (SCI) 177
NIA *see* National Institute on Aging
NIH News in Health
publications
acupuncture 370n
good posture for better health 58n
yoga for back pain 367n
nivolumab, defined 493
NLM *see* U.S. National Library of Medicine
NMRI *see* nuclear magnetic resonance imaging
nociceptors
physical therapy 314
understanding pain 12
North American Spine Society (NASS), contact 502
nonsteroidal anti-inflammatory drugs (NSAIDs)
ankylosing spondylitis 206
Klippel-Feil syndrome (KFS) 318
pain relievers 328
skeletal deformities 191
spinal fusion surgery 405
spinal manipulation 351
spinal stenosis 238
Tarlov cyst 294
treatment for back pain 51
whiplash 140
nonsurgical treatment
back pain 24
cervical disc disease 298
kyphosis 191
neck pain 43
slipped (herniated) disc 226

nonsurgical treatment, *continued*
spinal fracture 148
spinal stenosis 238
spondylolisthesis 308
norepinephrine, pain management 14
nuclear magnetic resonance imaging (NMRI)
hypopharyngeal cancer 441
metastatic squamous neck cancer 425
nasopharyngeal cancer 432
oropharyngeal cancer 450
spinal cord tumors 416
nucleoplasty
described 398
low back pain 54
nucleus pulposus
cervical disc disease 391
defined 6
disc regeneration 400
numbness and tingling
back pain 26
sacroiliac joint syndrome 303
nutrition
defined 493
healthy back 39
nutritional supplements, scoliosis 198

O

OA *see* osteoarthritis
obesity
arthritis 82
back pain 21
defined 493
intervertebral disc disease (IVDD) 220
lordosis 193
spina bifida 250
spinal cord injury (SCI) 181
see also overweight
occipital-cervical spine injuries, cervical fracture 141
occupational risk factors
ergonomics for computer workstations 92
low back pain 37
Occupational Safety and Health Administration (OSHA)
publications
back disorders and injuries 84n
computer workstations eTool 92n
safe patient-handling programs 101n
ODI *see* Oswestry Disability Index
Office of Disability Employment Policy (ODEP), contact 505
Office of the Assistant Secretary for Planning and Evaluation (ASPE)
publication
back injury among caregivers 101n
Office on Women's Health (OWH)
publication
backpack safety 121n
"Office Technology and Musculoskeletal Disorders: Building an Ecological Model" (CDC) 92n
oligodendrocytes, spinal cord injury (SCI) 177
Omnigraphics
publications
anatomy and functions of the spine 3n
back and neck braces 345n
back pain during pregnancy 125n
cervical disc disease 297n
chronic myofascial pain 312n
first chiropractic visit 360n
kyphosis 188n
lordosis 192n
minimally invasive spinal surgery 387n
neck pain 41n
neck surgery 391n
physical therapy for back and neck disorders 341n
Pilates 133n
sacroiliac joint syndrome 302n
slipped (herniated) disc 223n
spinal fusion surgery 403n
spinal injections 337n
spondylolisthesis 305n

Omnigraphics
publications, *continued*
thoracic and lumbar spine fractures 145n
torticollis 309n
opioid receptors, pain transmission 14
opioids
low back pain 51
managing chronic pain 323
pain management 14
oropharyngeal cancer
defined 493
overview 447–57
"Oropharyngeal Cancer Treatment (Adult) (PDQ®)—Patient Version" (NCI) 447n
orthopedists
RICE 20
spina bifida 256
osteoarthritis (OA)
arthritis 201
overview 211–7
work-related musculoskeletal disorders (WMSDs) 81
see also arthritis
"Osteoarthritis" (NIAMS) 211n
"Osteoarthritis (OA)" (CDC) 211n
osteomyelitis, infections 35
osteophytes, spinal stenosis 234
osteoporosis
back pain 23
cervical fracture 142
defined 493
low back surgery 397
overview 151–72
skeletal deformities 189
spondylolisthesis 306
thoracic spine mobilizations 474
"Osteoporosis" (NIAMS) 151n
osteotomy, osteoarthritis (OA) 214
Oswestry Disability Index (ODI), minimally invasive spine surgery 471
"Outcome Analysis for Minimally Invasive Spine Surgery" (NIH) 471n
over-the-counter (OTC)
cervical disc disease 299
chiropractic care 359
defined 493
over-the-counter (OTC), *continued*
herniated disc 226
medications for spinal pain 327
neck surgery 392
nonsteroidal anti-inflammatory drugs (NSAIDs) 207
nonsurgical treatment 43
sacroiliac joint syndrome 304
spina bifida 250
understanding pain 18
overweight
aerobic exercise 108
defined 493
low back pain 37
neutral spine posture 60
osteoarthritis (OA) 212
skeletal deformities 193
see also obesity
oxaprozin, nonsteroidal anti-inflammatory drugs (NSAIDs) 334
oxycodone
back pain treated 51
pain relievers 328

P

Paget disease
arthritis 236
skeletal deformities 189
pain
ankylosing spondylitis 205
backpack overload 122
chiropractic visit 360
chronic myofascial pain (CMP) 312
ergonomics 71
facet joints 6
imaging tests 226
neck surgery 391
nonsurgical treatment 44
opioids 325
osteoarthritis (OA) 212
osteoporosis 167
overview 11–20
physical therapy 342
spinal fusion surgery 405
Tarlov cyst 294
tethered spinal cord syndrome 271
see also chronic pain
Pain Connection, contact 502

"Pain: Hope through Research" (NINDS) 11n
pain management
  chronic pain 325
  EXPAREL 469
  Tarlov cyst 294
  understanding pain 17
pain pathway, anatomy of pain 12
pain relievers
  lumbar spinal surgery 396
  myofascial pain syndrome 313
  osteoarthritis (OA) 214
  spinal pain 327
  understanding pain 18
  yoga 368
painkillers
  neurochemistry of pain 14
  spinal pain medications 327
papillomavirus, defined 494
paralysis
  cauda equina syndrome (CES) 245
  cervical fracture 141
  research studies 481
  spina bifida 252
  spinal cord injury (SCI) 182
  tumors and cysts 279
paraplegia, defined 174
pars interarticularis, spondylolisthesis 306
patient-controlled analgesia (PCA), EXPAREL 469
patient handling injuries, preventing back injury 102
patrick test, sacroiliac joint syndrome 303
PCA *see* patient-controlled analgesia
pedicles
  spinal stenosis 231
  vertebra 5
pelvic floor muscles, ergonomics 73
pelvis
  ankylosing spondylitis 205
  back braces 346
  bone grafts 405
  low back pain 35
  neck surgery 391
  neutral spine posture 60
  pregnancy 125
  sacroiliac joint syndrome 302
pelvis, *continued*
  scoliosis 197
  spinal stenosis 229
  thoracic and lumbar spine 146
peptides, neurochemistry of pain 14
perception (hearing), defined 494
peripheral nerve stimulation, pain 19
peripheral nerves
  anatomy of spine 8
  cell replacement 479
  transcutaneous electrical nerve stimulation (TENS) 53
  understanding pain 19
peripheral nervous system (PNS)
  carpal tunnel syndrome (CTS) 79
  cauda equina syndrome (CES) 245
  inflammation and pain 16
persistent pain *see* chronic pain
personal protective equipment (PPE), musculoskeletal disorders 83
philadelphia collar, cervical braces 345
physiatrists
  ankylosing spondylitis 208
  osteoarthritis (OA) 215
  osteoporosis 164
physical activity, defined 494
physical examination
  cervical disc disease 298
  chiropractic care 357
  herniated disc 225
  neck pain 43
  scoliosis 197
  skeletal deformities 190
  spinal stenosis 237
  spondylolisthesis 307
  see also medical history
physical therapy
  back pain 50
  cervical disc disease 299
  cognitive-behavioral therapy 366
  epidural stimulation 481
  ergonomics 75
  intervertebral disc disease (IVDD) 221
  low back surgery 401
  metastatic squamous neck cancer 428

physical therapy, *continued*
minimally invasive spine surgery 388
myofascial pain 314
neck injuries 141
nonsurgical treatments 191
overview 341–4
pinched nerve 244
spinal cord injury (SCI) 180
spinal stenosis 31
thoracic spine mobilizations 473
tumors and cysts 288
understanding pain 20
"Physical Therapy for Back and Neck Disorders" (Omnigraphics) 341n
Pilates
ergonomics 73
overview 133–6
"Pilates Promotes Back Health" (Omnigraphics) 133n
"Pinched Nerve Information Page" (NINDS) 244n
pinched nerves, overview 244
placebo
acupuncture 371
defined 494
nonsteroidal anti-inflammatory drugs (NSAIDs) 335
spinal manipulation 351
understanding pain 20
plasticity
pain 16
research studies 476
pneumonia, spinal cord injury (SCI) 181
PNS *see* peripheral nervous system
positron emission tomography (PET) scan
hypopharyngeal cancer 440
metastatic squamous neck cancer 425
nasopharyngeal cancer 432
oropharyngeal cancer 449
tumors and cysts 281
"Post-Operative Pain Management Following Spine Surgery (EXPAREL)" (NIH) 469n
posterior cervical fusion (PCF)
defined 44
posterior cervical fusion (PCF), *continued*
minimally invasive spine surgery 472
posterior cervical laminectomy, defined 393
posterior pelvic pain, pregnancy 125
posture
anatomy of spine 3
arthritis 81
back pain 22
back pain prevention 91
backpack safety 122
childhood brain 413
ergonomic 111
inflammatory joint disease 209
kyphosis 188
neck pain 41
osteoporosis 153
overview 58–65
physical therapy 341
spondylolisthesis 307
tumors and cysts 279
yoga 135
pregnancy
back pain 23, 125
defined 494
EXPAREL 470
osteoporosis 169
Pilates 135
sacroiliac joint syndrome 302
spina bifida 249
tethered spinal cord syndrome 271
pregnant women
back pain 125
Pilates 135
posture 58
pressure sores, spinal cord injury (SCI) 181
prevention, defined 494
prognosis, defined 494
prostaglandins, nonsteroidal anti-inflammatory drugs (NSAIDs) 333
prostheses
osteoarthritis (OA) 214
spinal cord injury (SCI) 179
protein, defined 494
pseudarthrosis, spinal fusion surgery 406
puberty, defined 494

Q

QOL *see* quality of life
quadriplegia, spinal cord injury (SCI) 174
quality of life (QOL)
  chronic pain 323
  osteoporosis 151
  posture 58
  spina bifida 257
  spinal cord injury (SCI) 181
  spinal tumors and cysts 288
"Questions to Ask Your Doctor" (AHRQ) 383n

R

radiation, defined 494
radiation therapy
  brain and spinal cord tumors 282, 420
  hypopharyngeal cancer 444
  metastatic squamous neck cancer 428
  oropharyngeal cancer 455
radiculopathy
  electrodiagnostics 48
  EXPAREL 470
  lower back pain 34
  overview 243–6
radiofrequency denervation
  surgical procedures 398
  treatment for back pain 54
randomized controlled trial
  low back surgery 401
  treatment for back pain 53
RANK ligand (RANKL) inhibitor, osteoporosis 162
receptors
  chronic pain 12
  osteoporosis 162
  prescription medications 328
  research studies 478
regeneration
  chronic low back pain 400
  described 477
  spinal cord injury (SCI) 179
rehabilitation
  ankylosing spondylitis 208
rehabilitation
  back belts 118
  brain and spinal cord tumors 282
  cell replacement 480
  nasopharyngeal cancer 435
  neck injuries 143
  oropharyngeal cancer 454
  osteoporosis 160
  spina bifida 266
  spinal cord injury (SCI) 181
  spinal fusion surgery 406
  understanding pain 20
Rehabilitation Services Administration (RSA), contact 505
reproductive function, spinal cord injury (SCI) 183
rest, ice, compression, and elevation (RICE), described 20
rheumatoid arthritis (RA)
  defined 494
  EXPAREL 470
  inflammatory joint disease 201
  musculoskeletal disorders 81
  nonsteroidal anti-inflammatory drugs (NSAIDs) 333
  placebo 20
  spinal stenosis 235
ribs
  anatomy of spine 3
  ankylosing spondylitis 204
  bone allograft 407
  cell replacement 482
  Klippel-Feil syndrome (KFS) 316
rigid braces, described 347
robotics
  oropharyngeal cancer 455
  research studies 483
rofecoxib, nonsteroidal anti-inflammatory drugs (NSAIDs) 355
rotation fractures, thoracic and lumbar spine 147
roundback *see* kyphosis
ruptured disc *see* herniated disc

S

sacroiliac joint syndrome, overview 302–5

"Sacroiliac Joint Syndrome" (Omnigraphics) 302n
sacroiliitis, low back pain 35
sacrum
 ankylosing spondylitis (AS) 204
 sacroiliac joint syndrome 302
 spinal cord injury (SCI) 174
 spinal stenosis 230
 Tarlov cysts 293
"Safe Lifting Techniques" (USDA) 88n
"Safe Patient Handling Programs" (OSHA) 101n
SBAA *see* Spina Bifida Association of America
scar tissue
 congenital torticollis 310
 syringomyelia 292
 tethered spinal cord syndrome 271
Scheuermann kyphosis, described 188
sciatica
 chiropractic care 358
 intervertebral disc disease (IVDD) 219
 low back pain 35
 pregnancy 125
 smoking 22
 spinal injections 338
 spinal stenosis 232
SCIs *see* spinal cord injuries
scoliosis
 back pain 23
 Klippel-Feil syndrome (KFS) 316
 overview 196–8
 spina bifida 252
 spinal fusion surgery 404
 spinal stenosis 233
 syringomyelia 290
 tethered spinal cord syndrome 271
"Scoliosis in Children and Adolescents" (NIAMS) 196n
Scoliosis Research Society (SRS), contact 502
sedentary lifestyles, low back pain 33
sexual function
 spina bifida 265
 spinal cord injury (SCI) 181
 spinal stenosis 233
 syringomyelia 290
shock absorbers *see* intervertebral discs
short-term pain *see* acute pain
shunts, spina bifida 252
single photon emission computed tomography (SPECT), central nervous system (CNS) tumors 281
skeletal irregularities, low back pain 35
slipped disc
 overview 223–7
 spinal fusion surgery 403
 spinal injections 338
"Slipped (Herniated) Disc" (Omnigraphics) 223n
smell, defined 494
smoking
 back pain 22
 central nervous system (CNS) tumors 277
 cervical disc disease 297
 hypopharyngeal cancer 439
 intervertebral disc disease (IVDD) 220
 low back pain 39
 neck pain 44
 oropharyngeal cancer 448
 osteoporosis 155
sodium, defined 494
soft collar, cervical braces 345
SOMI *see* sterno-occipital mandibular immobilization device
spasm
 back pain 22
 cervical fracture 142
 chronic myofascial pain 314
 lordosis 193
 slipped disc 226
 spondylolisthesis 307
spasticity
 central nervous system (CNS) tumors 280
 spinal cord injury (SCI) 181
SPECT *see* single photon emission computed tomography
spina bifida
 cauda equina syndrome (CES) 245
 defined 495
 Klippel-Feil syndrome (KFS) 316

spina bifida, *continued*
kyphosis 189
overview 248–70
"Spina Bifida" (CDC) 248n, 254n
Spina Bifida Association of America (SBAA), contact 502
spinal canal
cauda equina syndrome (CES) 245
chiropractic care 358
lumbar spinal surgery 398
minimally invasive spine surgery (MISS) 388
neck surgery 391
spinal cord tumors 276
spinal manipulation 350
spinal stenosis 232
spondylolisthesis 308
syringomyelia 289
spinal column
low back pain 35
lumbar surgery 396
osteoarthritis 213
tethered spinal cord syndrome 271
thoracic and lumbar spine fractures 145
spinal cord injury (SCI)
overview 173–83
research studies 475
syringomyelia 289
tethered spinal cord syndrome 271
"Spinal Cord Injury (SCI): Condition Information" (NICHD) 173n
"Spinal Cord Injury: Hope through Research" (NINDS) 475n
Spinal Cord Injury Model System (SCIMS) Information Network, contact 503
Spinal Cord Society (SCS), contact 503
spinal cord stimulation, pain management 19
spinal cord tumors *see* spinal tumors
spinal decompression
back pain 53
described 397
minimally invasive spine surgery (MISS) 388
spinal fusion surgery, overview 403–6
"Spinal Fusion Surgery" (Omnigraphics) 403n
spinal injections, overview 337–40
"Spinal Injections" (Omnigraphics) 337n
"Spinal Manipulation for Low Back Pain" (NCCIH) 349n
"Spinal Manipulation or Home Exercise More Effective Than Medication for Acute Neck Pain, Study Finds" (NCCIH) 353n
spinal stenosis
back pain 23
Klippel-Feil syndrome (KFS) 318
low back pain 35
lumbar surgery 396
minimally invasive spine surgery (MISS) 388
overview 229–41
spinal fusion surgery 404
"Spinal Stenosis" (NIAMS) 229n
"Spinal Stenosis" (NIH) 29n
spinal tap *see* lumbar puncture
spinal traction, described 343
SPINE-health, contact 502
Spine Intervention Society (SIS), contact 502
SpineSource, Inc., contact 502
SpineUniverse, contact 502
Spondylitis Association of America (SAA), contact 502
spondyloarthritis, lower back pain 36
spondylolisthesis
back braces 347
back pain 23
kyphosis 189
lordosis 193
lumbar surgery 397
overview 305–9
spinal fusion surgery 404
spinal stenosis 234
"Spondylolisthesis" (Omnigraphics) 305n
spondylolysis, minimally invasive spine surgery (MISS) 388
SSI *see* surgical site infection
sterno-occipital mandibular immobilization device (SOMI), cervical braces 346
steroids
back pain 52

steroids, *continued*
brain and spinal cord tumors 282
defined 495
nonsteroidal anti-inflammatory drugs (NSAIDs) 334
spinal injections 337
stress
ankylosing spondylitis (AS) 209
back pain 23
chronic myofascial pain (CMP) 312
lordosis 192
minimally invasive spine surgery (MISS) 388
neck pain 41
osteoarthritis (OA) 212
sacroiliac joint syndrome 305
spina bifida 266
spinal stenosis 234
stroke
chiropractic care 358
defined 495
nonsteroidal anti-inflammatory drugs (NSAIDs) 334
osteoarthritis (OA) 216
subaxial cervical spine injuries, cervical fracture 141
sulfasalazine, ankylosing spondylitis (AS) 207
surgical site infection (SSI), surgery 379
swayback *see* lordosis
synovium, spinal stenosis 231
syringomyelia
Klippel-Feil syndrome (KFS) 316
overview 288–92
tethered spinal cord syndrome 271
"Syringomyelia Fact Sheet" (NINDS) 288n
syrinx, syringomyelia 288

T

tachykinins, pain management 14
tai chi
back pain 28
defined 495
tailbone
posterior pelvic pain 125
sacroiliac joint syndrome 302
spinal cord injury (SCI) 174
targeted therapy, oropharyngeal cancer 456
Tarlov cysts, overview 293–5
"Tarlov Cysts" (GARD) 293n
TCM *see* traditional Chinese medicine
temporomandibular joint (TMJ), chiropractic care 358
tendons
ankylosing spondylitis (AS) 204
back belts 118
back disorders 85
depicted *200*
intervertebral disc disease (IVDD) 220
low back pain 48
musculoskeletal disorders (MSDs) 78
TENS, defined 495
TENS *see* transcutaneous electrical nerve stimulation
tethered spinal cord syndrome, overview 271–2
"Tethered Spinal Cord Syndrome Information Page" (NINDS) 271n
tetraplegia, spinal cord injury (SCI) 174
thalamus, deep brain stimulation 19
thoracic spine
corset braces 346
fractures 145
kyphosis 188
thoracolumbar corset, spinal fractures 148
thorax, spinal cord injury (SCI) 175
throat
hypopharyngeal cancer 439
metastatic squamous neck cancer 424
oropharyngeal cancer 447
spinal fusion surgery 404
TLIF *see* transforaminal lumbar interbody fusion
tobacco
defined 495
hypopharyngeal cancer 439
osteoporosis 155
tolerance
back pain 51
torticollis 311

tongue, defined 495
tonsillectomy, metastatic squamous neck cancer 425
tonsils, oropharyngeal cancer 447
torticollis, overview 309–12
transcutaneous electrical nerve stimulation (TENS)
  back pain 25
  osteoarthritis (OA) 214
  Tarlov cysts 293
transforaminal lumbar interbody fusion (TLIF)
treadmills, osteoporosis 171
trochanteric belts, back braces 346
tumor growth, nasopharyngeal cancer 437
Tylenol (acetaminophen), spina bifida 250

U

ultrasound
  defined 250
  Klippel-Feil syndrome (KFS) 318
  myofascial pain 314
  physical therapy 342
  slipped disc 227
ultrasound imaging, defined 49
"Understanding Acupuncture" (*NIH News in Health*) 370n
United Spinal Association, contact 503
urinary tract infection (UTI)
  defined 495
  spina bifida 252
U.S. Department of Agriculture (USDA)
  publications
    driving ergonomics 111n
    safe lifting techniques 88n
U.S. Department of Veterans Affairs (VA)
  publication
    ergonomics 71n
U.S. Food and Drug Administration (FDA)
  contact 498
  publications
    M6-C™ artificial cervical disc 375n
U.S. Food and Drug Administration (FDA)
  publications, *continued*
    pain medicine 327n
    pain relievers 333n
U.S. National Library of Medicine (NLM), contact 498
UTI *see* urinary tract infection

V

valdecoxib, COX-2 selective inhibitors 335
VAS *see* visual analog scale
vehicle modifications, back injuries 104
vertebrae
  ankylosing spondylitis (AS) 203
  cervical disc disease 297
  cervical fracture 141
  intervertebral disc disease (IVDD) 219
  Klippel-Feil syndrome (KFS) 315
  kyphosis 188
  lordosis 193
  minimally invasive spinal surgery (MISS) 388
  neck surgery 391
  osteoporosis 153
  sacroiliac joint syndrome 302
  slipped disc 224
  spinal column 145
  spinal cord injury (SCI) 173
  spinal cord tumors 414
  spinal fusion surgery 403
  spinal injections 337
  spinal stenosis 229
  spondylolisthesis 306
vertebral arch, defined 231
vertebral column
  epidural injection 401
  spinal cord 7
  spinal stenosis 231
vertebroplasty
  back pain 53
  defined 26
  lumbar surgery 397
Vioxx (rofecoxib), COX-2 selective inhibitors 335

virus
arthritis 202
bone allograft 208
central nervous system (CNS) tumors 277
defined 495
intervertebral disc disease (IVDD) 220
visual analog scale, spine surgery 471
vitamin D
body maintenance 70
defined 495
healthy diet 28
osteoporosis 153
vitamins
chemotherapy 288
nutrition 159
spina bifida 250
vomiting
brain tumor signs 415
migraine 492
spinal injections 340
spinal tumors 279

W

weight loss
arthritis 202
back pain 26
chiropractic care 357
oropharyngeal cancer 448
"What Are Clinical Trials and Studies?" (NIA) 461n
"What to Expect at Your First Chiropractic Visit" (Omnigraphics) 360n
"What You Should Know before Your Surgery" (CDC) 379n
"When Your Back Hurts, Don't Let Back Pain Knock You Flat" (NIAMS) 29n
"Whiplash Information Page" (NINDS) 140n
whiplash injuries, facet joints 6
women
back belts 118
back pain 22
chronic myofascial pain 313
folic acid 265
women, *continued*
fractures 146
gender and pain 16
low back pain 33
osteoarthritis (OA) 212
osteoporosis 152
Pilates 135
posture 58
pregnancy 125
spina bifida 249
spinal injections 340
spinal stenosis 232
"Work-Related Musculoskeletal Disorders and Ergonomics" (CDC) 78n
workplace
back injuries 115
neck pain 43
spinal pain at work 80
work-related musculoskeletal disorders (WMSDs) 80
wrist stretch, workplace exercises 107

X

X-rays
arthritis 203
bone and joint scans 206
cervical disc disease 298
chiropractic care 357
defined 495
fluoroscopy 338
hypopharyngeal cancer 441
Klippel-Feil syndrome (KFS) 318
kyphosis 190
metastatic squamous neck cancer 428
nasopharyngeal cancer 436
neck pain 43
osteoarthritis (OA) 213
sacroiliac joint syndrome 303
slipped disc 226
spinal cord injury (SCI) 178
spinal cord tumors 420
spinal fusion surgery 404
spinal stenosis 237
spondylolisthesis 307

Y

yin and yang, acupuncture 370
yoga
  back health 135
  back pain 28
  chronic pain 325
  complementary and alternative
      medicine (CAM) 227
  defined 495
yoga, *continued*
  ergonomics 73
  low back pain 365
  posture 62
  pregnancy 127
  strengthening exercises 50
"Yoga May Help Treat Back Pain"
  (*NIH News in Health*) 367n
"Young Retail Workers"
  (CDC) 121n